PNEUMONIA ESSENTIALS

Edited by

Burke A. Cunha, MD, MACP

Chief, Infectious Disease Division
Winthrop-University Hospital
Mineola, New York
Professor of Medicine
State University of New York
School of Medicine
Stony Brook, New York

2008

PHYSICIANS' PRESS

Innovative Medical Publishing

ABOUT THE EDITOR

Burke A. Cunha, MD, is Chief, Infectious Disease Division at Winthrop-University Hospital, Mineola, New York; Professor of Medicine, State University of New York School of Medicine, Stony Brook, New York; and one of the world's leading authorities on the treatment of infectious diseases. During his 30-year career, he has contributed more than 1000 articles, 175 book chapters, and 15 books on infectious diseases to the medical literature, including the international bestseller, *Antibiotic Essentials*, now in its 7th edition. He has received numerous teaching awards, including the prestigious Aesculapius Award for outstanding teaching. He also serves on the editorial boards of more than two dozen medical journals, is Editor-in-Chief of *Infectious Disease Practice* and *Antibiotics for Clinicians*, and is Infectious Disease Editor-in-Chief for eMedicine on-line. Dr. Cunha is a Fellow of the Infectious Disease Society of America, American Academy of Microbiology, American College of Clinical Pharmacology, and American College of Chest Physicians. He has had a life-long interest in antimicrobial therapy in normal and compromised hosts, antibiotic pharmacokinetics/pharmacodynamics, pharmacoeconomics, and antibiotic resistance. Dr. Cunha is a Master of the American College of Physicians, awarded for achievements as a master clinician and teacher. He has had a life-long interest in antimicrobial therapy, fevers/FUO, nosocomial infections, infections in the compromised host, and pneumonias.

Be sure to visit www.physicianspress.com for a complete listing of medical titles, along with topical reviews, self-assessment questions, and other clinical information. Feel free to contact us by e-mail with comments or suggestions.

Additional copies of *Pneumonia Essentials* may be obtained at medical bookstores, or you may contact us directly at:

Physicians' Press
620 Cherry Avenue
Royal Oak, Michigan, 48073
Tel: (248) 616-3023
Fax: (248) 616-3003
www.physicianspress.com

Printed in the United States of America   ISBN: 978-1-890114-70-1

TABLE OF CONTENTS

CONTRIBUTORS

Burke A. Cunha, MD
Chief, Infectious Disease Division
Winthrop-University Hospital
Mineola, New York
Professor of Medicine
SUNY School of Medicine
Stony Brook, New York
*All Chapters except HIV Infection
and Pediatric Pneumonias*

Edward J. Bottone, PhD
Professor of Medicine
Professor of Microbiology
Professor of Pathology
Mount Sinai School of Medicine
New York, New York
Sputum Gram Stain

Daniel Caplivski, MD
Assistant Professor of Medicine
Infectious Disease Division
Mt. Sinai School of Medicine
New York, New York
Gram Stain Atlas

Dennis J. Cleri, MD
St. Francis Medical Center
Trenton, New Jersey
Professor of Medicine
Seton Hall University
School of Graduate Medical Education
Trenton, New Jersey
Bioterrorism

Mark S. Freed, MD
President and Editor-in-Chief
Physicians' Press
Royal Oak, Michigan
Overview of Pneumonia

Pierce Gardner, MD
John E. Fogarty International Center for Advanced
Study in the Health Sciences
Senior Advisor, Clinical Research and Training
National Institutes of Health
Bethesda, Maryland
Prophylaxis and Immunization

Douglas S. Katz, MD
Vice Chair for Clinical Research and Education
Director, Body CT
Winthrop-University Hospital
Mineola, New York
Professor of Clinical Radiology
State University of New York School of Medicine
Stony Brook, New York
Chest X-Ray Atlas

Leonard R. Krilov, MD
Chief, Pediatric Infectious Disease Division
Winthrop-University Hospital
Mineola, New York
Professor of Pediatrics
State University of New York
School of Medicine
Pediatric Pneumonias

James H. McGuire, MD
Director, International Health Division
Professor of Medicine
University of Maryland School of Medicine
Baltimore, Maryland
Parasites, Fungi, Unusual Organisms

George H. McCracken, Jr, MD
Distinguished Professor of Pediatric Infectious
Disease and the Sarah M. and Charles E. Seay
Chair in Pediatric Infectious Disease
University of Texas Southwestern Medical Center
Dallas, Texas
Pediatric Pneumonias

Robert Moore, MD
Chairman, Department of Radiology
Stony Brook University Hospital, Stony Brook,
New York, Professor of Radiology
State University of New York School of Medicine
Stony Brook, New York
Chest X-Ray Atlas

John H. Rex, MD
Vice-President and Medical Director for Infection
AstraZeneca Pharmaceuticals, Macclesfield, UK
Adjunct Professor of Medicine, University of
Texas Medical School, Houston, Texas
Antifungal Therapy

CONTRIBUTORS

Paul E. Sax, MD
Director, HIV Program
Brigham and Women's Hospital
Assistant Professor of Medicine
Harvard Medical School
Boston, Massachusetts
HIV Infection and Pneumonia

David Schlossberg, MD
Tuberculosis Control Program
Philadelphia Department of Health
Professor of Medicine
Temple University School of Medicine
Philadelphia, Pennsylvania
Tuberculosis

Paul E. Schoch, PhD
Director, Clinical Microbiology Laboratory
Winthrop-University Hospital
Mineola, New York
Medical Microbiology

Daniel S. Siegal, MD
Department of Radiology
Mount Auburn Hospital
Harvard Medical School
Boston, Massachusetts
Chest X-Ray Atlas

Damary C. Torres, PharmD
Clinical Pharmacy Specialist
Winthrop-University Hospital
Mineola, New York
Associate Clinical Professor of Pharmacy
College of Pharmacy, St. John's University
Queens, New York
Antimicrobial Drug Summaries

Kenneth F. Wagner, DO
Attending Physician, Infectious Disease
Consultant, National Naval Medical Center
Associate Professor of Medicine, Uniformed
Services, University of the Health Sciences
F. Edward Hebert School of Medicine
Bethesda, Maryland
Parasites, Fungi, Unusual Organisms

for

noble and beautiful

Marie

"Beauty is truth, and

Truth beauty"

Keats

ACKNOWLEDGMENTS

To accomplish the task of presenting the data compiled in this reference, a small, dedicated team of professionals was assembled. This team focused their energy and discipline for many months into typing, revising, designing, illustrating, and formatting the many chapters that make up this text. I wish to acknowledge Monica Crowder Kaufman and Lisa Lusardi Haave for their important contributions. I would also like to thank the many contributors who graciously contributed their time and energy, Mark Freed, MD, President and Editor-in-Chief of Physicians' Press, for his vision, commitment, and guidance, Norman Lyle for cover design, and the staff at Dickinson Press for their printing expertise.

Burke A. Cunha, MD

NOTICE

ABBREVIATIONS

ABE	acute bacterial endocarditis	gm	gram
ABM	acute bacterial meningitis	GU	genitourinary
AECB	acute bacterial exacerbation of chronic bronchitis	HAP	hospital-acquired pneumonia
		HA-MRSA	hospital-acquired MRSA
AFB	acid fast bacilli	HHV-6	human herpes virus 6
ARDS	adult respiratory distress syndrome	HLA	histocompatibility antigen
AV	arteriovenous	HSV	herpes simplex virus
BAL	bronchoalveolar lavage	I & D	incision and drainage
BMT	bone marrow transplant	IFA	immunofluorescent antibody
BOOP	bronchiolitis obliterans with organizing pneumonia	IgA	immunoglobulin A
		IgG	immunoglobulin G
CABG	coronary artery bypass grafting	IgM	immunoglobulin M
CAP	community-acquired pneumonia	ILI	influenza-like illness
CA-MRSA	community-acquired MRSA	INH	isoniazid
CCU	critical care unit	IT	intrathecal
CD_4	CD_4 T-cell lymphocyte	IV/PO	IV or PO
CIE	counter-immunoelectrophoresis	IV	intravenous
CLL	chronic lymphocytic leukemia	IVDA	intravenous drug abuser
CMV	cytomegalovirus	kg	kilogram
CNS	central nervous system	L	liter
CPK	creatine phosphokinase	LDH	lactate dehydrogenase
CrCl	creatinine clearance	LFT	liver function test
CSF	cerebrospinal fluid	LLQ	left lower quadrant
CT	computerized tomography	LUQ	left upper quadrant
CXR	chest x-ray	MAI	Mycobacterium avium-intracellulare
DFA	direct fluorescent antibody	mcg	microgram
DIC	disseminated intravascular coagulation	mcL	microliter
		MDR	multidrug resistant
DM	diabetes mellitus	MDRSP	multidrug resistant S. pneumoniae
DNA	deoxyribonucleic acid	mg	milligram
e.g.	for example	MI	myocardial infarction
EEG	electroencephalogram	MIC	minimum inhibitory concentration
EIA	enzyme immunoassay	min	minute
ELISA	enzyme-linked immunosorbent assay	mL	milliliter
EMB	ethambutol	MRI	magnetic resonance imaging
ENT	ear, nose, throat	MRSA	methicillin-resistant S. aureus
Enterobacteriaceae: Citrobacter, Edwardsiella, Enterobacter, E. coli, Klebsiella, Proteus, Providencia, Shigella, Salmonella, Serratia, Hafnia, Morganella, Yersinia		MRSE	methicillin-resistant S. epidermidis
		MRSP	macrolide-resistant S. pneumoniae
		MSSA	methicillin-sensitive S. aureus
		MSSE	methicillin-sensitive S. epidermidis
		NHAP	nursing home acquired pneumonia
ESBLs	extended spectrum β-lactamases	NNRTI	non-nucleoside reverse transcriptase inhibitor
esp	especially		
ESR	erythrocyte sedimentation rate	NP	nosocomial pneumonia
ESRD	end-stage renal disease	NRTI	nucleoside reverse transcriptase inhibitor
ET	endotracheal		
FUO	fever of unknown origin	NSAID	nonsteroidal anti-inflammatory drug
g	gram	OI	opportunistic infection
GI	gastrointestinal	PBS	protected brush specimen

PCEC	purified chick embryo cells	RR	respiratory rate
PCN	penicillin	RUQ	right upper quadrant
PCP	Pneumocystis (jiroveci) carinii pneumonia	SBE	subacute bacterial endocarditis
		SGOT/SGPT	serum transaminases
PCR	polymerase chain reaction	SLE	systemic lupus erythematosus
PE	pulmonary embolism	SOT	solid organ transplant
PI	protease inhibitor	sp.	species
PML	progressive multifocal leukoencephalopathy	SPEP	serum protein electrophoresis
		SQ	subcutaneous
PMN	polymorphonuclear leucocytes	TB	tuberculosis
PPD	purified protein derivative	TID	three times per day
PO	oral	TMP	trimethoprim
PRSP	penicillin-resistant S. pneumoniae	TMP-SMX	trimethoprim-sulfamethoxazole
PVE	prosthetic valve endocarditis	TST	tuberculin skin test
PVL	Pantone Valentine Leukocidin	UTI	urinary tract infection
PZA	pyrazinamide	VAP	ventilator-associated pneumonia
q__h	every __ hours	VCA	viral capsid antigen
q__d	every __ days	VISA	vancomycin-intermediate S. aureus
qmonth	once a month	VRE	vancomycin-resistant enterococci
qweek	once a week	VRSA	vancomycin-resistant S. aureus
RBC	red blood cell	VZV	varicella zoster virus
RLQ	right lower quadrant	WBC	white blood cell
RMSF	Rocky Mountain spotted fever	yrs	years
RNA	ribonucleic acid		

Chapter 1

Overview of Pneumonia

Mark S. Freed, MD
Burke A. Cunha, MD

OVERVIEW OF PNEUMONIA

Pneumonia is one of the most common medical problems encountered in clinical practice and the leading fatal infectious disease worldwide. In the United States alone, 4 million individuals develop pneumonia each year and 1 million individuals require hospitalization, resulting in 75,000 deaths and $10 billion in health care expenditures. Despite the ability of antimicrobial therapy to augment normal host defenses and prevent/control infection, prescribing errors are common, including treatment of colonization, suboptimal empiric therapy, inappropriate combination therapy, dosing and duration errors, and mismanagement of apparent antibiotic failure. Inadequate consideration of antibiotic resistance potential, tissue penetration, drug interactions, side effects, and cost also limits the effectiveness of antimicrobial therapy. *Pneumonia Essentials* is a concise, practical, and authoritative guide to the diagnosis, evaluation, treatment, and prevention of community-acquired pneumonia (CAP), nursing home-acquired pneumonia (NHAP), nosocomial (hospital-acquired) pneumonia (NP), tuberculosis (TB), chronic pneumonias, and pneumonias in the immunocompromised host.

A. Description. Pneumonia is an infectious/inflammatory disorder of the lung parenchyma. Most patients present with fever, chills, pulmonary symptoms (cough, dyspnea, sputum production, pleuritic chest pain), and one or more infiltrates/opacities on chest x-ray (Table 1.1). Elderly patients may present with malaise, anorexia, confusion, and diarrhea rather than prominent pulmonary symptoms, and the chest x-ray may be relatively normal in the hyperacute stage of pneumonia, in patients with marked leukopenia, and in certain types of pneumonia (e.g., Pneumocystis carinii pneumonia, Mycoplasma pneumonia). Pathologically, the pulmonary alveoli and/or interstitium are filled with white blood cells, red blood cells, and fibrin; lung weight is increased; and the responsible microbe can be recovered by stain or culture.

Table 1.1. Clinical Manifestations of Pneumonia

- Constitutional symptoms (e.g., fever, chills)
- Pulmonary symptoms (cough, dyspnea, sputum production, pleuritic chest pain)
- Extrapulmonary findings suggest the presence of an atypical pathogen (e.g., otitis/myringitis with mycoplasma, rash [Horder's spots] with psittacosis, loose stools/diarrhea with Legionella)
- Other manifestations
  - ▸ Related to complications of pneumonia (e.g., hemoptysis from vascular invasion, endocarditis/meningitis from bacteremia, stress ulcer/GI bleed)
  - ▸ Related to exacerbation/worsening of comorbid conditions (e.g., heart failure, angina, acute MI, renal insufficiency, pulmonary decompensation, hyperglycemia)

B. Classification. Pneumonia can be broadly classified into community-acquired pneumonia (CAP), nursing home-acquired pneumonia (NHAP), or nosocomial (hospital-acquired) pneumonia (NP) (Figure 1.1). The various classifications have implications for the etiologic diagnosis, evaluation, therapy, and prognosis. Pneumonia can also be classified by severity of illness, location of treatment, rapidity of onset, pathogen, and host immune status (Table 1.2).

1. Community-Acquired Pneumonia (CAP). CAP is usually classified into ambulatory or hospitalized pneumonia and typical or atypical pneumonia. Typical CAP presents without extrapulmonary findings (e.g., myringitis, pharyngitis, rash). Atypical CAP presents with extrapulmonary findings and can further be classified into zoonotic or nonzoonotic pneumonia based on the presence of a zoonotic vector. Features of nonzoonotic and zoonotic atypical pneumonias are described in Tables 4.1 and 4.4, respectively.

2. Nursing Home-Acquired Pneumonia (NHAP). NHAP may resemble CAP or HAP and occur sporadically or as part of a nursing home outbreak.

3. Nosocomial (Hospital-Acquired) Pneumonia (NP). NP is usually classified into ventilator-associated pneumonia (VAP) or non-ventilator-associated pneumonia.

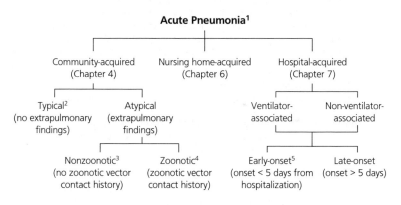

Figure 1.1. General Classification of Acute Pneumonia

1. Further classification into host immune status, rapidity of onset, and severity has implications for etiologic diagnosis, evaluation, and therapy
2. The most common CAP pathogens are shown in Table 1.4
3. The most common nonzoonotic atypical pneumonia pathogens in normal hosts include M. pneumoniae, C. pneumoniae, and Legionella spp.
4. The most common zoonotic pathogens in normal hosts include C. psittaci (psittacosis), C. burnetii (Q fever), and F. tularensis (tularemia)
5. Nearly all cases of pneumonia appearing during the first 5 days of hospitalization represent incubating community-acquired pneumonia

C. **Epidemiology.** A variety of bacteria, viruses, fungi, mycobacteria, chlamydia, parasites, and rickettsia can cause pneumonia (Table 1.3). Usual CAP pathogens are shown in Table 1.4, and common sites of acquisition of pneumonia pathogens (ambulatory, hospital, ICU) are shown in Table 1.5. *Single pathogens, not copathogens, cause CAP.* (Patients presenting with "multiple bacterial pathogens" are seen only with aspiration pneumonia or lung abscess.) In normal hosts with CAP, apparent multiple/copathogens (except for MSSA/MRSA with viral influenza) almost always is based on combined serologic and microbiologic data. In compromised hosts, pulmonary pathogens usually present sequentially, not simultaneously, as copathogens. Specific patient subsets are predisposed to certain pathogens and types of pneumonia, as suggested by the history, physical examination, laboratory testing, chest x-ray, and sputum Gram stain (Table 1.6, Chapter 2). Factors associated with severe CAP are shown in Table 1.7; general features of bacterial, viral, and fungal pneumonias are shown in Table 1.9; and detailed descriptions of important pneumonia pathogens are provided in Chapters 4-11.

D. **Pathogenesis**. The ability of a microbe to cause infection depends on the balance between inoculum size, virulence, and the adequacy of host defenses (Table 1.10). Several microbes have developed their own strategies to antagonize host defense mechanisms (Table 1.11). The primary modes of acquisition of pneumonia include aspiration of nasopharyngeal/gastric flora, inhalation of airborne pathogens, direct spread from a contiguous infected site, and hematogenous spread from a distant infected site (Table 1.12).

E. **Diagnosis and Evaluation (Figure 1.2)**
  1. **Initial Evaluation.** A history, physical examination, laboratory testing, chest x-ray, and sputum Gram stain is indicated for nearly all individuals with suspected pneumonia. This information is used to confirm the diagnosis, identify early complications, assess comorbid medical conditions, and arrive at a presumptive etiologic diagnosis. Patients are then triaged to home vs. hospital care, and empiric antimicrobial therapy is started. Diagnostic clues to the etiology of pneumonia may be evident from the history, physical examination, laboratory testing, patient subset, Gram stain, and chest x-ray (Chapters 2, 3, 11). Detailed information about specific pneumonia pathogens is provided in Chapters 4-11.
  2. **Noninfectious Mimics**. Several noninfectious medical conditions can present with pulmonary symptoms, fever, and chest x-ray opacities/infiltrates that mimic pneumonia (Table 1.13). Pulmonary symptoms in the absence of an opacity/infiltrate on chest x-ray are usually due to acute bronchitis/acute exacerbation of chronic bronchitis (AECB), tracheobronchitis, or asthma. See also chest x-ray atlas (Chapter 11).
  3. **Outpatient vs. Hospital Management.** The decision to treat pneumonia in an ambulatory vs. hospital setting is based on the presence of risk factors that limit the safety/effectiveness of outpatient management, the Pneumonia Severity

Index, and clinical judgement (Tables 1.14, 1.15).

4. **Identification of Presumed Pathogen/Syndrome.** Several methods can be used to identify the pneumonia pathogen, including culture (blood, sputum, pleural fluid/tissue, lower respiratory tract specimen, lung tissue); IgM response or 4-fold rise in antibody titer to a microbial antigen; antigen detection (urine, blood, pleural fluid); or amplification of microbial DNA/RNA (PCR) obtained from blood, sputum, pleural fluid, tissue, or the nasopharynx. Various collection procedures, cultures, stains, DNA probes, and serology tests are available (Chapter 14). Findings that confirm the etiologic diagnosis of pneumonia are shown in Table 1.16.

5. **In-hospital Evaluation**. In-hospital evaluation is aimed at identifying the pneumonia pathogen, detecting pulmonary and systemic complications, and evaluating the status of comorbid medical conditions. All patients require a chest x-ray, arterial blood gas (ABG), complete blood count (CBC), chemistry profile (electrolytes, liver/renal function tests), blood cultures x 2 (prior to antibiotics), and sputum Gram stain/culture (Tables 1.17, 1.18). Select patients require AFB stain/culture, Legionella testing, specific serologies, or pleural fluid analysis (Table 1.17). More aggressive techniques may be useful for patients admitted into the ICU, including bronchoscopy with bronchoalveolar lavage, protected bronchial brush specimens, and transbronchial biopsy.

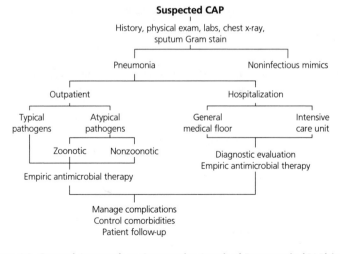

Figure 1.2. General Approach to Community-Acquired Pneumonia (CAP) in Normal Hosts (see text pp. 6-8 for details)

F. Empiric Antimicrobial Therapy. Antimicrobial therapy is directed against the presumed pneumonia pathogen (Chapters 4-10). Considerations related to drug selection, route of administration (IV vs. PO therapy), and duration of therapy are listed in Table 1.19 and detailed in Chapter 15. In general, PO therapy is recommended for patients able to take/absorb PO drugs. When IV therapy is indicated, the patient is usually switched to PO therapy after clinical improvement, typically within 72 hours. Adjunctive therapeutic measures are sometimes required, including supplemental oxygen (to maintain pO_2 saturation > 90%), bronchodilators, and suction/chest PT to mobilize/facilitate the clearance of respiratory secretions. Instructions for ambulatory patients treated for CAP are shown in Table 1.20.

G. Complications of Pneumonia. The majority of normal hosts with CAP treated with appropriate antimicrobial therapy on an ambulatory basis have an uncomplicated course and excellent prognosis (mortality < 1%). However, complications do occur, particularly in elderly patients, immunocompromised hosts, and individuals with underlying medical conditions, which may threaten survival. Complications include pulmonary complications (e.g., vascular invasion with infarction, bronchopulmonary fistula, pleural adhesions), systemic complications (e.g., bacteremia), exacerbation of comorbid conditions (e.g., diabetes mellitus), other complications related to the acute illness (e.g., stress ulcer), and failure to respond to therapy (Table 1.21). Management of major complications is described in Chapter 12.

H. Failure to Respond to Therapy. The usual response to antimicrobial therapy is shown in Table 1.22. A small minority of patients (< 5%) fail to respond to therapy due to a variety of causes (Tables 1.23 and 15.9).

I. Follow-up. Parameters for hospital discharge are shown in Table 1.19. A repeat chest x-ray may be obtained at 4-6 weeks (younger nonsmokers) or 8-12 weeks (elderly patients with COPD) to confirm radiographic resolution and exclude underlying pulmonary pathology (e.g., post-obstructive pneumonia due to lung cancer), which may occur in 2% of cases.

J. Prognosis. Pneumonia is the most fatal infectious disease worldwide and accounts for 75,000 deaths each year in the U.S. alone. Low mortality rates (< 1%) occur in otherwise healthy patients treated in the ambulatory setting. Higher mortality rates (8%) occur in hospitalized patients with mortality rates of 30-50% in ICU patients. Prognosis depends on the pulmonary pathogen, underlying cardiopulmonary and immune status, and other factors (Table 1.24).

K. Prevention. Preventive measures are highly effective at reducing the incidence and severity of pneumonia. Immunizations and chemoprophylaxis are reviewed in Chapter 13, and measures to reduce the incidence of hospital–acquired pneumonia are described in Chapter 7.

Table 1.2. Classification/Stratification of Pneumonia

Location of acquisition	Community-acquired (CAP)
	Nursing home-acquired (NHAP)
	Nosocomial (hospital-acquired) pneumonia (NP)
	    Ventilator-associated pneumonia (VAP)
	    Non-ventilator-associated pneumonia

Presence of extrapulmonary findings	Typical (extrapulmonary findings absent) Atypical (extrapulmonary findings present)
Presence/absence of zoonotic vector (if extrapulmonary findings)	Zoonotic (e.g., psittacosis, Q fever, tularemia) Non-zoonotic (e.g., Legionella, C. pneumoniae, M. pneumoniae)
Severity of illness	Mild, moderate, severe
Location of treatment	Home (ambulatory) Nursing home Hospital - general medical floor Hospital - intensive care unit
Rapidity of onset	Acute, subacute, chronic
Pathogen	General class (bacterial, viral, fungal, chlamydial, parasitic, mycobacterial) Specific pathogen (e.g., pneumococcus, S. aureus, mycoplasma)
Host immune status	Normal Immunocompromised (impaired cell-mediated immunity, impaired humoral immunity, or both)

Table 1.3. Pneumonia Pathogens

Bacterial	Fungal	Atypical Pathogens
Common:	Usually in normal hosts	Chlamydophilia (Chlamydia)
Streptococcus pneumoniae	Histoplasma capsulatum	pneumoniae
Haemophilus influenzae	Blastomyces dermatitidis	Legionella spp.
Moraxella catarrhalis	Coccidioides immitis	Mycoplasma pneumoniae
Oral anaerobic bacteria	Actinomyces sp.	Coxiella burnetii (Q fever)
(aspiration):		Chlamydia psittaci
Bacteroides spp.	Usually in compromised hosts	Chlamydia trachomatis
Fusobacterium spp.	Cryptococcus neoformans	(neonates only)
Peptostreptococcus spp.	Nocardia asteroides	Francisella tularensis
Peptococcus spp.	Sporothrix schenckii	Mycobacterium tuberculosis
Prevotella spp.	Penicillium marneffei	Nontuberculous mycobacteria
Streptococcus pyogenes	Aspergillus sp.	
Escherichia coli	Zygomycetes	**Viral**
Klebsiella pneumoniae	Pseudallescheria boydii	Children
		Respiratory syncytial virus (RSV)
		Parainfluenza virus (types 1, 2, 3)
	Parasitic	Adenovirus (types 1, 2, 3)
Uncommon:	Pneumocystis (jiroveci) carinii	Influenza B virus
Acinetobacter baumanii	Strongyloides stercoralis	
Actinomyces sp.	Paragonimus westermani	Adults (common):
Eikenella corrodens	Toxoplasma gondii	Influenza A virus
Neisseria meningitidis		Influenza B virus
Nocardia sp.		Adenovirus types 4 and 7
Pasteurella multocida		(military recruits)
Proteus spp.		
Serratia marcescens		Adults (uncommon):
Pseudomonas aeruginosa		Adenovirus (types 1, 2, 3, 5)
Pseudomonas		Varicella-zoster virus (VZV)
pseudomallei		Cytomegalovirus (CMV)
Yersinia pestis		Herpes simplex virus (HSV-1)
Staphylococcus aureus		Respiratory syncytial virus (RSV)
(MSSA/MRSA)		Parainfluenza virus
		Measles virus
		Hantavirus

Table 1.4. Usual Pathogens of Community-Acquired Pneumonia[†]

Pathogen	Approximate Frequency
S. pneumoniae	30-40%
H. influenzae	5%
M. catarrhalis	5%
Atypical pathogens	10-20%
Legionella	5%
M. pneumoniae	5%
C. pneumoniae	5%
Viruses (influenza, parainfluenza, adenovirus)	10%
Aspiration pneumonia	5-10%
S. aureus (MSSA/MRSA)*	3%
Group A strep, N. meningitidis	3%
Gram-negative bacilli	3%
No specific pathogen demonstrated (standard testing)	30-40%

* Virtually all cases occur with influenza pneumonia, including community-acquired MRSA (PVL-positive) strains

† Co-pathogens in CAP are rare (except for S. aureus CAP with viral influenza)

Table 1.5. Common Sites of Acquisition of Community-Acquired Pneumonia

Pathogen	Ambulatory	Hospital	Intensive care unit
S. pneumoniae*	x		x
M. pneumoniae	x		x
C. pneumoniae	x		
H. influenzae	x	x	x
M. catarrhalis	x		
Influenza[†]	x	x	x
PCP	x	x	x
Viruses		x	x
Aerobic gram-negative bacilli		x	x
M. tuberculosis	x	x	

* S. pneumoniae is the most common pneumonia pathogen and accounts for 50% of all cases of pneumonia admitted to the hospital

† Including avian influenza

Table 1.6. Clues to Suggest a Specific Pneumonia Pathogen*

- History: age, animal contact, travel history, immune status, alcohol history, comorbid conditions (e.g., COPD, bronchiectasis)
- Physical findings
- Laboratory tests
- Sputum color, odor, consistency
- Gram stain/other stains
- Chest x-ray: pattern, location, progression/resolution of infiltrates
- Geographic location
- Season
- Pleural fluid analysis

* Also see Chapters 2, 3, 11

Table 1.7. Factors Associated With Severe CAP

Category	Factors
Pathogen factors	Inoculum size, encapsulated organisms (K. pneumoniae), intracellular organisms (Legionella), inherent virulence (plague, SARS, hantavirus, influenza/PVL-positive CA-MRSA)
Pulmonary factors	Decreased functional lung capacity (emphysema), advanced lung disease (chronic bronchitis)
Cardiac factors	Congestive heart failure, severe valvular disease, cardiomyopathy, coronary artery disease
Systemic factors	Advanced age (CNS/esophageal dysfunction), hepatic insufficiency, renal insufficiency
Host defense factors	
Impaired B-lymphocyte function (humoral immunity)	SLE, multiple myeloma, cirrhosis, hyposplenia,* asplenia
Impaired T-lymphocyte function (cell-mediated immunity)	T-cell lymphomas, high dose/chronic steroid therapy, immunosuppressive therapy, HIV
Impaired combined B/T-lymphocyte function	CLL, SLE with flare/immunosuppressive therapy, advanced age

* See Table 1.8 for disorders associated with impaired splenic function

Table 1.8. Conditions Associated With Impaired Splenic Function/Humoral (B-Lymphocyte) Immunity

- Amyloidosis
- Celiac disease
- Chronic active hepatitis
- Chronic alcoholism
- Congenital asplenia
- Fanconi syndrome
- Hyposplenism of old age
- IgA deficiency
- Intestinal lymphangiectasia

- IV gamma globulin therapy
- Myeloproliferative disorders
- Non-Hodgkin lymphoma
- Regional enteritis
- Waldenstrom macroglobulinemia
- Rheumatoid arthritis
- Sézary syndrome
- Sickle cell trait/disease

- Splenectomy
- Splenic infarcts
- Splenic malignancies
- Steroid therapy
- SLE
- Systemic mastocytosis
- Systemic necrotizing vasculitis
- Thyroiditis
- Ulcerative colitis

Table 1.9. General Features of Viral, Bacterial, and Fungal Pneumonias

Feature	Viral Pneumonia	Bacterial Pneumonia	Fungal Pneumonia
Onset	Insidious*	Abrupt	Subacute/chronic
Antecedent URI	Common	Less common	Uncommon
Appearance	Nontoxemic	Toxemic	Nontoxemic
Rigors	Uncommon	Common	Uncommon
Cough	Nonproductive	Productive	Often productive
Sputum	None/mucoid	Purulent	Purulent (if present)
Pleuritic pain	Rare (influenza only)	Often Present	Sometimes present

URI = upper respiratory illness
* Excluding influenza, SARS, avian influenza, hantavirus
Adapted from: Brandstetter RD (ed). Pulmonary Medicine. Medical Economics Books, Oradell, NJ, 1989.

Table 1.10. Host Defense Mechanisms Against Pneumonia

System	Host Defenses	Mechanism of Lung Defense
Physical defenses	Nose	Filtering of larger particulate matter
	Cough; mucociliary escalator	Bulk clearance of microbes in secretions
Nonspecific cellular and humoral factors	Immunoglobulins (principally IgA); complement; antiproteases; opsonins	Binding of microbes to facilitate removal by the mucociliary escalator, ingestion and destruction by alveolar macrophages, or removal via pulmonary lymphatics
	Lactoferrin	Depletion of essential nutrients from some bacteria
	Alveolar macrophage	Endocytosis of bacteria and release of toxic oxygen, nitrogen radicals and lysosomal enzymes; direct and antibody-dependent cytotoxicity; secretion of IFN-γ, TNF
	Neutrophil	Endocytosis; generation of oxygen and nitrogen radicals, lactoferrin, lysozyme
Specific immune response	Specific antibody production; macrophage-T-lymphocyte interaction; recruitment of neutrophils, lymphocytes, natural killer cells	Enhanced production of variety of cytokines, including IFN-γ, IL-2, IL-12, TNF-β, IgA, IgG, IgM

Adapted from: Crapo JD, Glassroth J, Karlinsky JB, King TE. Baum's Textbook of Pulmonary Diseases, 7th ed. Philadelphia, Lippincott Williams & Wilkins, 2004. Murray JF, Nadel JA. Textbook of Respiratory Medicine, 3rd ed. Philadelphia, W.B. Saunders Company, 2000.

Table 1.11. Microbial Strategies Against Host Defense

Strategy	Pathogen	Mediators/Mechanisms
Inhibit cilia	P. aeruginosa	Phenazine pigments
	S. pneumoniae	Pneumolysin
	H. influenzae	Unidentified low-molecular-weight compound
Damage cilia	P. aeruginosa	Pyocyanin (a phenazine pigment)
	S. pneumoniae	Pneumolysin
	H. influenzae	Lipopolysaccharide (endotoxin)
Adhere to mucus	H. influenzae, P. aeruginosa	Pili, fibrils
Penetrate mucus and adhere	Influenza viruses	Viral neuraminidases
Inhibit inflammatory cells	H. influenzae	Culture filtrates inhibit neutrophil migration
	Respiratory viruses	May induce host damage to phagocytes
Avoid humoral defenses	Legionella, fungi, mycobacteria, respiratory viruses	Intracellular survival

Adapted from: same as Table 1.10.

Table 1.12. Mode of Acquisition of Pneumonia

- Microaspiration of nasopharyngeal secretions/pathogens
- Aspiration of gastric acid/pathogens (e.g., post-op, CNS/swallowing disorders)
- Inhalation of infected droplets (e.g., Legionnaires' disease, viral influenza, TB)
- Hematogenous spread from distant infected site (e.g., E. coli UTI)
- Direct contiguous spread (e.g., from mediastinitis)

Table 1.13. Noninfectious Mimics of Pneumonia*

Congestive heart failure
Atelectasis
Pulmonary embolus/infarction
Bronchogenic carcinoma
Metastatic carcinoma
Lymphangitic carcinomatosis
Lymphoma
Collagen vascular disease (esp. SLE, rheumatoid arthritis)
Sarcoidosis
Eosinophilic pneumonia
Pulmonary interstitial fibrosis
Hypersensitivity pneumonitis
Goodpasture's Syndrome/Wegener's granulomatosis
Drug-induced pulmonary disease (e.g., busulfan, bleomycin, cyclophosphamide, methotrexate, nitrofurantoin, sulfasalazine, amiodarone, gold salts)
Noncardiogenic pulmonary edema (e.g., salicylates, narcotics, chlordiazepoxide)
Bronchiolitis obliterans with organizing pneumonia (BOOP)
Septic pulmonary emboli (right-sided ABE)

* Also see chest x-ray atlas (Chapter 11) for differential diagnostic clues based on history, physical examination, labs, and chest x-ray.

Table 1.14. Triage of Pneumonia to Home vs. Hospital Care Based on the Pneumonia Outcomes Research Team (PORT) Score

Characteristic	Points*	Characteristic	Points*
Demographic factor		Physical examination finding	
Male	Age (years)	Altered mental status[+]	+20
Female	Age (years) –10	Respiratory rate > 30 breaths/min	+20
Nursing home resident	+10	Systolic blood pressure < 90 mmHg	+20
		Temperature < 35° C or > 40° C	+15
		Pulse > 125 beats/min	+10
Comorbid illnesses		Laboratory or radiographic finding	
Neoplastic disease[†]	+30	Arterial pH < 7.35	+30
Liver disease[‡]	+20	Blood urea nitrogen > 30 mg/dL	+20
Congestive heart	+10	Sodium < 130 mEq/L	+20
failure[¶]	+10	Glucose > 250 mg/dL	+10
Cerebrovascular	+10	Hematocrit < 30%	+10
disease[§]		Arterial partial pressure of oxygen	
Renal disease**		< 60 mmHg[++]	+10
		Pleural effusion	+10

Risk Class	No. of Points	Mortality (%)	Recommended Site of Care
I	No predictors	0.1	Outpatient
II	≤ 70	0.6	Outpatient
III	71-90	2.8	Outpatient
IV	91-130	8.2	Hospital
V	> 130	29.2	Hospital

*   *A total point score for a given patient is obtained by adding the patient's age in years (age – 10, for females) plus the points for each patient characteristic* (e.g., for a 70-year-old male with heart failure and pH of 7.3, point score = 70 + 10 + 30 = 110 (risk class IV). Home care is recommended for risk classes I, II, III; hospital care is recommended for risk class IV, V.

†   Any cancer except basal or squamous cell cancer of the skin that was active at the time of presentation or diagnosed within 1 year of presentation.

‡   A clinical or histologic diagnosis of cirrhosis or other form of chronic liver disease such as chronic active hepatitis.

¶   Systolic or diastolic ventricular dysfunction documented by history and physical examination, chest x-ray, echocardiography, Muga scanning, or left ventriculography

§   A clinical diagnosis of stroke, transient ischemic attack, or stroke documented by MRI or computed tomography.

** A history of chronic renal disease or abnormal BUN and creatinine.

+   Disorientation (to person, place, or time, not known to be chronic), stupor or coma.

++ In the Pneumonia Patient Outcome Research Team cohort study, an oxygen saturation value < 90% on pulse oximetry or intubation before admission was also considered abnormal.

Adapted from: Fine, et al. Pneumonia Patient Outcome Research Team cohort study. N Engl J Med 336:243, 1997.

Table 1.15. Management of CAP in Immunocompetent Adults: Recommendations from the Infectious Diseases Society of America (IDSA)

- Initial site of treatment should be based on (1) assessment of preexisting conditions that compromise safety of home care; (2) calculation of the pneumonia PORT (Pneumonia Outcome Research Team) Severity Index with recommendation for home care for risk classes I, II, and III (Table 1.14); and (3) clinical judgment

- Hospitalized patients treated with IV antibiotics may be changed to oral antibiotics when the patient is clinically improving, able to ingest drugs, hemodynamically stable, and has a functioning GI tract

- Discharge criteria: During the 24 hour prior to discharge to home, the patient should have no more than 1 of the following characteristics (unless this represents the baseline status): temperature > 37.8°C; pulse > 100 beats/min; respiratory rate > 24 breaths/min; systolic blood pressure < 90 mmHg; arterial oxygen saturation < 90%; inability to maintain oral intake

Adapted from: IDSA Practice Guidelines. Clin Infect Dis 37:1405-1433, 2003

Table 1.16. Criterion for Establishing an Etiologic Diagnosis of Pneumonia*

- Blood culture positive for a pulmonary pathogen

- Pleural fluid culture positive for a pulmonary pathogen

- Isolation of Legionella pneumophila or positive urinary antigen test for Legionella (L. pneumophila serogroup 1 only)

- Sputum positive DFA for Legionella

- Legionella antibody titer ≥1:256 (acute titer) or ≥ 4-fold increase from acute to convalescent titers (4-6 weeks later)

- Presence of Pneumocystis (carinii) jiroveci in induced sputum or in bronchoalveolar lavage fluid

- Elevated IgM or ≥ 4-fold rise in IgG antibody titer to pulmonary pathogen

- Urine positive for S. pneumoniae or H. influenzae antigen

DFA = direct fluorescence antibody test
* Definite pneumonia pathogen is identified in 60% of cases

Table 1.17. Tests for Evaluation of Pneumonia

Subset	Test	Comments
All patients	Chest x-ray	Used to confirm diagnosis of pneumonia, detect associated lung diseases, implicate a pathogen (in some), assess severity, and use as baseline to assess response. Repeat at 4-6 weeks in patients > 40 years and at 8-12 weeks in elderly or COPD to ensure resolution and exclude noninfectious mimics of pneumonia (e.g., lung cancer)
	Sputum Gram stain/culture*	CAP: optional for outpatients; recommended for hospitalized patients. May also obtain sputum via tracheostomy/nasotracheal aspirates, induced sputum (recommended for M. tuberculosis and PCP). Ensure adequate specimen.[†] Single predominant organism in good specimen is diagnostic. Sputum of no value in AECB. NP: sputum is unhelpful/misleading (indicates colonization, not infection)
Hospitalized patients	Lab tests[‡]	Used to assess comorbid medical disorders. May suggest a pathogen in some
	Blood cultures x 2 (preferably before treatment)	Positive cultures; usually S. pneumoniae, H. influenza, E. coli (excluding s. aureus/IV line/venipuncture related organisms)
Select patients	AFB staining/culture	Obtain in seriously ill patients without an alternative diagnosis if clinical features suggest TB or in outbreak settings, especially if > 40 years or immunocompromised
	Legionella testing	Obtain in those with extrapulmonary findings, especially relative bradycardia ± mental status changes, ↓ PO_4 /↑ LFTs, or nonresponsive to beta-lactams
	Thoracentesis with Gram stain, culture, pH, WBC count/differential	Recommended if moderate-large pleural effusion present
	Sputum cytology	May detect bronchogenic cancer (post-obstructive pneumonia)
	Serological testing	Available for all atypical pathogens, bioterrorist agents, influenza, hantavirus, SARS

* Preferably obtain specimen before antibiotic therapy. Inability to obtain specimens for diagnostic studies should not delay antibiotic treatment of ill patients
† Only 30% of elderly patients produce adequate sputum
‡ CBC with differential, electrolytes, LFTs, BUN/creatinine
Adapted from: IDSA Practice Guidelines. Clin Infect Dis 31:347-382, 2000.

Table 1.18. Laboratory Tests for Hospitalized Patients with Community-Acquired Pneumonia

- Chest x-ray
- Blood cultures x 2 (preferably before therapy)
- Complete blood count (including platelet count), liver function tests, BUN/creatinine, electrolytes (including $PO_4^=$), urinalysis
- Sputum Gram stain and culture. If TB suspected, acid-fast stain and culture. If Legionella suspected, ESR, CRP, CPK, ferritin, Legionella sputum DFA and urinary antigen assay. If mycoplasma suspected, cold agglutinins
- Pleural fluid analysis: white cell count and differential, LDH, pH, lactic acid, protein, glucose; Gram stain, acid-fast stain; culture for bacteria (aerobes/anaerobes), fungi, AFB

Adapted from: Bartlett JG. Approach to the Patient with Pneumonia. In Gorbach, Bartlett, Blacklow (eds). Infectious Disease, 2nd edition, W.B. Saunders, Philadelphia, PA.

Table 1.19. Considerations for Antimicrobial Therapy for CAP

Issue	Comment
Need for chest x-ray and Gram stain	A chest x-ray is recommended for all patients. Chest x-ray confirms diagnosis, excludes noninfectious mimics, and often suggests pathogen (see also chest x-ray atlas, Chapter 11). Gram stain of good sputum specimen demonstrating single predominant organism confirms pathogen (see also Chapter 3)
Outpatient vs. inpatient	Decision is based on Pneumonia Severity Index (Table 1.14) and clinical judgement regarding advisability/availability of home care
Choice of therapy	Empiric therapy is directed against the most likely pneumonia pathogen based on history, physical examination, chest x-ray, sputum Gram stain (Chapters 2, 3, 11). Coverage against typical/atypical pathogens is recommended. Subsequent antimicrobial therapy may require adjustment based on culture and sensitivity testing
Oral therapy	Oral therapy can be used for ambulatory patients and hospitalized patients with non-severe CAP
Switch from IV to PO therapy	May be treated entirely IV, PO, or IV/PO. Switch to PO therapy is recommended for patients after defervescence and improvement in clinical status/respiratory symptoms (usually within 72 hours) who can take/absorb PO medication (by mouth or NG/PEG tube)
Duration of therapy	In normal/healthy hosts, most CAPs can be treated with 5-10 days of antimicrobial therapy. Longer duration of therapy may be needed for some pathogens (e.g., Legionella) and in immunocompromised hosts.
Discharge from hospital	Patients should demonstrate clinical stability (T < 37.5°C x 1 day, O_2 saturation > 90%, RR < 24/min, ability to eat/drink), no other complications or complications under control (e.g., MI, arrhythmia, PE, heart failure, empyema, lung abscess), and stable/controlled comorbid medical disorders

Table 1.20. Instructions for Ambulatory Patients Treated for CAP

- Maintain good hydration (caution in patients with heart failure)
- Avoid cough suppressants, cigarettes
- Follow-up call at 5-7 days
- Follow-up office visit at 5-7 days for persistent fever, dyspnea, cough, or chest pain
- Follow-up chest x-ray to exclude bronchial obstruction (lung cancer) at 4-6 weeks (young adult) or at 8-12 weeks (elderly patient, COPD, or multilobar involvement)

Table 1.21. Complications of Pneumonia

- Pulmonary complications: empyema, lung abscess/cavitation, bronchopleural fistula, necrotizing pneumonia, pulmonary infarction, bronchiolitis obliterans (BOOP), ARDS
- Systemic complications: sepsis in asplenics, bacteremia with metastatic infection (e.g., meningitis, endocarditis, septic arthritis)
- Exacerbation of comorbid medical disorders: heart failure, coronary heart disease, diabetes mellitus, COPD
- Complications related to mechanical ventilation: pneumothorax, subcutaneous emphysema, ARDS
- Pulmonary drug reactions
- Other unrelated complications: stress ulcer/GI bleed, DVT/pulmonary embolism
- Failure to respond to therapy (see Table 1.23)

Table 1.22. Usual Response to Therapy for CAP

Sections	Comment
Outpatient (young, healthy adults)	• Most return to work at < 1 week and fully recover by 2 weeks • 2-4% manifest progressive symptoms or worsening of medical disorders (coronary heart disease, heart failure, asthma, COPD)
Hospitalized patients	• Most require 3-7 days for clinical stability; 2 days for pulse ≤ 100/min; and 3 days for respiratory rate ≤ 24/min, O_2 saturation ≥ 90%, temperature ≤ 37.2°C (99°F) • 70% develop complications (e.g., respiratory failure, heart failure, MI, arrhythmia, shock, GI bleed, renal insufficiency) • Once clinically stable, deterioration is uncommon • Mortality ~ 8% (usually due to respiratory failure, heart disease, complication of infection) • Mortality rates up to 30-50% have been reported in high-risk patient populations (e.g., severe cardiopulmonary disease, immunocompromised host, ventilator-associated pneumonia) or for virulent pathogens (e.g., P. aeruginosa)

Table 1.23. Causes of Failure to Respond to Treatment for CAP/NHAP/NP

Category	Causes
Persistent fever *Treatment problem*	• Inadequate time for clinical improvement (fever usually decreases within 72 hours; pulmonary symptoms usually improve in 3-5 days; chest x-ray shows some improvement/no progression at one week) • Error in drug selection (incorrect/inadequate spectrum or inadequate activity) • Underdosing of antibiotic • Drug side effects • Drug-drug interactions (antibiotic inactivation/antagonism) • Antibiotic resistance (rarely a cause)
Diagnostic problem	• Viral or fungal pneumonia unresponsive to antibiotics (obtain cultures/specific serology) • TB unresponsive to antibiotics (obtain sputum AFB smears/cultures) • Noninfectious mimic of pneumonia (e.g., heart failure, lymphoma, bronchogenic carcinoma, sarcoidosis, pulmonary embolism/hemorrhage, SLE pneumonitis, radiation/chemical pneumonitis, drug fever, pulmonary drug reactions)
Host problem	• Obstruction of bronchus (e.g., bronchogenic carcinoma), sequestered lung
Initial improvement followed by recrudescence of fever	• Drug fever secondary to medications (usual) or antibiotics (less common) • Septic complication (lung abscess, empyema, complicated parapneumonic effusion) • Non-septic complication (acute gout, acute MI, acute pulmonary embolism, C. difficile diarrhea/colitis, etc.)

Table 1.24. Factors Related to Poor Prognosis for Patients with Pneumonia

Age > 65 years

Coexisting Disease
  Diabetes
  Renal failure
  Coronary heart disease
  Heart failure
  COPD
  Chronic alcoholism
  Hospitalization within one year previously
  Immunosuppression
  Malignancy
  Hyposplenism/asplenia

Physical Examination Abnormality
  Respiratory rate > 30/min
  Systolic blood pressure < 90 mmHg or diastolic blood pressure < 60 mmHg
  Temperature > 38.3°C or hypothermia
  Altered mental status not drug induced (lethargy, stupor, disorientation, coma)
  Extrapulmonary site of infection (e.g., meningitis)

Laboratory Abnormality
  White cell count < 4000/mm^3 or > 30,000/mm^3
  pO_2 < 60 mmHg or pCO_2 > 48 mmHg on room air
  Renal insufficiency (creatinine > 1.7 mg/dL)
  Albumin < 3.0 mg/dL
  Hematocrit < 30%

Virulent Pathogen
  Streptococcus pneumoniae (serotype 3)
  Legionella sp.
  Klebsiella pneumoniae
  Escherichia coli
  Staphylococcus aureus
  Pseudomonas aeruginosa

Chest X-Ray Abnormality
  Multilobar pneumonia
  Rapid progression of pneumonia
  Persistent pleural effusion/empyema

Adapted from: Fine, et al. Pneumonia Patient Outcome Research Team cohort study. N Engl J Med 336:243, 1997. Fine et al. Prognosis and outcomes of patients with community-acquired pneumonia. JAMA 274:134-141, 1995.

REFERENCES AND SUGGESTED READINGS

Chang M, Rozenfeld M, Cunha BA. Community-acquired pneumonia: pneumocystis carinii vs. mycobacterium tuberculosis (TB). Infectious Disease Practice 27:253-4, 2003.

Cotton LM, Strampfer MJ, Cunha BA. Legionella and mycoplasma pneumonia: a community hospital experience. Clinics in Chest Medicine 8:441-53, 1987.

Cunha BA, Quintiliani R. The atypical pneumonias, a diagnostic and therapeutic approach. Postgraduate Medicine 66:95-102, 1979.

Cunha BA. Ambulatory community acquired pneumonia: the predominance of atypical pathogens. European Journal of Clinical Microbiology and Infectious Disease 2:579-83, 2003.

Cunha BA. Antimicrobial resistance: strategies for control. Medical Clinics of North America 84:1407-27, 2000.

Cunha BA. Chlamydia pneumoniae community-acquired pneumonia. Emergency Medicine 32:15-9, 2000.

Cunha BA. Diagnostic significance of relative bradycardia. Clinical Microbiology & Infectious Disease 6:633-4, 2000.

Cunha BA. Community-acquired pneumonia: diagnostic and therapeutic considerations Medical Clinics of North America 85:43-77, 2001.

Cunha BA. Community-acquired pneumonias (Part I) differential diagnosis. Postgraduate Medicine 82:126-140, 1987.

Cunha BA. Community-acquired pneumonias (Part II) complications and empiric therapy. Postgraduate Medicine 82:149-162, 1987.

Cunha BA. Community-acquired pneumonia in HIV patients. Clinical Infectious Diseases 28:410-1, 1999.

Cunha BA. Community-acquired pneumonia in patients with HIV. Infections in Medicine 16:798-800, 1999.

Cunha BA. Community-acquired pneumonias: reality revisited. American Journal of Medicine 108:436-37, 2000.

Cunha BA. Diagnostic and therapeutic approach to the atypical pneumonias. Postgraduate Medicine 90:89-101, 1991.

Cunha BA. Empiric oral monotherapy for hospitalized patients with community-acquired pneumonia. An idea whose time has come. European Journal of Clinical Microbiology and Infectious Disease 23:78-81, 2004.

Cunha BA. Penicillin resistant pneumococci. Postgraduate Medicine 113:42-54, 2003.

Cunha BA. Severe acute respiratory syndrome (SARS) - a clinical perspective. Infectious Diseases Practice 27:191-6, 2003.

Cunha BA. Severe community-acquired pneumonia: determinants of severity and approach to therapy. Infections in Medicine 22:53-8, 2005.

Cunha BA. Slowly and non-resolving pneumonias. Drugs for Today 36:829-34, 2000.

Cunha BA. The antibiotic treatment of community-acquired, atypical, and nosocomial pneumonias. Medical Clinics of North America 79:581-598, 1995.

Cunha BA. The chlamydia pneumonias. Infectious Disease Practice 24:80-6, 2000.

Cunha BA. Viral influenza and its complications. Emergency Medicine 32:56-67, 2000.

Ly HT, Thermidor M, Cunha BA. Pneumocystis carinii community-acquired pneumonia in a non-HIV patient. Heart & Lung 32:261-4, 2004.

Mohan S, Nair V, Cunha BA. Post-viral influenza pneumococcal pneumonia in an intravenous drug abuser (IVDA). Heart & Lung 34:222-6, 2005.

Prince SE, Dominger KA, Cunha BA, et al. Klebsiella pneumoniae pneumonia. Heart & Lung 26:413-7, 1997.

Tarver RD, Teague SD, Heitkamp DE, et al. Radiology of community-acquired pneumonia. Radiol Clin North Am 43:497-512, 2005.

GUIDELINES

Bartlett JG, Dowell SF, Mandell LA, File Jr TM, Musher DM, Fine MJ. Practice guidelines for the management of community-acquired pneumonia in adults. Infectious Diseases Society of America. Clin Infect Dis 31:347-82, 2000 .

Mandell LA. Guidelines for community-acquired pneumonia: a tale of 3 countries. Clin Infect Dis 31:422-5, 2000.

Mandell LA, Wunderink RG, Anzueto A, et al. Infectious Diseases Society of American/American Thoracic Society consensus guidelines on the management of community-acquired pneumonia in adults. Clin Infect Dis 44:S27-S72, 2007.

Nathwani D, Rubinstein E, Barlow G, Davey P. Do guidelines for community-acquired pneumonia improve the cost-effectiveness of hospital care? Clin Infect Dis 32:728-41, 2001.

Yu VL, Ramirez J, Roig J, et al. Legionnaires disease and the updated IDSA guidelines for community-acquired pneumonia. Clin Infect Dis. 39:1734-7, 2004.

TEXTBOOKS

Baddour L, Gorback SL (eds). Therapy of Infectious Diseases. Saunders, Philadelphia, Pennsylvania, 2003.

Balows A, Hausler WJ, Jr., Ohashi M, Turano A (eds). Laboratory Diagnosis of Infectious Diseases. Principles and Practice (vol 1). Springer-Verlag, New York, 1988.

Brandstetter RD (ed). Pulmonary Medicine. Medical Economics Books, Oradell, New Jersey, 1989.

Bryskier A (ed). Antimicrobial Agents. ASM Press, Washington, D.C., 2005.

Cimolai N (ed). Laboratory Diagnosis of Bacterial Infections. Marcel Dekker, New York, 2001.

Cunha BA. Atypical pneumonias. In Conn RD, Borer WZ, Snyder JW (eds.) Current Diagnosis 9. WB Saunders, Philadelphia, 1996.

Cunha BA. Bacterial pneumonias. In Rakel RE (ed): Current Therapy-1999, 54th Edition. W.B. Saunders Co., Philadelphia, Pennsylvania, 1999.

Finch RG, Greenwood D, Norrby SR, Whitley RJ (eds). Antibiotic and Chemotherapy, 8th Edition. Churchill Livingstone, Edinburgh, Scotland, 2003.

Glauser MP, Pizzo PA (eds). Management of Infection in Immunocompromised Patients. W.B. Saunders, London, England, 2000.

Gorbach SL, Bartlett JG, Blacklow NR (eds). Infectious Diseases, 3rd Edition. Lippincott, Williams & Wilkins, Philadelphia, 2004.

Karetzky M, Cunha BA, Brandstetter RD. The Pneumonias. Springer-Verlag, New York, 1993.

Levison ME (ed). The Pneumonias: Clinical Approaches to Infectious Diseases of the Lower Respiratory Tract. John Wright, PSG, Littleton, MA, 1984.

Loeb M, Smieja M, Smaill F (eds). Evidence-Based Infectious Diseases. BMJ Publishing Group, Ltd., London, England, 2004.

Madkour MM (ed). Tuberculosis. Springer-Verlag, Berlin Germany, 2004.

Mandell GL, Bennett JE, Dolin R (eds). Mandell, Douglas and Bennett's Principles and Practice of Infectious Disease, 6th Edition. Elsevier, Philadelphia, 2005.

Niederman MS (ed). Severe Pneumonia. Taylor & Francis Group, Boca Raton, Florida, 2005.

Pilch RF, Ziliinskas RA (eds). Encyclopedia of Bioterrorism Defense. Wiley-Liss, Hoboken, New Jersey, 2005.

Rubin RH, Young LS, (eds). Clinical Approach to Infection in the Compromised Host, 3rd Edition, Plenum Medical Book Co., New York, 1994.

Root RK (ed). Clinical Infectious Disease: A Practical Approach. Oxford University Press, New York, 1999.

Sarosi GA, Davies SF (eds). Fungal Diseases of the Lung. Grune & Stratton, New York, 1986.

Schlossberg D (ed). Medical Interventions for Bioterrorism and Emerging Infections. Handbooks in Healthcare Co., Newtown, Pennsylvania, 2004.

Schlossberg D (ed). Tuberculosis & Nontuberculous Mycobacterial Infections, 5th Edition. McGraw-Hill, New York, 2006.

Singh N, Aguado JM (eds). Infectious Complications in Transplant Patients. Kluwer Academic Publishers, Boston, 2000.

Chapter 2

Pneumonia Clues Based on History, Physical Examination, Laboratory Tests, and Chest X-Ray

Burke A. Cunha, MD

Table 2.1. Pneumonia Clues Based on Patient Subsets

Subset	Likely Pathogens
Normal hosts	S. pneumoniae, H. influenzae, M. catarrhalis
Children/young adults	Mycoplasma pneumoniae, C. pneumoniae, viral pneumonia
Elderly	S. pneumoniae, H. influenzae, K. pneumoniae, Legionella, influenza, aspiration pneumonia/anaerobic lung abscess, M. tuberculosis
Alcoholism (chronic)	S. pneumoniae, K. pneumoniae, M. tuberculosis, aspiration pneumonia/anaerobic lung abscess
Diabetes, SLE chronic renal failure	S. pneumoniae, H. influenzae, M. catarrhalis, E. coli
Construction	Legionella, aspergillosis
Soil exposure	Histoplasmosis, blastomycosis
Bird exposure	Psittacosis, cryptococcosis, avian influenza
Cat/sheep exposure	Q fever
Deer/rabbit exposure	Tularemia
Chronic care facilities	S. pneumoniae, H. influenzae, K. pneumoniae, M. tuberculosis, C. pneumoniae, influenza, MDR gram-negative bacilli
IV drug abusers	S. aureus, P. aeruginosa; actually septic pulmonary emboli, not CAP
HIV	PCP, M. tuberculosis/MAI, Salmonella, Legionella, CMV, Rhodococcus equi, histoplasmosis, S. pneumoniae, K. pneumoniae, H. influenzae
Leukopenia (prolonged/profound)	Aspergillus, mucormycosis
Organ transplant	CMV, Herpes simplex virus, aspergillus, cryptococcosis, PCP
Foreign travel	M. tuberculosis, Q fever, melioidosis, paragonimiasis, amebic cysts, hydatid cysts, SARS, avian influenza
Asplenia/hyposplenia	S. pneumoniae, H. influenzae, N. meningitidis
Uremia	M. tuberculosis
COPD	S. pneumoniae, H. influenzae, M. catarrhalis
Cystic fibrosis/chronic bronchiectasis	P. aeruginosa, S maltophilia, B. cepacia

Table 2.1. Pneumonia Clues Based on Patient Subsets (cont'd)

Subset	Likely Pathogens
Post-viral influenza	S. pneumoniae, H. influenzae
Silicosis/coal mining	M. tuberculosis
Sarcoidosis	M. tuberculosis
Lymphoma/malignancy	M. tuberculosis
Rodent exposure	Hantavirus, tularemia, SARS, plague
Chickenpox exposure	Varicella
Corticosteroid therapy	M. tuberculosis, aspergillosis
Urinary tract infection	E. coli
Periodontal disease	Actinomycosis, aspiration pneumonia/anaerobic lung abscess

Adapted from: Cunha BA. Pneumonia Clues. In: Keretsky M, Cunha BA, Brandstetter R (eds). The Pneumonias. Medec Books, Oradell, NJ, 1993.

Table 2.2. Pneumonia Clues Based on History of Exposure

Exposure	Presumptive Diagnosis
Environmental contact	
Soil/plant	Legionnaires' disease, histoplasmosis, blastomycosis, sporotrichosis
Silicosis	Tuberculosis
Zoonotic contact	
Bird	Psittacosis, blastomycosis, histoplasmosis, cryptococcosis, SARS, avian influenza
Cat	Tularemia, Q fever
Rabbit/deer	Tularemia
Dog	Dirofilaria immitis
Small rodents	Plague, hantavirus, SARS
Human (sick person) contact	Influenza, adenovirus, TB, SARS, avian influenza, pneumonic plague

Adapted from: Cunha BA. Pneumonia Clues. In: Keretsky M, Cunha BA, Brandstetter R (eds). The Pneumonias. Medec Books, Oradell, NJ, 1993.

Table 2.3. Pneumonia Clues Based on Seasonal Incidence and Clinical Setting*

Pathogen	Seasonal Incidence	Clinical Setting	Clinical Clues
Common Pathogens			
S. pneumoniae	All year; winter	Elderly, smokers, cardiopulmonary disease, alcoholism	RLL segmental/lobar infiltrates/consolidation. Little/no pleural effusion; empyema not uncommon
H. influenzae	All year; winter	Same as S. pneumoniae	RLL segmental/lobar infiltrates/consolidation. Small/moderate pleural effusion
M. catarrhalis	All year	COPD	No lobar predilection. No pleural effusion
L. pneumophila	All year; summer/fall; outbreaks	Construction sites, air-cooling apparatus	Rapidly progressive asymmetrical infiltrates. Relative bradycardia. Watery diarrhea ± abdominal pain. Mental confusion
M. pneumoniae	All year; winter	Multiple members of household ill, often at 3-4 week intervals	Pharyngitis, otitis/bullous myringitis, dry hacking cough > 1 week. No relative bradycardia. Watery diarrhea. No mental confusion
C. pneumoniae	All year; winter	Young adults, person-to-person spread	Pharyngitis. Mycoplasma-like illness with laryngitis. No relative bradycardia. No mental confusion
Anaerobes	All year	Aspiration	Poor dentition, difficulty swallowing. Infiltrates in dependent lobe(s)

Table 2.3. Pneumonia Clues Based on Seasonal Incidence and Clinical Setting* (cont'd)

Pathogen	Seasonal Incidence	Clinical Setting	Clinical Clues
Uncommon Pathogens (< 1% incidence)			
Psittacosis	All year	Exposure to birds, esp. parrots, turkeys, pigeons (20% have no bird exposure)	Headache, splenomegaly, epistaxis, relative bradycardia
Q fever	All year	Contact with sheep, goats, cattle, cats, esp. at parturition	Headache, splenomegaly, relative bradycardia
Tularemia (pulmonary)	All year	Handling infected rodents, rabbits	Purplish/bluish painful ulcer, regional adenopathy
Plague (pneumonia)	Spring to fall	Handling infected rodents, humans, cats	Delirium, sepsis, buboes
Other Pathogens			
Respiratory syncytial virus (RSV)	Winter	Contact with children with bronchiolitis	Croup-like presentation
Influenza	Winter/spring	Closed populations, intrahousehold spread	Severe headache, severe prostration, severe myalgias
Parainfluenza 1, 2, 3	All year	Croup in household	Conjunctivitis
Adenovirus	Winter	Closed populations	Conjunctivitis, sore throat
Hantavirus	All year	Close contact with deer mice	Severe myalgias, pulmonary edema
Avian influenza	All year	Infected persons/birds	Rapid onset severe myalgias/dyspnea
SARS	All year	Infected persons/ Asian travel	Rapid onset severe myalgias/dyspnea
PCP	All year	HIV, chronic steroids, organ transplants	Progressive dyspnea x 1 week, ↑ LDH

* Acute tuberculosis and some fungal pneumonias may be indistinguishable from early stages of acute bacterial pneumonia

Adapted from: Koster FT, Barker LR. Respiratory Tract Infections. In Barker LR, Burton JR, Zieve PD (eds). Principles of Ambulatory Medicine, 5th edition, Williams and Wilkins, Baltimore, MD.

Table 2.4. Pneumonia Clues Based on Symptoms

Symptom	Presumptive Diagnosis
Cough (nonproductive)	Mycoplasma, Legionella, Q fever, C. pneumoniae, tularemia, viral pneumonia, viral influenza
Chest pain (pleuritic)	Bacterial pneumonia, viral influenza
Dyspnea (severe)	Viral pneumonia, PCP, severe bacterial pneumonia
Night sweats	M. tuberculosis, histoplasmosis
Abdominal pain	Legionella
Ear pain	Mycoplasma, C. pneumoniae
Sore throat	Mycoplasma, C. pneumoniae, viral influenza, SARS, group A streptococci, adenovirus
Hoarseness Acute	Viral influenza, C. pneumoniae
Chronic	M. tuberculosis
Watery diarrhea	Mycoplasma, Legionella
Headache (severe)	Psittacosis, Q fever, viral influenza
Mental confusion	Legionella, Mycoplasma (only with meningoencephalitis)
Muscle aches (severe)	Coccidioidomycosis, viral influenza, SARS, hantavirus
Nosebleeds	Psittacosis

Adapted from: Cunha BA. Pneumonia Clues. In: Keretsky M, Cunha BA, Brandstetter R (eds). The Pneumonias. Medec Books, Oradell, NJ, 1993.

Table 2.5. Pneumonia Clues Based on Physical Findings

Physical Finding	Suggested Pathogen/Infection
HEENT	
Facial macules (Horder's spots)	Psittacosis
Seborrheic dermatitis (severe)	PCP (HIV)
Conjunctivitis	Adenovirus, pertussis, C. pneumoniae, influenza
Otitis/bullous myringitis	Mycoplasma
Pharyngitis (non-exudative)	Mycoplasma, C. pneumoniae, viral infection, adenovirus, Group A streptococci
Nose ulcer	Histoplasmosis
Tongue ulcer	Histoplasmosis
Oral ulcers (severe)	PCP (HIV), histoplasmosis, S. pneumoniae (SLE)
Hairy leukoplakia	PCP
Perioral ulcers of Stevens-Johnson syndrome	Mycoplasma
Choroidal tubercules	Miliary tuberculosis
Sinusitis	S. pneumoniae, H. influenzae, M. catarrhalis
Herpes labialis	S. pneumoniae
Periodontal disease	Aspiration pneumonia
Oral thrush	PCP
Laryngitis	Tuberculosis, C. pneumoniae, respiratory viruses
Scarlatiniform rash	Group A streptococci
Heart	
Relative bradycardia	Legionella, psittacosis, Q fever
Culture-negative endocarditis	Q fever, Legionella, Aspergillus
Cardiomegaly (myocarditis)	Influenza, mycoplasma, psittacosis, Legionella, hantavirus
Chest	
Erythema multiforme	Mycoplasma
Chest wall sinuses	Actinomycosis, M. tuberculosis, lung abscess, empyema, carcinoma
Seborrheic dermatitis (severe)	PCP
Scarlatiniform rash	Group A streptococci
Abdomen	
Hyposplenia/asplenia	S. pneumoniae, H. influenzae, K. pneumoniae
Hepatosplenomegaly	M. tuberculosis, histoplasmosis, Q fever, psittacosis, S. pneumoniae (chronic alcoholics, SLE, CLL, B-cell lymphomas)
Splenomegaly	S. pneumoniae (chronic cirrhosis, SLE, CLL, B-cell lymphomas)

Table 2.5. Pneumonia Clues Based on Physical Findings (cont'd)

Physical Finding	Suggested Pathogen/Infection
Extremities	
Erythema multiforme	Mycoplasma, HSV-1
Erythema nodosum	Coccidioidomycosis, histoplasmosis, blastomycosis, M. tuberculosis, Group A streptococci
Ecthyma gangrenosum	Pseudomonas, Serratia marcescens
Skin ulcers	Blastomycosis, sporotrichosis, tularemia, histoplasmosis
Vesicular lesions	VZV
Obscure phlebitis	Psittacosis
Generalized adenopathy	Miliary tuberculosis, HIV, Group A streptococci
Folliculitis of legs	HIV (PCP)
Urticaria	Atypical measles
Ulcerative lymphangitis	Sporotrichosis
Eschar	Tularemia, anthrax
Genitourinary system	
Epididymoorchitis	Tuberculosis, blastomycosis, lymphoma

HEENT = head, eyes, ears, nose, and throat.
Adapted from: Cunha BA. Pneumonia Clues. In: Keretsky M, Cunha BA, Brandstetter R (eds). The Pneumonias. Medec Books, Oradell, NJ, 1993.

Table 2.6. Pneumonia Clues Based on Laboratory Testing

Finding	Suggested Pathogen/Condition
Leukopenia	Influenza, HIV (PCP), miliary tuberculosis, drug induced, SLE, disseminated histoplasmosis, fulminant (pneumococcal), Staphylococcus pneumonia
Eosinophilia	Bronchopulmonary aspergillosis, drug-induced, sarcoidosis, PIE syndrome, coccidioidomycosis, lymphoma, vasculitis, hypersensitivity pneumonitis, Wegener's granulomatosis, Strongyloides stercoralis (hyperinfection syndrome)
Basophilia	Lymphoma, VZV, sarcoidosis
Polyclonal gammopathy	Sarcoidosis, HIV (PCP)
Abnormal liver function tests	Lymphoma, miliary tuberculosis, drug-induced, adenoviruses, Legionnaires' disease, Q fever, psittacosis, SARS
Monocytosis	Tuberculosis, SLE
Thrombocytopenia	Sarcoidosis, SLE, lymphoma, miliary tuberculosis, influenza, adenovirus, hantavirus, SARS, HIV (PCP), drug-induced

Adapted from: Cunha BA. Pneumonia Clues. In: Keretsky M, Cunha BA, Brandstetter R (eds). The Pneumonias. Medec Books, Oradell, NJ, 1993.

Table 2.7. Pneumonia Clues Based on Sputum Characteristics

Sputum Characteristic	Usual Pathogen/Infection
Foul smell	Oral anaerobes (aspiration)
Creamy yellow or salmon color	Staphylococcus aureus
Currant-jelly color	S. pneumoniae, Klebsiella
Raspberry-syrup color	Pneumonic plague
Red color (pseudohemoptysis)	Serratia marcescens (pigmented strains)
Blood-streaked (hemoptysis)	Klebsiella, influenza, TB, pneumonic plague
No PMNs	Psittacosis, Q fever, Legionella, Mycoplasma, C. pneumoniae
Eosinophils	Strongyloides stercoralis (hyperinfection syndrome) helminths (pulmonary migration phase)
Mononuclear cells	Legionella, Mycoplasma, C. pneumoniae
Mixed flora	Aspiration pneumonia, AECB, poor sputum specimen (contamination with oral epithelial cells)

Adapted from: Cunha BA. Pneumonia Clues. In: Keretsky M, Cunha BA, Brandstetter R (eds). The Pneumonias. Medec Books, Oradell, NJ, 1993.

Table 2.8. Pneumonia Clues Based on Sputum Gram Stain

Gram Stain	Pathogen	Other Characteristics
Gram Positive		
Diplococci	Streptococcus pneumoniae	Coffee-bean configuration (lancet-shaped)
Cocci in grape-like clusters	Staphylococcus aureus	May be seen in combination with short chains or pairs
Cocci in short chains or pairs	Group A streptococci	Length correlates with virulence; smaller streptococci more virulent
Comma-shaped	Nocardia	Sometimes appear like "Chinese letters" on Gram stain
Gram Negative		
Coccobacillary (pleomorphic)	Hemophilus influenzae	Encapsulated
Bacilli	Klebsiella	Plump and encapsulated
Diplococci	Neisseria meningitidis Branhamella catarrhalis	Kidney-bean–shaped (not lancet–shaped)

Adapted from: Cunha BA. Pneumonia Clues. In: Keretsky M, Cunha BA, Brandstetter R (eds). The Pneumonias. Medec Books, Oradell, NJ, 1993.

Table 2.9. Pneumonia Clues Based on Infiltrate Location

Infiltrate	Infectious Causes	Noninfectious Causes
Upper lung zones	Tuberculosis Histoplasmosis Coccidioidomycosis Atypical tuberculosis Klebsiella Proteus Legionella	Eosinophilic granuloma Silicosis Bronchial adenoma Loeffler's syndrome Extrinsic allergic alveolitis Sarcoidosis Radiation pneumonitis Ankylosing spondylitis
Mid-lung zones	S. pneumoniae H. influenzae Legionella	Metastatic carcinoma Bronchial adenoma Eosinophilic granuloma Lymphoma Idiopathic pulmonary hemosiderosis Goodpasture's syndrome Sarcoidosis Extrinsic allergic alveolitis Silicosis Hypersensitivity pneumonitis
Lower lung zone	Cryptococcosis Sporotrichosis Mycoplasma Melioidosis H. influenzae S. pneumoniae Group A streptococci E. coli Tularemia Q fever Psittacosis Legionella C. pneumoniae Amebiasis Hydatid cysts Aspiration pneumonia/abscess	Idiopathic pulmonary hemosiderosis (IPH) Metastatic carcinoma Goodpasture's syndrome Wegener's granulomatosis Drug-induced pulmonary disease Extrinsic allergic alveolitis Arteriovenous malformation Pulmonary embolus/infarct Rheumatoid nodules Fibrosing alveolitis

Adapted from: Cunha BA. Pneumonia Clues. In: Keretsky M, Cunha BA, Brandstetter R (eds). The Pneumonias. Medec Books, Oradell, NJ, 1993.

Table 2.10. Pneumonia Clues Based on Progression/Resolution of Infiltrates

Infiltrate	Infectious Causes	Noninfectious Causes
Rapidly progressive	Legionnaires' disease Pneumonic plague Adenovirus Hantavirus Influenza Avian influenza SARS Aspiration pneumonia S. aureus Gram-negative pneumonia	Congestive heart failure Noncardiogenic pulmonary edema ARDS Systemic lupus erythematosus
Rapidly resolving	None	Pulmonary edema/CHF "Vanishing tumor" (localized CHF) Acute pulmonary drug reactions Acute eosinophilic pneumonias SLE
Slowly resolving	Recurrent aspiration Lung abscess Legionnaires' disease Tuberculosis Nocardia Actinomycosis Fungal pneumonias (systemic mycoses) S. pneumoniae PCP Postobstructive pneumonia/carcinoma Inadequate/inappropriate therapy	Pulmonary emboli/infarction Bronchogenic carcinoma Lymphoma Chronic pulmonary drug reactions Bronchopulmonary aspergillosis Wegener's granulomatosis Rheumatoid lung Sarcoidosis ARDS BOOP

Adapted from: Cunha BA. Pneumonia Clues. In: Keretsky M, Cunha BA, Brandstetter R (eds). The Pneumonias. Medec Books, Oradell, NJ, 1993.

Table 2.11. Pneumonia Clues Based on Pleural Effusion Characteristics

Pleural Fluid	Infectious Causes	Noninfectious Causes
Bloody*	Tularemia Anthrax	Mesothelioma Pulmonary infarct Carcinoma (pulmonary/metastatic) Lymphoma Trauma
Yellow/whitish	Empyema Hydatid cyst	Chylous effusion
Brownish	Empyema Amebic cyst	Parapneumonic effusion
Yellow-green	None	Rheumatoid lung
pH ≤ 7.3	Empyema Tuberculosis	Bronchogenic carcinoma (rarely) Rheumatoid lung SLE
↓ Glucose	Tuberculosis Bacterial Cryptococcosis Coccidiomycosis Mycoplasma Empyema	Carcinoma Rheumatoid lung Lymphoma Esophageal rupture Parapneumonic effusion
↑ Protein	Tuberculosis	Carcinoma Lymphoma Rheumatoid lung
↑ Amylase	None	Pancreatitis/pseudocyst Adenocarcinoma Esophageal rupture
Extracellular debris	Abscesses Anaerobic empyema	Rheumatoid lung
PMNs	Bacteria Cryptococcosis Coccidiomycosis Empyema Tuberculosis (early)	Pancreatitis Subdiaphragmatic abscess (sympathetic effusion) CHF Idiopathic
Lymphocytes	Tuberculosis	Carcinoma Lymphoma Rheumatoid lung SLE

Table 2.11. Pneumonia Clues Based on Pleural Effusion Characteristics

Pleural Fluid	Infectious Causes	Noninfectious Causes
Eosinophils	Strongyloides stercoralis (hyperinfection syndrome) Paragonimiasis	Lymphoma Churg-Strauss granulomatosis Mesothelioma Carcinoma Pulmonary drug reactions Pneumothorax Chest tube Air/blood in pleural space

* TB effusion is not grossly blood but usually contains RBCs

Table 2.12. Pneumonia Clues Based on Size of Pleural Effusion on Chest X-Ray*

Effusion	Infectious Causes	Noninfectious Causes
None/very small	S. pneumoniae[†] Mycoplasma	–
Small/moderate	H. influenzae Tularemia[‡] Legionella Anthrax Hantavirus Adenovirus	Primary tuberculosis (not reactivation TB) Acute pancreatitis Pulmonary infarct[‡] Meigs' Syndrome Drugs (nitrofurantoin, methysergide, drug-induced SLE) SLE Rheumatoid lung Cirrhosis or ascites[¶] Heart failure[¶] Nephrosis[¶] Hypoalbuminemia[¶]
Large	Group A streptococci[§] Coccidiomycosis	Malignancy[§,#]

* Bilateral pleural effusions are almost never infectious in origin
† Empyema likely if effusion is present
‡ Bloody pleural effusion is characteristic
§ Serosanguineous pleural effusion is characteristic
¶ Pleural fluid is a transudate
# Trachea is not deviated to opposite side in malignant pleural effusion
Adapted from: Cunha BA. Pneumonia Clues. In: Keretsky M, Cunha BA, Brandstetter R (eds). The Pneumonias. Medec Books, Oradell, NJ, 1993.

Table 2.13. Pleural Effusion Profiles in Various Diseases

Pleural Fluid	Infectious		Noninfectious		Rheumatoid Effusion	SLE
	TB	Empyema	Malignancy	Mesothelioma		
WBCs (per mm³)	< 5000; lymphocyte predominance	> 10,000; PMN predominance	< 10,000; lymphocyte predominance	↑ PMNs/ lymphocytes	> 10,000; lymphocyte predominance	> 10,000; lymphocyte predominance
Eosinophils	–	–	+	±	–	–
RBCs (per mm³)	< 10,000	–	> 100,000	–	–	–
pH	< 7.3	< 7.3	> 7.3	> 7.3	< 7.3	< 7.3
Glucose	↓↓	Normal/↓	↓	Normal/↓	↓↓↓	Normal
Rheumatoid factor	↑	–	↑	–	↑	±
Other	< 1% mesothelial cells; pleural biopsy/culture (+) for AFB	Purulent; foul odor (2° to anaerobic organisms)	↑LDH₄/LDH₅; ↓ α-2 globulins; ↑ amylase; cytology (+) for malignant cells	Very viscous	Turbid, greenish yellow; ↓ C₃; ↑↑ protein; epithelioid cells; degenerated PMNs/ amorphous cellular debris	↑ pleural fluid ANA is diagnostic; ↓ pleural fluid C₃

+ present; – absent; ± present or absent; ↑ increased; ↓ decreased; (+) positive

---

REFERENCES AND SUGGESTED READINGS

Cunha BA. Clinical significance of pleural fluid transudates and exudates (Part I). Infectious Disease Practice 22:15, 1998.

Cunha BA. The diagnostic significance of transudates and exudates (Part II). Infectious Disease Practice 22:31, 1998.

Cunha BA. Community-acquired pneumonia-Pearls. Infections in Medicine 20:27-30, 2003.

Walsh RD, Cunha BA. Diagnostic significance of the sputum gram's stain in pneumonia. Hospital Physician 28:37-44, 1992.

TEXTBOOKS

Cunha BA. Pneumonias - Pearls and Pitfalls. In Branstetter R (ed). Textbook of Pulmonary Medicine. Medical Economics, Oradell, 1988.

Keretsky M, Cunha BA, Brandstetter R (eds). The Pneumonias. Medec Books, Oradell, New Jersey, 1993.

Light RW. Pleural Diseases. 3rd Ed, Baltimore, Williams & Wilkins, 1995.

Chapter 3

Sputum Gram Stain In Pneumonias

Paul E. Schoch, PhD
Edward J. Buttone, PhD
Burke A. Cunha, MD

SPUTUM GRAM STAIN

A. **Description.** The Gram stain, developed over 100 years ago, remains a rapid and accurate diagnostic technique that provides presumptive etiologic diagnosis in properly selected patients currently unavailable by any other means.

B. **Utility.** A well-collected, good quality sputum specimen has excellent sensitivity and specificity provided that there is little/no squamous epithelial contamination from mucous membranes and that a single predominant organism is present. The Gram stain is most useful diagnostically in patients with community-acquired pneumonia (CAP) with a productive cough. In contrast, it has little diagnostic value in patients with acute exacerbation of chronic bronchitis (AECB) who develop CAP, aspiration pneumonia, nursing home acquired pneumonia (NHAP), or nosocomial pneumonia (NP) (Table 3.1).

   1. **AECB.** Patients with chronic bronchitis have purulent sputum that is chronically colonized by normal oral/respiratory flora. In these cases, the Gram stain adds no useful diagnostic information as organisms demonstrated on Gram stain/culture are regularly reported as "normal flora" with multiple organisms. Moreover, the Gram stain may provide misleading diagnostic information in patients with AECB who develop CAP and should not be part of the diagnostic work-up.

   2. **Nosocomial Pneumonia (NP).** Nosocomial pneumonia develops after 5 or more days in the hospital. During hospitalization, patients' normal respiratory flora becomes colonized by aerobic gram-negative bacilli of the hospital microbiologic mileau. In addition, respiratory secretions of ventilated patients become colonized as a function of time in the ICU/use of broad-spectrum antimicrobial therapy and are not necessarily reflective of lower respiratory tract flora/pathogens. As such, the organism(s) Gram stained/cultured from respiratory secretions in NP rarely indicate the true pathogen and should not be used to guide antimicrobial therapy. Specifically, neither the recovery of Staphylococcus aureus (MSSA/MRSA) or Pseudomonas aeruginosa from the respiratory secretions of ventilated patients with fever, leucocytosis and pulmonary infiltrates is diagnostic of S. aureus/P. aeruginosa NP unless accompanied by characteristic clinical findings of a rapidly progressive necrotizing pneumonia (fulminant clinical course accompanied by rapid cavitation within 72 hours after the onset of NP). Diagnosis can only be made with certainty by demonstrating these organisms actively invading lung tissue via lung biopsy.

Table 3.1. Situations in Which the Sputum Gram Stain is Unhelpful

CAP with:	• COPD (chronic bronchitis always has mixed/normal flora)
	• Neutropenia (no PMNs in sputum)
	• Aspiration pneumonia (normal throat flora)
Nosocomial pneumonia	• Particularly in intubated patients, respiratory secretions are often colonized with hospital flora (P. aeruginosa, Enterobacter, S. maltophilia, B. cepacia, S. aureus [MSSA/MRSA])

C. **Technique (Table 3.2).** For a Gram stain of sputum to be useful in CAP, the specimen must be collected in a way that minimizes squamous epithelial contamination from skin/mucous membranes; lower respiratory tract specimens with abundant PMNs are optimal. Dentures should be removed and the mouth rinsed with water before the specimen is collected. Sputum should be obtained by instructing patients to take a deep cough, preferably before antibiotic therapy, although inability to obtain specimens for diagnostic studies should not delay antibiotic treatment in ill patients. (Sputum may also be obtained via tracheostomy/nasotracheal aspirates or induced sputum [recommended for M. tuberculosis, PCP]). The sputum sample should be spread thinly on a clean glass slide and allowed to air dry. It should then be gently flamed (heat-fixed) using a Bunsen burner. Thick sputum smears do not decolorize properly and may be difficult to interpret. The Gram stain should be scanned microscopically to assure that the specimen is of high quality before attempting Gram stain interpretation (Table 3.3). Gram stained smears of sputum should first be examined under low power (10x) to identify optimally stained areas for evaluation under high power oil immersion microscopy (100x). The best specimens contain abundant PMNs on low power without squamous epithelial contamination. If the specimen is of poor quality under light microscopy, it is not cost effective to interpret the smear or send the sputum for culture.

D. **Interpretation.** PMN nuclei stain pink, Gram-positive organisms stain blue, and Gram-negative organisms stain red. Overdecolorization of Gram stain results in organisms that all appear to be Gram-negative, while underdecolorization results in organisms that all appear to be Gram-positive. Pneumonia clues based on the sputum characteristics and Gram stain are shown in Tables 2.7, 2.8, and 3.4. Pneumonia isolates arranged by Gram stain, morphology, and oxygen requirements are shown in Table 3.5.

Table 3.2. Technique for Gram Stain

Sputum Gram Stain

- Place specimen on slide
- Heat fix smear on slide by passing it quickly over a flame
- Place crystal violet solution on slide for 20 seconds
- Wash gently with water
- Apply Gram iodine solution to slide for 20 seconds
- Decolorize the slide quickly in solution of acetone/ethanol
- Wash slide gently with water
- Counterstain slide with safranin for 10 seconds
- Wash gently with water; air dry or blot dry with bibulous paper

Interpretation: Gram-negative organisms stain red; gram-positive organisms stain blue. Bacteroides sp. stain weakly pink. Fungi stain deep blue.

Table 3.3. Sputum Gram Stain Grading Criteria

1. Purulent portions of the specimen should be selected for Gram stain preparation
2. The slide should be stained according to Gram stain protocol (Table 3.2).
3. Using the low power objective (10X), evaluate the specimen for the presence of squamous epithelial cells and PMNs. The quality of the specimen is reported as "GOOD" or "UNSATISFACTORY" and is determined by estimating the average number of cells per LOW POWER FIELD only. The specimen is scored as follows:

> 10-25 PMNs . . . . +1
> \> 25 PMNs . . . . +2
> Mucous threads (add only if > 25 PMNs) . . . . . . +1
> 10-25 squamous epithelial cells . . . . –1
> \> 25 squamous epithelial cells . . . . –2

4. A score of +1, +2 or +3 is adequate for culture. A score of 0, –1 or –2 is inadequate.
5. When a specimen is unsatisfactory, a new specimen should be obtained/submitted.
6. When a specimen is of good quality, the organisms present must be evaluated further using the following criteria for quantitation of cells and microorganisms using the oil immersion (100x) lens:

> 0 (none) . . . . 0 per 15-20 fields examined
> Rare to occasional . . . . 1 per 10-20 fields examined
> 1 + ... 1-5 per 5-10 fields examined
> 2 + ... 1-20 per nearly all fields examined
> 3 + ... 20-50 per nearly all fields examined
> 4 + ... 50 per nearly all fields examined

Adapted from: Barlett JG, Ryan KJ, Smith TF, et al. Cumitech: 7A, Laboratory Diagnosis of the Lower Respiratory Tract Infections. American Society for Microbiology. Washington, D.C., 1987. Isenberg, HD (ed). Clinical Microbiology Procedures Handbook. American Society for Microbiology, 1.3.1-1.3.6, 1994.

Table 3.4. Pneumonia Clues Based on Sputum Gram Stain*

Organism	Gram Stain	Comments
S. pneumoniae	Lancet-shaped Gram-positive diplococci	Bullet-shaped diplococci (not streptococci)
Staphylococci	Gram-positive cocci (grape-like clusters)	Clusters predominant. Short chains or pairs may also be present
Group A streptococci	Gram-positive cocci (short chains or pairs)	Clusters not present
Nocardia Actinomyces	Beaded/filamentous branching gram-positive bacilli	Coccobacillary forms common
Rhodococcus equi	Filamentous Gram-positive bacilli/cocci	Fragments into Gram-positive bacilli/cocci
Bacillus anthracis	Gram-positive bacilli	Blunt-ended. Long chains
Anaerobic oropharyngeal flora (contaminated sputum specimen)	Gram-positive/negative cocci/bacilli	Filamentous. Fragments into Gram-positive bacilli/cocci
Anaerobic oropharyngeal flora (aspiration pneumonia/ lung abscess)	Gram-positive/negative cocci/bacilli	Anaerobic oral flora gram stain poorly. Gram-variable organisms
H. influenzae	Pleomorphic Gram-negative coccobacillary organisms	May resemble pneumococci. May be encapsulated. Lightly stained on Gram staining
Klebsiella	Gram-negative bacilli	Plump and encapsulated
P. aeruginosa	Gram-negative bacilli	Thin and often arranged in end-to-end pairs. Bipolar staining
Moraxella (Branhamella) catarrhalis Neisseria meningitidis	Gram-negative diplococci	Kidney bean-shaped diplococci

* Presumptive diagnosis based on Gram stain of a good quality sputum specimen in patients with acute pneumonia

Table 3.5. Pneumonia Isolates by Gram Stain, Morphology, and Oxygen Requirements

AEROBIC ISOLATES	

GRAM-POSITIVE COCCI (CLUSTERS)
Staphylococcus aureus
  (MSSA/MRSA/VISA/VRSA))
 	
GRAM-POSITIVE COCCI (CHAINS)
Group A streptococci
Streptococcus viridans group
  (S. mitior, milleri, mitis, mutans, oralis,
  sanguis, parasanguis, salivarius)
 	
GRAM-POSITIVE COCCI (PAIRS)
Streptococcus pneumoniae
 	
GRAM-NEGATIVE COCCI (PAIRS)
Moraxella (Branhamella) catarrhalis
Neisseria meningitidis
 	
GRAM-POSITIVE BACILLI
Arcanobacterium (Corynebacterium)
  haemolyticum
Bacillus anthracis
Corynebacterium diphtheriae
Nocardia asteroides, braziliensis
Rhodococcus equi
	GRAM-NEGATIVE BACILLI
	Acinetobacter baumannii, lwoffi,
	  calcoaceticus, haemolyticus[§]
	Actinobacillus actinomycetemcomitans
	Alcaligenes (Achromobacter) xylosoxidans
	Bordetella pertussis
	Burkholderia (Pseudomonas) cepacia
	Burkholderia (Pseudomonas) pseudomallei
	Citrobacter diversus, freundii, koseri*
	Enterobacter agglomerans, aerogenes,
	  cloacae*
	Escherichia coli*
	Francisella tularensis[§]
	Hemophilus influenzae, parainfluenzae,
	  aphrophilus, paraphrophilus
	Klebsiella pneumoniae, oxytoca*
	Pasteurella multocida
	Proteus mirabilis, penneri, vulgaris*
	Pseudomonas aeruginosa
	Salmonella typhi, non-typhi*
	Serratia marcescens*
	Stenotrophomonas (Xanthomonas,
	  Pseudomonas) maltophilia[§]

CAPNOPHILIC ISOLATES	
GRAM-NEGATIVE BACILLI Eikenella corrodens[†]	Capnophaga

ANAEROBIC ISOLATES	
GRAM-POSITIVE COCCI Peptococcus Peptostreptococcus **GRAM-POSITIVE BACILLI** Actinomyces israelii, odontolyticus[‡] Lactobacillus sp.[‡]	**GRAM-NEGATIVE BACILLI** Fusobacterium nucleatum Prevotella (Bacteroides) bivia Prevotella (Bacteroides) melaninogenicus, intermedius

* Enterobacteriaceae (oxidase negative, catalase positive)
† Capnophilic organisms grow best under increased CO_2 tension
‡ Microaerophilic organisms - grow best under decreased O_2 concentration
§ Oxidase negative

Chapter 4

Treatment of Community-Acquired Pneumonia (CAP)

Burke A. Cunha, MD
Dennis J. Cleri, MD
David Schlossberg, MD

This chapter is organized by clinical syndrome, patient subset, and in some cases, specific organism. Clinical summaries immediately follow each treatment grid. The information presented pertains to infectious diseases and antimicrobial agents in adults. Therapeutic recommendations are based on antimicrobial effectiveness, reliability, cost, safety, and resistance potential. Switching to a more specific/narrow spectrum antimicrobial is not more effective than well-chosen empiric/initial therapy and usually results in increased cost and more side effects and drug interactions. The antimicrobial dosages in this section represent the usual dosages for normal renal and hepatic function. _For any treatment category (i.e., preferred IV therapy, alternate IV therapy, PO therapy), recommended drugs are equally effective and not ranked by priority_. **Dosage adjustments, side effects, drug interactions, and other important prescribing information are described in the individual drug summaries in Chapter 16.** Use of any drug should be preceded by careful review of the package insert, which provides indications and dosing approved by the U.S. Food and Drug Administration. _"IV-to-PO Switch"_ in the last column of the shaded title bar in each treatment grid indicates the clinical syndrome should be treated either by IV therapy alone or IV followed by PO therapy, but _not_ by PO therapy alone. _"PO Therapy or IV-to-PO Switch"_ indicates the clinical syndrome can be treated by IV therapy alone, PO therapy alone, or IV followed by PO therapy (unless otherwise indicated in the footnotes under each treatment grid). Most patients on IV therapy should be switched to PO equivalent therapy after clinical improvement.

Community-Acquired Pneumonia (CAP): Pathogen Unknown

Subset	Usual Pathogens*	IV Therapy	PO Therapy or IV-to-PO Switch
Pathogen unknown	S. pneumoniae¶ H. influenzae M. catarrhalis Legionella sp. Mycoplasma pneumoniae Chlamydophilia (Chlamydia) pneumoniae	Levofloxacin 750 mg (IV) q24h x 5 days **or** Moxifloxacin 400 mg (IV) q24h x 1-2 weeks **or combination therapy with** Ertapenem 1 gm (IV) q24h x 1-2 weeks **or** Ceftriaxone 1 gm (IV) q24h x 1-2 weeks **plus either** Doxycycline‡ (IV) x 1-2 weeks **or** Azithromycin 500 mg (IV) q24h x 1-2 weeks (minimum of 2 doses before switching to PO therapy)	Levofloxacin 750 mg (PO) q24h x 5 days **or** Quinolone† (PO) q24h x 1-2 weeks **or** Telithromycin 800 mg (PO) q24h x 7-10 days **or** Doxycycline‡ (PO) x 1-2 weeks **or** Macrolide†† (PO) q24h x 1-2 weeks

Duration of therapy represents total time IV, PO, or IV + PO. Most patients on IV therapy able to take PO meds should be switched to PO therapy after clinical improvement
*   *Compromised hosts may require longer courses of therapy*
†   *Levofloxacin 500 mg or moxifloxacin 400 mg or gemifloxacin 320 mg*
†† *Azithromycin 500 mg or clarithromycin XL 1 gm*
¶   *Macrolides should not be used in areas where macrolide-resistant S. pneumoniae (MRSP) or multidrug-resistant S. pneumoniae (MDRSP) strains are prevalent*
‡   *Doxycycline 200 mg (IV or PO) q12h x 3 days, then 100 mg (IV or PO) q12h x 4-11 days. Loading dose is not needed PO if given IV with the same drug*

Clinical Presentation: Fever, cough, respiratory symptoms, chest x-ray consistent with pneumonia. Typical CAPs (S. pneumoniae, H. influenzae, M. catarrhalis) present only with pneumonia without extrapulmonary findings. Atypical CAPs (Legionella, M. pneumoniae, C. pneumoniae) present with pneumonia plus extra-pulmonary findings (e.g., myringitis, pharyngitis, rash). See pp. 48-62 for detailed information about individual pneumonia pathogens

Diagnosis: Identification of organism on sputum gram stain/culture. Same organism is found in blood if blood cultures are positive. Also see Chapter 11 for typical chest x-ray patterns

Diagnostic Considerations: Sputum is useful if a single organism predominates and is not contaminated by saliva. Purulent sputum, pleuritic chest pain, pleural effusion favor typical pathogens; extra-pulmonary findings favor atypical pathogens

Pitfalls: Obtain chest x-ray to verify the diagnosis and rule out non-infectious mimics (e.g., heart failure)

Therapeutic Considerations: Do not switch to narrow-spectrum antibiotic after organism is identified on gram stain/blood culture. Pathogen identification is important for prognostic and public health reasons, not for therapy. Macrolide-resistant S. pneumoniae (MRSP) is an important clinical problem (prevalence ≥ 30%). Severity of CAP is related to the degree of cardiopulmonary/immune dysfunction and impacts the length of hospital stay, not the therapeutic approach or antibiotic choice

Prognosis: Related to cardiopulmonary status and splenic function

Typical Bacterial Pneumonia

Subset	Usual Pathogens*	IV Therapy	PO Therapy or IV-to-PO Switch
Typical bacterial pathogens	S. pneumoniae¶ H. influenzae M. catarrhalis	Levofloxacin 750 mg (IV) q24h x 5 days **or** Moxifloxacin 400 mg (IV) q24h x 1-2 weeks **or** Ertapenem 1 gm (IV) q24h x 1-2 weeks **or** Ceftriaxone 1 gm (IV) q24h x 1-2 weeks **or** Doxycycline‡ (IV) x 1-2 weeks **or** Tigecycline 100 mg (IV) x 1 dose, then 50 mg (IV) q12h x 1-2 weeks	Levofloxacin 750 mg (PO) q24h x 5 days **or** Quinolone† (PO) q24h x 1-2 weeks **or** Telithromycin 800 mg (PO) q24h x 7-10 days **or** Doxycycline‡ (PO) x 1-2 weeks **or** Macrolide†† (PO) q24h x 1-2 weeks **or** Amoxicillin/clavulanic acid XR 2 tablets (PO) q12h x 7-10 days **or** Cephalosporin** (PO) q12h x 1-2 weeks
	K. pneumoniae	See next page	See next page

Duration of therapy represents total time IV, PO, or IV + PO. Most patients on IV therapy able to take PO meds should be switched to PO therapy after clinical improvement

* Compromised hosts may require longer courses of therapy

† Levofloxacin 500 mg or moxifloxacin 400 mg or gemifloxacin 320 mg

†† Azithromycin 500 mg or clarithromycin XL 1 gm

¶ Macrolides should not be used in areas where macrolide-resistant S. pneumoniae (MRSP) or multidrug-resistant S. pneumoniae (MDRSP) strains are prevalent

‡ Doxycycline 200 mg (IV or PO) q12h x 3 days, then 100 mg (IV or PO) q12h x 4-11 days. Loading dose is not needed PO if given IV with the same drug

** Cefdinir 300 mg or cefditoren 400 mg or cefixime 400 mg or cefpodoxime 200 mg

Typical Bacterial Pneumonia (cont'd)

Subset	Usual Pathogens*	IV Therapy	PO Therapy or IV-to-PO Switch
Typical bacterial pathogens (cont'd)	K. pneumoniae	Meropenem 1 gm (IV) q8h x 2 weeks **or** Ertapenem 1 gm (IV) q24h x 2 weeks **or** Levofloxacin 750 mg (IV) q24h x 5 days **or** Moxifloxacin 400 mg (IV) q24h x 2 weeks **or** Ceftriaxone 1 gm (IV) q24 x 2 weeks	Levofloxacin 750 mg (PO) q24h x 5 days **or** Moxifloxacin 400 mg (PO) q24h x 2 weeks **or** Gemifloxacin 320 mg (PO) q24h x 2 weeks

Duration of therapy represents total time IV, PO, or IV + PO. Most patients on IV therapy able to take PO meds should be switched to PO therapy after clinical improvement

*   *Compromised hosts may require longer courses of therapy*
†   *Levofloxacin 500 mg or moxifloxacin 400 mg or gemifloxacin 320 mg*
††   *Azithromycin 500 mg or clarithromycin XL 1 gm*
¶   *Macrolides should not be used in areas where macrolide-resistant S. pneumoniae (MRSP) or multidrug-resistant S. pneumoniae (MDRSP) strains are prevalent*
‡   *Doxycycline 200 mg (IV or PO) q12h x 3 days, then 100 mg (IV or PO) q12h x 4-11 days. Loading dose is not needed PO if given IV with the same drug*
**   *Cefdinir 300 mg or cefditoren 400 mg or cefixime 400 mg or cefpodoxime 200 mg*

Streptococcus pneumoniae

Epidemiology: S. pneumoniae is a lancet-shaped gram-positive diplococcus that is part of the normal oropharyngeal flora and is the most common cause of CAP in patients requiring hospitalization. More than 500,000 cases develop each year in the United States alone. As with H. influenzae and N. meningitidis, oropharyngeal carriage is increased during the winter months. S. pneumoniae may be transmitted from carriers, resulting in sporadic cases in the general population or in outbreaks in closed populations (orphanages, military training camps, schools, day-care centers). Pneumococcal virulence is related to the size of the polysaccharide capsule: the large the capsule, the more virulent the strain (type 3 is more virulent than types 1, 2). Ninety capsular serotypes have been described, and serotype prevalence varies by age/location. In children, types 1,4,5,6A,6B,9V,14,18C,19A,19F and 23F cause invasive infection. In adults, types 3,7F,9V,14 and 23F are the most common serotypes, and types 3,6B, and 19F are common in fatal infections.

Clinical Presentation: The onset of pneumococcal pneumonia is abrupt with high fever (≥ 102°F) and a single shaking chill followed by a productive cough (purulent sputum that is often rust colored), dyspnea ± pleuritic chest pain. S. pneumoniae is the only CAP pathogen in normal hosts associated with herpes labialis. Coinfections are extremely rare. As with other typical CAP pathogens, extrapulmonary features are not usually part of the clinical presentation. However, bacteremia occurs in about 12% of cases and infrequent metastatic septic complications may develop secondary to bacteremia/contiguous spread, including suppurative pericarditis (contiguous spread), and septic arthritis, ABE, or ABM (hematogenous spread). The triad of pneumococcal CAP, endocarditis, and meningitis in chronic alcoholics is well known. Patients with asplenia are particularly sensitive to S. pneumoniae infection and usually present with overwhelming pneumococcal sepsis (shock, hypotension, purpura fulminans, DIC), and patients with hyposplenism may present with severe CAP. Rarely extra-pulmonary features may occur in HIV infection and the elderly (mental confusion), and some elderly patients may develop RUQ pain/jaundice. The classic chest x-ray shows segmental/lobar consolidation with air bronchograms, although bronchopneumonia or interstitial infiltrates may also occur. A "bulging fissure" sign is not an uncommon manifestation of increased lobar volume. Pleural reaction is not uncommon with S. pneumoniae CAP, and empyema develops in 0.5-1%. However, a moderate or large pleural effusion argues against the diagnosis of S. pneumoniae, and S. pneumoniae CAP does not cavitate. Bronchopleural fistula/lung abscesses are rare. As with H. influenzae, S. pneumoniae CAP predominantly affects the right lower lobe.

Diagnostic Considerations: S. pneumoniae may be demonstrated by sputum Gram stain/culture, although false-positives and false-negative occurs. S. pneumoniae appears as lancet-shaped, gram-positive diplococci (coffee bean appearance) surrounded by a capsule (clear zone around diplococci on Gram stain), which may be confused with poorly decolorized gram-negative diplococci (M. catarrhalis, N. meningitidis). S. pneumoniae is a bacteremic organism and many patients with S. pneumoniae CAP have positive blood cultures. Established diagnosis can be made by recovery of the organism from the blood, pleural fluid, or transtracheal/transthoracic needle aspirate. Diagnosis may also be made by the presence of pneumococcal urinary antigen after excluding other sites of S. pneumoniae infection (e.g., sinusitis).

Pitfalls: Overdecolorization of sputum Gram stain specimens may be misidentified as gram-negative diplococci (M. catarrhalis, N. meningitides). The diagnosis of S. pneumoniae CAP should be questioned if extrapulmonary findings are present (excluding septic metastatic complications). "Pneumococcal pneumonia" with cavitation is likely to be K. pneumoniae CAP since cavitation rarely, if ever, occurs with S. pneumoniae. Because S. pneumoniae CAP is associated with little or no pleural effusion, a moderate or large pleural effusion should suggest an alternate pathogen/diagnosis (Group A streptococci/bronchogenic carcinoma). In chronic alcoholics with the classical triad of pneumococcal ABM, ABE, and CAP, the cardiac/CNS manifestations that occur during therapy are often overshadowed by the pneumonia. Patients with pneumococcal pneumonia typically manifest one of three fever defervescence patterns. Most often, following appropriate antimicrobial therapy, there is a rapid defervescence of fever during the first 1-2 days. Other patients manifest an initial rapid decrease in temperature followed by a secondary increase in temperature 3-5 days later (second most common pattern). Lastly, some patients may defervesce slowly over a week with a "hectic/septic" fever pattern (least common pattern), and this pattern is typical in patients with impaired immunity (HIV, CLL, multiple myeloma, SLE, chronic alcoholism, hyposplenism). Excluding these fever defervescence patterns, recrudescence of fever ≥ 1 week on appropriate antimicrobial therapy is suggestive of drug fever (relative bradycardia), empyema, or a metastatic septic complication (ABM, septic joint, ABE).

Therapeutic Considerations: Nearly all pneumococci remain susceptible to beta-lactam antibiotics, including many strains of S. pneumoniae that show "decreased sensitivity" to penicillin. Highly penicillin-resistant strains (PRSP) of S. pneumoniae (MIC ≥ 10 mcg/ml) fortunately remain rare; such strains may be effectively treated with respiratory quinolones, telithromycin, ertapenem, meropenem, daptomycin, linezolid, vancomycin, or quinupristin/dalfopristin. Macrolides and TMP-SMX are associated with increasing prevalence of penicillin-resistant S. pneumoniae (PRSP) and multidrug-resistant S. pneumoniae (MDRSP). Macrolide-resistant S. pneumonia (MRSP) is an important clinical problem (prevalence ≥ 30%). MDRSP is treated with the same antibiotics as for highly PRSP. Patients with metastatic septic complications should be treated with antibiotics that penetrate the site of infection in therapeutic concentrations. For S. pneumoniae in the CNS, meropenem (meningeal doses), ceftriaxone, cefepime (meningeal doses), or linezolid are optimal. The same antibiotics/dose may be used for pneumococcal septic arthritis or pneumococcal ABE. Patients with pneumococcal septic arthritis also usually require closed drainage for eradication of the infection, and patients with pneumococcal ABE may require valve replacement or develop perivalvular disease that may require drainage. Therapy is usually continued for 1-2 weeks. Longer duration of therapy may be required in compromised hosts.

Prognosis: The prognosis in pneumococcal CAP is related to the degree of impaired humoral immunity, capsular size/type (mortality rates up to 30% with type 3), and underlying cardiopulmonary status of the host. Risk factors for adverse outcome are shown in Table 1.24. Most healthy younger adults feel better/defervesce in 3-5 days, although chest x-ray abnormalities may persist for 4-12 weeks. S. pneumoniae CAP is usually severe in patients with hyposplenism, COPD, chronic alcoholism, or HIV. Remarkably, S. pneumoniae lung lesions heal completely after appropriate antimicrobial therapy without sequelae/diminished lung function. Prognosis is guarded in patients with metastatic septic complications (purulent pericarditis, ABE, ABM, septic arthritis) and is poorest in patients with asplenia and overwhelming pneumococcal sepsis. Pneumococcal pneumonia has been termed the "captain of death" and the "old man's friend" because it is frequently fatal in elderly patients with decreased humoral immunity/severe cardiopulmonary disease. The overall mortality rate in hospitalized patients is 12%.

Prevention: A polyvalent vaccine against the 23 pneumococcal strains responsible for ~ 90% of infections is effective (Chapter 13).

Haemophilus influenzae

Epidemiology: H. influenzae is a pleomorphic gram-negative bacillus responsible for ~ 5% of CAPs. Patients predisposed to H. influenzae include chronic alcoholics, smokers, asthmatics, and those with bronchogenic carcinoma, COPD, or chronic bronchiectasis. A minority of patients with H. influenzae CAP are normal hosts. H. influenzae CAP has a bimodal age distribution, being most common in young children and the elderly.

Clinical Presentation: In children, typical presenting symptoms include the acute onset of fever and cough; some may have pleuritic chest pain, which may be proceeded by coryza, and some may have a subacute onset. In adults, typical presenting symptoms include the subacute onset of fever ± chills and productive cough. Accompanying pleuritic chest pain and shortness of breath are usually related to underlying pulmonary disease. As with other causes of typical CAP, extra-pulmonary organ involvement does not occur. Physical exam usually reveals rales over the affected segment/lobe without signs of consolidation. Chest x-ray demonstrates a patchy bronchopneumonia (most common in adults) or a unilateral focal segmental/lobar consolidation without cavitation (most common in children). Mild/moderate sized pleural effusion (exudative) on the side of the infiltrate is typical, especially in children, while empyema and lung necrosis/abscess are rare. The right lower lobe is the most common location for H. influenzae CAP.

Diagnostic Considerations: H. influenzae is a fastidious gram-negative bacillus that grows on chocolate agar but not on blood agar. H. influenzae is part of the normal oropharyngeal flora. Recovery of H. influenzae from sputum (i.e., not contaminated by saliva) in a patient with CAP is presumptive evidence of H. influenzae CAP. H. influenzae is also a bacteremic organism, and blood cultures are positive in 72% of patients with segmental pneumonia and 28% of patients with bronchopneumonia. The diagnosis may also be made by demonstrating H. influenzae antigen in the urine, or by Gram stain/culture of pleural fluid. Both typable and non-typable strains cause CAP.

Pitfalls: The recovery of H. influenzae from the nasopharynx/mouth indicates oropharyngeal colonization, not H. influenzae CAP. CAP with a massive pleural effusion/hydrothorax argues against the diagnosis of H. influenzae and suggests the possibility of Group A streptococcus. Because H. influenzae CAP does not cavitate, a lobar infiltrate that cavitates in 3-5 days should suggest K. pneumoniae rather than H. influenzae or S. pneumoniae. H. influenzae appears as small, encapsulated, pleomorphic gram-negative bacilli on sputum Gram stain and should not be confused with gram-negative diplococci (M. catarrhalis, N. meningitidis), which are common oropharyngeal colonizers. If present, pleural effusions are exudative and contain the organism. Empyema should suggest an alternate diagnosis (K. pneumoniae, S. pneumoniae). Gram stain of the sputum showing encapsulated gram-negative plump/pleomorphic gram-negative bacilli limits diagnostic possibilities to H. influenzae or K. pneumoniae; both are common in chronic alcoholics and may be differentiated by culture/susceptibility testing. Dual infections due to co-pathogens are rare.

Therapeutic Considerations: H. influenzae CAP is sensitive to a wide array of antimicrobial agents depending upon whether the strain is ampicillin sensitive or resistant. Ampicillin-sensitive strains may be treated with a beta-lactam, doxycycline, respiratory quinolone, telithromycin, or amoxicillin/clavulanic acid. First generation cephalosporins and macrolides have limited activity against H. influenzae (azithromycin > clarithromycin > erythromycin). Encapsulated and non-encapsulated strains of H. influenzae are equally sensitive to the antibiotics mentioned.

Prognosis: H. influenzae CAP is usually mild/moderate, and prognosis is good in children and in non-elderly immunocompetent adults. Severe CAP may develop in the elderly, those with severe underlying lung disease (COPD/bronchiectasis), and those with chronic alcoholism. Prognosis is guarded in patients with septic metastatic complications (e.g., meningitis), which are unusual.

Moraxella (Branhamella) catarrhalis

Epidemiology: M. catarrhalis is a gram-negative bacillus responsible for < 2% of CAPs. It is particularly common in elderly smokers with COPD (chronic bronchitis), and only 10% of patients with M. catarrhalis CAP are normal hosts and children. M. catarrhalis is the most common cause of CAP in patients with AECB requiring hospital admission, although it more frequently causes bronchitis, tracheobronchitis, or AECB. M. catarrhalis is acquired as with other bacterial pneumonias via inhalation/aspiration, and the incidence is highest during the winter months. M. catarrhalis is not a particularly virulent pulmonary pathogen, but may present as severe CAP in patients with decreased lung function. M. catarrhalis also causes nursing home-acquired pneumonia, but is not a cause of hospital-acquired pneumonia (excluding smokers/COPD).

Clinical Presentation: The onset of M. catarrhalis CAP is typically subacute and follows bronchitis or AECB in smokers/COPD patients. Patients with M. catarrhalis CAP present with a productive cough and purulent sputum, like S. pneumoniae or H. influenzae, and can be readily differentiated by sputum Gram stain. Chills are infrequent, and the febrile response is variable but without relative bradycardia. As with other causes of typical CAP, there are no extra-pulmonary findings, and myalgias/arthralgias are not part of the clinical presentation. On chest x-ray, there is usually consolidation superimposed on COPD findings, and cavitation/pleural effusion are rare. On laboratory testing, a modest leukocytosis is usually present.

Diagnostic Considerations: Diagnosis is made by sputum Gram stain/culture. Sputum Gram stain reveals gram-negative diplococci, and sputum culture demonstrates aerobic, oxidase-positive, non-motile gram-negative diplococci. M. catarrhalis is not a bacteremic pathogen so blood cultures are usually negative.

Pitfalls: Because the sputum Gram stain in patients with COPD (chronic bronchitis) usually shows no predominant organism/normal flora, Gram stain/culture are unhelpful in this setting (Table 3.1). If M. catarrhalis grows from a purulent sputum specimen in a patient without an infiltrate on chest x-ray, the patient has bronchitis, tracheobronchitis or AECB, but not CAP. M. catarrhalis may resemble overly decolorized S. pneumoniae on Gram stain, but M. catarrhalis diplococci are kidney-bean shaped in contrast to the lancet-shaped diplococci of S. pneumoniae. M. catarrhalis may also resemble N. meningitidis, but may be differentiated from N. meningitides by its inability to produce acid from glucose, lactose, maltose, and sucrose.

Therapeutic Considerations: Virtually all strains of M. catarrhalis are potent beta-lactamase producers; therefore, susceptibility testing is not routinely performed. M. catarrhalis is susceptible to quinolones, doxycycline, beta-lactams (beta-lactamase stable), macrolides, telithromycin, and TMP-SMX. It is resistant to penicillin, ampicillin, and amoxicillin (inactivated by beta-lactamases). Amoxicillin/clavulanic acid preparations (beta-lactamase resistant beta-lactams) are effective. Treatment is usually for 1-2 weeks.

Prognosis: Prognosis is related to the extent of pre-existing lung disease. Clinical resolution is slow because of limited functional lung capacity.

Streptococcus pyogenes (Group A Streptococci)

Epidemiology: Group A streptococcus is an uncommon cause of CAP which may develop in normal individuals, in military recruits in training camps, in the setting of closed chest trauma, or secondary to an acute extra-pulmonary illness. Some patients give a history of an antecedent upper respiratory tract infection, and antecedent streptococcal pharyngitis is present in about two-thirds of patients.

Clinical Presentation: Symptom onset is acute, with high fever ($\geq 102^\circ$ F), shaking chills, and cough. Pleuritic chest pain and dyspnea are common. Auscultation reveals localized rales, and a moderate/large pleural effusion is usually evident on chest x-ray.

Diagnostic Considerations: CAP with a moderate/large pleural effusion (which may obscure associated lobar infiltrate/consolidation) should be considered to be Group A streptococcal CAP until proven otherwise. Thoracentesis typically shows serosanguineous pleural effusion fluid; if empyema is present, the fluid is acidic/purulent. The diagnosis is confirmed by demonstrating Group A streptococci by Gram stain/culture of pleural effusion or empyema fluid. Blood cultures are positive in 10-15%. Less commonly, an elevated ASO titer can be used to confirm the diagnosis. As with all serological tests, false negatives may occur if the ASO titer is ordered too early. An otherwise unexplained increase in ASO titers without pulmonary findings consistent with Group A streptococcal pneumonia is of no clinical significance.

Pitfalls: Any patient presenting with CAP and a large pleural effusion should be considered to have Group A streptococcal pneumonia until proven otherwise. The associated infiltrate, which may be obscured by the large pleural effusion, does not cavitate. Patients with a large serosanguineous pleural effusion may have bronchogenic carcinoma, but patients with bronchogenic carcinoma will not have the systemic/pulmonary signs and symptoms of Group A streptococcal pneumonia. Although preceded by pharyngitis in two-thirds of cases, only 20% of patients with Group A streptococcal CAP have sputum Gram stain/culture positive for the organism. Streptococci may be misidentified in Gram stain of sputum/pleural fluid as diplococci if the organism becomes fragmented during Gram stain preparation. Group A streptococci on a properly prepared Gram stain always appears in chains, and chain length is inversely proportional to virulence. Some diplococci may appear on Gram stain, but longer chains are always present in Group A streptococcal CAP. In contrast, S. pneumoniae never appears in chains longer than diplococci. Preliminary identification of Group A streptococci on cultures is with a bacitracin disk; final identification is made with streptococcal antisera. Although Group A streptococcal CAP is often associated with a stormy course and slow defervescence, antibiotics should not be changed during therapy. Leukocytosis and new temperature spikes occurring after clinical defervescence suggests pleural effusion, which may need to be drained.

Therapeutic Considerations: Patients with Group A streptococcal pneumonia usually require ≥ 1 week to defervesce. Recrudescence of fever or subsequent increase in WBC count during therapy suggests empyema. Antimicrobial therapy is required for at least 2 weeks, and several additional weeks may be required for complicated cases (empyema).

Prognosis: Prognosis is related to the extent of empyema and rapidity of empyema drainage. A prolonged febrile/stormy course is to be expected, but is not necessarily associated with a bad prognosis.

Klebsiella pneumoniae

Epidemiology: K. pneumoniae accounts for about 1% of CAP and occurs almost exclusively in chronic alcoholics with advanced cirrhosis. Rarely, patients with COPD or diabetes mellitus are affected. It is also a cause of nosocomial pneumonia, as Klebsiella is a common colonizer in oropharyngeal secretions of hospitalized patients, particularly alcoholics and diabetics. There is no occupational or seasonal predilection. K. pneumoniae may be acquired via aerosolized droplet infection or aspiration of oropharyngeal secretions, and presents as a bacterial lobar pneumonia without extra-pulmonary features.

Clinical Presentation: Patients are acutely ill with abrupt onset of high fever (> 102° F), chills, and a productive cough. Chest pain and dyspnea are common, and cyanosis may be present. In some patients, the sputum is thin and resembles "currant red jelly." In others, the sputum is tenacious and bright red (mixture of pus/blood). Hemoptysis without purulent sputum is less common. On auscultation, there are signs of lobar consolidation. On chest x-ray, K. pneumoniae has an upper lobe predilection ("bulging fissure" sign), but may involve any lobe, and multilobar involvement is common. Cavitation at 5-7 days is characteristic of K. pneumoniae CAP, and abscesses develop in ≤ 50% of patients. Empyema is present in ≤ 30% of patients. Because chronic alcoholics are compromised hosts and because the thick capsule of Klebsiella is resistant to phagocytosis, K. pneumoniae typically presents as severe CAP.

Diagnostic Considerations: K. pneumoniae is likely in chronic alcoholics with lobar pneumonia that cavitates in 5-7 days. Gram stain of the sputum shows abundant PMNs with multiple plump gram-negative encapsulated bacilli. The capsule of K. pneumoniae is thick and a key virulence factor. Diagnosis is made by culture of the organism from the sputum/blood in a patient with clinical/chest x-ray findings as described above. Blood cultures are positive in 25%.

Pitfalls: K. pneumoniae CAP resembles S. pneumoniae CAP. However, S. pneumoniae does not cavitate and K. pneumoniae regularly cavitates in 5-7 days. K. pneumoniae may also cause a chronic cavitary pneumonia with low-grade fevers, cough, purulent sputum, and weight loss. Chronic K. pneumoniae CAP is characterized by thin-walled cavities, rather than thick-walled cavities as with acute Klebsiella CAP. The differential diagnosis of chronic K. pneumoniae CAP includes tuberculosis and melioidosis.

Therapeutic Considerations: Non-ESBL producing strains of K. pneumoniae are sensitive to cephalosporins and quinolones. ESBL producing strains of K. pneumoniae are sensitive to carbapenems. Because K. pneumoniae CAP presents as a severe necrotizing pneumonia in compromised hosts (chronic alcoholics), it is prudent to begin empiric therapy with a carbapenem, which will be active against both ESBL and non-ESBL producing strains. Strains of K. pneumoniae that are cefotetan-susceptible and ceftazidime-resistant should be tested for ESBL production. TMP-SMX and anti-pseudomonal penicillins have suboptimal anti-K. pneumoniae activity. MDR K. pneumoniae may be treated with colistin, polymyxin B, or tigecycline.

Prognosis: Prognosis is related to the extent of lung damage and severity of liver disease (chronic cirrhosis). Prognosis is poor in patients who develop lung abscesses, bronchopleural fistulas, or pulmonary gangrene.

Nonzoonotic Atypical Pneumonia

Subset	Usual Pathogens*	Preferred IV Therapy	Alternate IV Therapy	PO Therapy or IV-to-PO Switch
Non-zoonotic pathogens (no zoonotic vector)	Legionella sp.‡ Mycoplasma pneumoniae‡ C. pneumoniae‡	Levofloxacin 500 mg (IV) q24h x 1-2 weeks **or** Moxifloxacin 400 mg (IV) q24h x 1-2 weeks **or** Doxycycline 200 mg (IV) q12h x 3 days, then 100 mg (IV) q12h x 4-11 days	Azithromycin 500 mg (IV) q24h x 1-2 weeks (minimum of 2 doses before switching to PO therapy)	Levofloxacin 500 mg (PO) q24h x 1-2 weeks **or** Moxifloxacin 400 mg (PO) q24h x 1-2 weeks **or** Gemifloxacin 320 mg (PO) q24h x 1-2 weeks **or** Doxycycline 200 mg (PO) q12h x 3 days, then 100 mg (PO) q12h x 4-11 days** **or** Clarithromycin XL 1 gm (PO) q24h x 1-2 weeks **or** Azithromycin 500 mg (PO) q24h x 1-2 weeks

Duration of therapy represents total time IV, PO, or IV + PO
*   *Compromised hosts may require longer courses of therapy*
**   *Loading dose is not needed PO if given IV with the same drug*
‡   *May require prolonged therapy: Legionella (4 weeks); Mycoplasma (2-3 weeks); Chlamydia (2-3 weeks)*

Nonzoonotic Atypical Pathogens (Legionella sp., M. pneumoniae, C. pneumoniae)

Diagnostic Considerations: Each atypical pathogen has a different and characteristic pattern of extrapulmonary organ involvement (Table 4.1).
Pitfalls: Failure to respond to beta-lactams should suggest diagnosis of atypical CAP.
Therapeutic Considerations: Treat Legionella x 4 weeks. Treat Mycoplasma or Chlamydia x 2 weeks.
Prognosis: Related to severity of underlying cardiopulmonary disease.

Legionnaires' Disease

Epidemiology: Legionnaires' disease is caused by any one of a variety of Legionella species, L. pneumophila being the most common species with over a dozen serotypes. Other common Legionella species include L. bozemanii, L. dumoffii, L. gormanii, L. micdadei, L. longbeachae, L. jordanis, L. oakridgensis, L. wadsworthii, and L. feeleii. Unlike other pulmonary pathogens, the natural habitat of Legionella species is aquatic: Legionella organisms live in a fresh water environment and survive in a symbiotic relationship with freshwater amoeba. Legionella infection may be introduced into humans via droplet aerosolization of Legionella-contaminated water supplies (e.g., cooling towers, water systems, whirlpools, showers, air conditioners, respiratory therapy devices). Legionnaires' disease can occur in isolated cases or in outbreaks (community-acquired or nosocomial), which involves exposure to contaminated environmental/hospital water sources. Legionella has a seasonal predisposition and is most common in the fall/winter. Legionella is rare in young children, uncommon in young adults, and is most common in adult/elderly patients. Individuals with impaired cell-mediated immunity (↓ T-lymphocyte function) are most susceptible, but normal hosts can be infected as well.

Clinical Presentation: Most patients with Legionella CAP require hospitalization, as Legionella is more severe than M. pneumoniae or C. pneumoniae CAP in normal hosts. Symptom onset is usually acute, with high fever (≥ 102° F) and relative bradycardia. Myalgias and chills are not uncommon. Like other atypical pneumonias, Legionella is characterized by its pattern of extra-pulmonary manifestations (Tables 4.1, 4.2), which is the key to diagnosis. Endocarditis, myocarditis, and glomerulonephritis may also occur but are rare. Legionella may also present as worsening/unresponsive CAP to beta-lactam therapy. On chest x-ray, Legionella is recognized not by the appearance of the infiltrate, which can be variable, but by its rapid, asymmetric progression. There is no lobar predominance with Legionella CAP, bilateral involvement is usual, consolidation/pleural effusion are not uncommon, and cavitation is rare. Specific Legionella testing is indicated in patients with fever ≥ 102°F plus relative bradycardia (if not on verapamil, diltiazem or beta blockers or have arrhythmias/heart block), mental confusion, watery diarrhea, abdominal pain, mild/transient ↑ SGOT/SGPT, early/transient ↓ serum phosphorus, ↑ CPK, ↑↑↑ CRP (> 30), and no cold agglutinins.

Diagnostic Considerations: A presumptive diagnosis may be made by a syndromic weighted clinical point score system (Table 4.3). Lack of response to beta lactam therapy in a CAP patient should also suggest the possibility of Legionella and prompt specific testing. The diagnosis is confirmed by Legionella DFA of sputum/respiratory secretions or by Legionella IGA titers; a single titer ≥ 1:256 or ≥ 4 fold increase between acute and convalescent titer is diagnostic. Legionella may also be cultured on CYE agar from sputum respiratory secretions, pleural effusion, or lung tissue. Legionella pneumophila (serotype 1) may also be diagnosed by urinary antigen test. PCR is not available in all clinical laboratories.

Pitfalls: Failure to consider the diagnosis Legionella CAP is common, as the constellation of signs/symptoms are often overlooked and no individual finding is pathognomonic. The pattern of extrapulmonary organ involvement differentiates Legionella from other causes of CAP. Hyponatremia is common in Legionella CAP but is non-specific and present in many pulmonary disorders. Decreased serum phosphorus is a less common but more specific finding for Legionella. Findings suggestive of an alternate (non-Legionella) cause of CAP include ↑ cold agglutinin titer, normal SGOT/SGPT, normal serum phosphorus, normal CPK level, normal/modestly elevated CRP, upper respiratory tract involvement (non-exudative pharyngitis, laryngitis, otitis), or E. multiforme. A zoonotic contact history argues against Legionella, but contact with an infected individual or water source should raise suspicion of possible Legionella CAP. Legionella DFA of sputum/respiratory secretions is positive early and rapidly becomes negative with treatment. IFA serological testing, as with other pathogens, may be falsely negative if ordered too early (usually at the time of clinical presentation), and antimicrobial therapy may eliminate/blunt IFA titers and making confirmation of the diagnosis (serologically) difficult/impossible. Legionella urinary antigen testing is useful but has limitations, as it is not always positive when the patient presents early, and it detects only Legionella pneumophila (serotype 1) and not other Legionella species. Legionella urinary antigen testing is most useful as a retrospective confirmatory test. As with all serological tests, a negative DFA, IFA, or Legionella urinary antigen test does not rule out Legionnaires' disease. Legionella requires special culture media (CYE agar) and does not grow on standard laboratory media.

Therapeutic Considerations: Antimicrobial agents with the highest degree of anti-Legionella activity (active against all species) are quinolones, telithromycin, doxycycline, and macrolides (excluding erythromycin). Rifampin has in vitro anti-Legionella activity, but as part of combination therapy (erythromycin + rifampin) has not been shown to offer any advantage over well selected monotherapy (quinolone, telithromycin, doxycycline). Legionella does not respond to beta-lactams and only somewhat to erythromycin. Patients treated with a quinolone, telithromycin, or doxycycline typically defervesce slowly over 5-7 days. During this time, temperatures decrease gradually, relative bradycardia disappears, and pulmonary symptoms decrease. Therapy is usually continued for 2-4 weeks depending upon clinical severity/host factors.

Prognosis: In young immunocompetent hosts with good cardiopulmonary function, prognosis is good with early therapy. Prognosis is guarded in elderly hosts with impaired cellular immunity (HIV, organ transplants, corticosteroid therapy) and in those severe cardiopulmonary disease (coronary artery disease, valvular heart disease, COPD, chronic bronchiectasis). Patients with severe CAP have a poor prognosis.

Mycoplasma pneumoniae

Epidemiology: M. pneumoniae is responsible for 5-15% of CAP, affects young adults and the elderly, and may require hospitalization. M. pneumoniae is spread from person-to-person via aerosolized droplets, and patients with mild/asymptomatic infection are important in transmission.

Clinical Presentation: Onset is subacute with a characteristic dry/non-productive cough that lasts for weeks, low-grade fever/chills, and mild myalgias. As with other atypical pneumonias, M. pneumoniae is characterized by its pattern of extra-pulmonary organ involvement, which may include sore throat (non-exudative pharyngitis), bullous myringitis, otitis media, rhinorrhea and/or watery loose stools/diarrhea (Table 4.1). Features that argue against the diagnosis of M. pneumoniae CAP include high fevers (> 102°F), relative bradycardia, laryngitis, abdominal pain, ↑ SGOT/SGPT, low serum phosphorus, or renal abnormalities. Chest x-ray shows ill-defined unilateral infiltrates without pleural effusion, consolidation or cavitation. As with other pulmonary pathogens, M. pneumoniae may present as severe CAP in compromised hosts, the elderly, and those with advanced lung disease (COPD).

Diagnostic Considerations: M. pneumoniae testing is recommended for patients with otherwise unexplained protracted nonproductive cough, low-grade fevers, loose stools/watery diarrhea, and an ill-defined infiltrate on chest x-ray. Cold agglutinin titers are elevated early/transiently (75%) and provide a rapid presumptive diagnosis; titers ≥ 1:64 in patients with CAP are due to M. pneumoniae. Serology is used to confirm acute infection. An elevated M. pneumoniae IgM ELISA titer suggests acute infection, but an elevated IgG titer indicates only past exposure; elevated IgM/IgG titers suggest recent infection. M. pneumoniae may be cultured from respiratory secretions on viral media (requires 1-2 weeks for growth). DNA probes and PCR are not available in most clinical laboratories.

Pitfalls: A dry, non-productive cough also suggests C. pneumoniae CAP, and CAP with loose/watery stools also may occur with Legionella. Before ascribing E. multiforme to M. pneumoniae, be sure that it is not due to other causes (e.g., drug induced). Features that argue against the diagnosis of M. pneumoniae include temperature > 102°F, relative bradycardia, moderate/large pleural effusion, consolidation/cavitation, otherwise unexplained abdominal pain, ↑SGOT/SGPT, low serum phosphorus. In a patient with CAP, otherwise unexplained abdominal pain should point to Legionella, not M. pneumoniae or C. pneumoniae. False-negative IgM tests occur if the initial titer is obtained too early or if convalescent titers are obtained before 6 weeks.

Therapeutic Considerations: Empiric therapy is initiated after a presumptive diagnosis is made based on the clinical presentation and elevated cold agglutinin titers. Doxycycline, macrolides, quinolones, or telithromycin result in rapid clinical response: patients feel better and temperatures decrease in < 72 hours, but dry cough usually continues for weeks after effective anti-mycoplasma therapy. Because Mycoplasma organisms reside on/in the bronchial epithelium, antimicrobial therapy should be continued for 2 weeks to eliminate carriage from oropharyngeal secretions to reduce the risk of transmission via aerosolized droplets.

Prognosis: M. pneumoniae is usually a mild, self-limiting illness in ambulatory immunocompetent adults. As with other pulmonary pathogens, M. pneumoniae may be severe in compromised hosts, the elderly, and those with advanced lung disease. Patients with M. pneumoniae and meningoencephalitis (headaches/stiff neck, mental confusion, very high cold agglutinin titers [usually ≥ 1:1024]) have a good prognosis, and CNS symptoms gradually resolve with therapy. The prognosis of M. pneumoniae complicated by transverse myelitis, brain stem/cerebellar ataxia, or Guillain-Barré syndrome is related to severity/duration of neurologic impairment. A protracted, dry cough may follow M. pneumoniae CAP, and some patients develop permanent post-M. pneumoniae asthma, especially those with inadequate duration or ineffective antimicrobial therapy.

Chlamydophilia (Chlamydia) pneumoniae

Epidemiology: C. pneumoniae is responsible for 5-10% of CAP and may occur as sporadic cases – C. pneumoniae outbreaks causing NHAP is not uncommon – or as part of an outbreak. C. pneumoniae is spread from person-to-person via aerosolized droplets, and the average incubation period between contact and primary infection is approximately 4 weeks. Patients with mild/asymptomatic infection are important in transmission. C. pneumoniae CAP is common in school age children/families, military recruits in training facilities, and the elderly. Unlike influenza or Legionella, there is no seasonal predisposition. Some patients with C. pneumoniae CAP develop a protracted dry cough and permanent asthma following acute infection.

Clinical Presentation: C. pneumoniae presents as a "mycoplasma-like" illness and ranges from mild to severe. Like other atypical CAPs, C. pneumoniae CAP is characterized by extra-pulmonary findings, particularly nasal discharge, sore throat, and hoarseness (Table 4.1). Sore throat precedes respiratory symptoms in 20-50%, and respiratory symptoms may precede the actual development of pneumonia by days-to-weeks. Temperature is usually ≤ 102° F and relative bradycardia is not present. Chest x-ray findings are typically that of a unilateral ill-defined infiltrate without consolidation, cavitation, or pleural effusion. Bilateral infiltrates are rare. C. pneumoniae testing is recommended in a CAP patient with low-grade fevers (≤ 102° F), dry/non-productive cough ± hoarseness, and an ill-defined unilateral infiltrate without pleural effusion, particularly in absence of cold agglutinins/elevated M. pneumoniae IgM titer.

Diagnostic Considerations: The diagnosis of C. pneumoniae CAP requires a single IgM titer of ≥ 1:16 or an IgG titer > 1:512 (ELISA or MIF). C. pneumoniae PCR testing is available in some centers. C. pneumoniae may be cultured from respiratory secretions using viral culture media.

Pitfalls: Features that argue against the diagnosis of C. pneumoniae CAP include the presence of relative bradycardia, high-grade fevers (≥ 102° F), ↑ SGOT/SGPT, ↓ serum phosphorus, ↑ cold agglutinins, or microscopic hematuria. IgG titers indicate past exposure, not current infection. ↑ IgM and ↑ IgG titers may be delayed for more than 3 and 6 weeks, respectively. As with all serological tests, false negatives may occur if IgM titers are obtained too early or if convalescent IgG titers are obtained < 3 weeks after the acute titer. Recovery of C. pneumoniae from respiratory secretions does not differentiate carriage from infection.

Therapeutic Considerations: Doxycycline, telithromycin, or quinolones are effective. C. pneumoniae is sensitive to erythromycin in vitro, but erythromycin is often ineffective in vivo. C. pneumoniae also responds to newer macrolides (clarithromycin/azithromycin). Therapy is usually for 1-2 weeks.

Prognosis: C. pneumoniae CAP is usually a mild/moderate pneumonia with an excellent prognosis. Severe CAP may occur in compromised hosts, the elderly, or those with severe lung disease (COPD, cystic fibrosis). Inadequate duration of therapy/ineffective antimicrobial therapy may result in permanent post-C. pneumoniae asthma.

Table 4.1. Diagnostic Features of Nonzoonotic Atypical Pneumonias

Key Characteristics	Mycoplasma pneumoniae	Legionnaires' Disease	C. (Chlamydia) pneumoniae
Symptoms			
Mental confusion	−	+	−
Prominent headache	−	±	−
Meningismus	−	−	−
Myalgias	±	±	±
Ear pain	+	−	±
Pleuritic pain	−	±	−
Abdominal pain	−	+	−
Diarrhea	+	+	−
Signs			
Rash	± a	−	−
Nonexudative pharyngitis	+	−	+
Hemoptysis	−	±	−
Lobar consolidation	−	±	−
Cardiac involvement	± b	−	−
Splenomegaly	−	−	−
Relative bradycardia	−	+	−
Chest X-Ray			
Infiltrate	Patchy	Patchy, consolidation	"Circumscribed" lesions
Bilateral hilar adenopathy	−	−	−
Pleural effusion	± (small)	±	−
Laboratory Abnormalities			
WBC count	↑ /N	↑	N
Hyponatremia	−	+	−
Hypophosphatemia	−	+	−
↑ AST/ALT (SGOT/SGPT)	−	+	−
↑ CPK	−	+	−
↑ CRP (> 30)	−	+	−
↑ Ferritin (> 500 ng/dL)	−	+	−
↑ Cold agglutinins (≥ 1:64)	+	−	−
Microscopic hematuria	−	+	−
Diagnostic Tests			
Direct isolation (culture)	±	± (CYE)	±
Serology (specific)	CF	IFA	CF
Legionella IFA titers	−	↑ ↑ ↑	−
Legionella DFA	−	+	−
Legionella urinary antigen	−	+††	−

ALT = alanine aminotransferase; AST = aspartate aminotransferase; CF = complement fixation; CYE = charcoal yeast agar; DFA/IFA = direct/indirect fluorescent antibody test; N = normal; WBC = white blood cell
+ = usually present; ± = sometimes present; − = usually absent
↑ = increased; ↓ = decreased; ↑ ↑ ↑ = markedly increased
a = erythema multiforme; b = myocarditis, heart block, or pericarditis
† = mental confusion only if meningoencephalitis habitus
†† = may not be positive early, but antigenuria persists for weeks. Useful only to diagnose L. pneumophila (serogroup 01), not other species/serogroups

Table 4.2. Clinical Features of Legionnaires' Disease

Organ Involvement	Common Features	Uncommon Features	Argues Against Legionnaires'
CNS	Mental confusion/ dullness, encephalopathic, headache	Lethargy	Meningeal signs, dizziness
HEENT	None	Vertigo	Sore throat, ear pain, bullous myringitis, otitis media
Cardiac	Relative bradycardia	Myocarditis	Splenomegaly
GI	Loose stools, watery diarrhea	Abdominal pain	Hepatic tenderness, RLQ pain, LUQ tenderness, peritoneal signs
Renal	Renal insufficiency	Decreased urine output, dark colored urine, acute renal failure	CVA tenderness, chronic renal failure
Laboratory CSF	Normal	Mild pleocytosis	RBCs, ↓ glucose, ↑ lactate
WBC count (blood)	Leukocytosis	Leukopenia	Thrombocytosis, thrombocytopenia
Gram stain (sputum)	Few mononuclear cells, no bacteria	PMN predominance, mixed flora	Purulent sputum, single predominant organism
Pleural fluid	Exudative pattern	↑ WBCs	RBCs, ↓ pH, ↓ glucose
SGOT/SGPT	Mildly elevated (2-5 x normal)	Moderately elevated (> 5 x normal)	Markedly elevated (> 10 x normal)
PO_4^-	Decreased transiently early	Decreased later	Increased
CPK	Increased early	Increased later	Normal value does not rule out Legionnaires'
CRP	> 30	< 30	Normal value does not rule out Legionnaires'
Ferritin	Highly increased early (> 500 ng/dL)	Increased (300-500 ng/dL)	Normal/slightly increased early. Normal value does not rule out Legionnaires'
Urine analysis	Proteinuria, microscopic hematuria	Myoglobinuria	Gross hematuria, pyuria, hemoglobinuria
Stool	Watery stools	Soft formed stools	Blood or mucus

CN = cranial nerve; CNS = central nervous system; CSF = cerebrospinal fluid; CVA = costovertebral angle; GI = gastrointestinal; HEENT = head, eyes, ears, nose and throat; LUQ = left upper quadrant; PVE = prosthetic valve endocarditis; RBC = red blood cell; RLQ = right lower quadrant; SBE = subacute bacterial endocarditis; WBC = white blood cell

Table 4.3. Modified Winthrop University Hospital Infectious Disease Division's Point System for Diagnosing Legionnaires' Disease in Adults

Presentation	Clinical Features*	Point Score
Headache	Acute onset	+ 1
Mental confusion/encephalopathic	Not drug-induced	+ 4
Lethargy	Acute onset	+ 3
Ear pain	Acute onset	– 3
Nonexudative pharyngitis/sore throat	Acute onset	– 3
Hoarseness	Acute onset	– 3
Sputum	Purulent	– 2
Hemoptysis	Mild/moderate	– 3
Chest pain	Pleuritic	– 2
Loose stools/watery diarrhea	Not drug-induced	+ 4
Abdominal pain	With/without diarrhea	+ 5
Relative bradycardia†	Temperature ≥ 102°F	+ 5
Lack of response to beta-lactams	After 72 hours	+ 5
Renal insufficiency	Otherwise unexplained	+ 3
Myocarditis	Otherwise unexplained	– 5
Splenomegaly	Otherwise unexplained	– 5
Laboratory Tests		
↓ pO_2 with ↑ A–a gradient (> 30)	Otherwise unexplained	– 5
↓ Na^+	Otherwise unexplained	+ 1
↓ PO_4^-	Otherwise unexplained	+ 5
↑ SGOT/SGPT (mild/transient)	Otherwise unexplained	+ 3
↑ Total bilirubin	Otherwise unexplained	+ 1
↑ CPK/aldolase	Otherwise unexplained	+ 4
↑ CRP (>30)	Otherwise unexplained	+ 4
↑ Cold agglutinin titer (≥ 1:64)	Otherwise unexplained	– 5
↑ Creatinine	Otherwise unexplained	+ 1
Microscopic hematuria	Otherwise unexplained	+ 2
Likelihood of Legionella		
Total Points	>10 Legionella likely 5-10 Legionella possible <5 Legionella unlikely	

* Acute onset, associated with pneumonia, and otherwise unexplained
† If not on beta blockers, diltiazem, verapamil; no arrhythmias or pacemaker

Zoonotic Atypical Pneumonia

Subset	Usual Pathogens*	Preferred IV Therapy	Alternate IV Therapy	PO Therapy or IV-to-PO Switch
Zoonotic pathogens (zoonotic vector)	C. psittaci (psittacosis) Coxiella burnetii (Q fever) Francisella tularensis (tularemia)	Doxycycline 200 mg (IV) q12h x 3 days, then 100 mg (IV) q12h x 11 days	Levofloxacin 500 mg (IV) x 2 weeks **or** Moxifloxacin 400 mg (IV) x 2 weeks	Doxycycline 200 mg (PO) q12h x 3 days, then 100 mg (PO) q12h x 11 days† **or** Levofloxacin 500 mg (PO) x 2 weeks **or** Moxifloxacin 400 mg (PO) x 2 weeks **or** Gemifloxacin 320 mg (PO) q24h x 2 weeks

Duration of therapy represents total time IV, PO, or IV + PO
* *Compromised hosts may require longer courses of therapy*
† *Loading dose is not needed PO if give IV with the same drug*

Clinical Presentation: CAP with extrapulmonary symptoms, signs, or laboratory abnormalities (Table 4.4)

Diagnostic Considerations: Zoonotic contact history is key to presumptive diagnosis: psittacosis (parrots and psittacine birds); Q fever (sheep, parturient cats); tularemia (rabbit, deer, deer fly bite). The diagnosis is confirmed by specific serological testing. Zoonotic CAP with splenomegaly/relative bradycardia suggests Q fever or psittacosis

Pitfalls: Organisms are difficult/dangerous to grow. Do not culture. Use serological tests for diagnosis

Therapeutic Considerations: Q fever endocarditis requires prolonged therapy

Prognosis: Good except for Q fever with complications (e.g., myocarditis, SBE)

Table 4.4. Diagnostic Features of Zoonotic Atypical Pneumonias

Key Characteristics	Psittacosis	Q Fever	Tularemia
Symptoms			
Mental confusion	–	–	–
Prominent headache	+	+	+
Meningismus	–	–	–
Myalgias	+	+	+
Ear pain	–	–	–
Pleuritic pain	±	±	±
Abdominal pain	–	–	–
Diarrhea	–	–	–
Signs			
Rash	± a	–	–
Nonexudative pharyngitis	–	–	±
Hemoptysis	–	–	±
Lobar consolidation	+	+	+
Cardiac involvement	±	±	–
Splenomegaly	+	+	–
Relative bradycardia	+	+	–
Chest X-Ray			
Infiltrate	Patchy consolidation	Patchy consolidation	"Ovoid bodies"
Bilateral hilar adenopathy	–	–	±
Pleural effusion	–	–	Bloody
Laboratory Abnormalities			
WBC count	↓	↑/N	↑/N
↓ Na^+	±	±	±
↓ PO_4^-	–	–	–
↑ AST/ALT (SGOT/SGPT)	+	+	–
↑ Cold agglutinins (≥ 1:64)	–	–	–
Microscopic hematuria			
Diagnostic Tests			
Direct isolation (culture)	–	–	–
Serology (specific)	CF	CF	TA

ALT = alanine aminotransferase; AST = aspartate aminotransferase; CF = complement fixation; IFA = indirect fluorescent antibody test; N = normal; TA = tube agglutination; WBC = white blood cell
+ = usually present; ± = sometimes present; – = usually absent
↑ = increased; ↓ = decreased; ↑↑↑ = markedly increased
a = Horder's spots

Viral Pneumonia

Subset	Usual Pathogens*	Preferred IV Therapy	Alternate IV Therapy	PO Therapy or IV-to-PO Switch
Influenza *Severe*	Influenza A Avian influenza A (H_5N_1)	Oseltamivir (Tamiflu) 75-150 mg (PO) q24h x 5 days **plus either** Rimantadine 100 mg (PO) q12h x 7-10 days **or** Amantadine 200 mg (PO) q24h x 7-10 days**		Start treatment as soon as possible after onset of symptoms, preferably within 2 days. Rimantadine/amantadine miss Influenza type B, which is usually a milder illness. Antiinfluenza drugs may be ineffective in severe influenza. Although amantadine resistance is now common, amantadine may be lifesaving by improving oxygenation
Mild/ moderate	Influenza A/B	Oseltamivir (Tamiflu) 75 mg (PO) q24h x 5 days	Zanamivir (Relenza) 10 mg (2 puffs via oral inhaler) q12h x 5 days	
Post-viral influenza	S. pneumoniae H. influenzae	Quinolone‡ (IV) q24h x 2 weeks **plus either** Nafcillin 2 gm (IV) q4h x 2 weeks **or** Clindamycin 600 mg (IV) q8h x 2 weeks	Ceftriaxone 1 gm (IV) q24h x 2 weeks **plus either** Vancomycin 1 gm (IV) q12h x 2 weeks **or** Linezolid 600 mg (IV) q12h x 2 weeks	Quinolone‡ (PO) q24h x 2 weeks
CAP and viral influenza	S. aureus (MSSA/CA-MRSA)	Linezolid 600 mg (IV) q12h x 2 weeks **or** Vancomycin 1 gm (IV) q12h x 2 weeks		Linezolid 600 mg (PO) q12h x 2 weeks **or** Minocycline 100 mg (PO) q12h x 2 weeks
SARS	SARS-associated coronavirus (SARS-CoV)	See therapeutic considerations, p. 69		

Duration of therapy represents total time IV, PO, or IV + PO
*   *Compromised hosts may require longer courses of therapy*
** *For avian influenza some recommend double dose amantadine/rimantadine*
‡   *Levofloxacin 500 mg or moxifloxacin 400 mg or gemifloxacin 320 mg*
Viral influenza may affect anyone in an unimmunized population but is most severe in the very young, second/third trimester of pregnancy, elderly, and immunosuppressed. The major causes include influenza virus, parainfluenza virus, adenovirus, RSV, hantaviruses, and CMV. Collectively, viruses account for ~ 10% of CAPs.

Viral Influenza

Clinical Presentation: Influenza virus is the most common cause of viral pneumonia. It is the only virus capable of worldwide epidemics and is estimated to cause 50,000 deaths each year. The peak incidence of influenza is late winter/early spring, and February is the usual peak month for influenza. The spectrum of infection ranges from a mild respiratory infection to fatal primary influenza pneumonia. Excluding epidemics/pandemics, influenza is relatively mild with high attack rates but low mortality rates. Epidemic or pandemic influenza due to highly virulent strains is associated with higher morbidity/mortality. Influenza C does not cause influenza but may cause a mild upper respiratory tract infection in children/adults. There are three types of influenza viruses (A, B, and C) which are single stranded of RNA respiratory viruses that differ in core proteins. Over 90% of influenza is caused by influenza A and 10% by influenza B. Influenza A may be severe, while influenza B is usually mild.

Clinical Presentation: Patients present with fever and shortness of breath ± pleuritic chest pain. The fever in viral influenza begins abruptly but decreases after 3 days (unless superimposed bacterial pneumonia). The severity of shortness of breath correlates with the oxygen diffusion defect. The incubation period of viral influenza is 2 days (range 1-4 days). Temperature at the onset is > 102°F accompanied by chills. Patients with primary influenza pneumonia usually present with a dry cough that may be blood tinged. Purulent sputum indicates superimposed bacterial pneumonia. Patients can often describe the precise hour that their illness began and rapidly become bedridden. The onset of influenza A is characterized by myalgias, particularly localized to the neck/back, and profound prostration. The severity and localization of these symptoms differentiate viral influenza A from the myalgias of ILIs. Retro-orbital pain is common and conjunctival suffusion differentiates influenza A from ILIs. Mild sore throat and hemoptysis may be present. Chest x-ray in mild cases is normal and in moderately severe cases, there may be patchy infiltrates. In severe Influenza A, the chest x-ray shows diffuse fluffy infiltrates within 48 hours. Purulent/blood tinged sputum, cyanosis, or vascular collapse indicates S. aureus pneumonia superimposed on influenza A pneumonia. Leukopenia is common with viral influenza; lymphopenia (relative/absolute) is a characteristic in severe influenza A.

Diagnostic Considerations: Chest x-ray shows minimal/no infiltrates early. Later, diffuse ill-defined infiltrates rapidly appear. The presence of focal/segmental infiltrates suggests superimposed bacterial pneumonia. If the patient presents with influenza pneumonia together with S. aureus pneumonia, the focal infiltrates on the chest x-ray will cavitate ≤ 72 hours. Such patients are critically ill with cyanosis/shock. Auscultation of the lungs in patients with primary influenza pneumonia are conspicuous by the absence of rales. (No adventitious sounds are present). Rales/pleural effusion suggests a superimposed bacterial pneumonia. Viral influenza may present as primary influenza pneumonia alone, as viral influenza together initially with S. aureus pneumonia, or as primary influenza pneumonia followed by bacterial pneumonia due to H. influenzae or S. pneumoniae (milder than influenza with S. aureus pneumonia). Patients with severe influenza pneumonia (without superimposed S. aureus pneumonia) are hypoxemic secondary to a severe oxygen diffusion defect. The degree of hypoxemia/↑ A-a are related to severity/mortality. In the pandemic of 1918, young, healthy military recruits died of hypoxemia from influenza pneumonia and relatively few died of superimposed bacterial pneumonia. With avian influenza A (H_5N_1), mortality has been due to influenza pneumonia without bacterial pneumonia. Influenza/avian influenza may be complicated by S. aureus (MSSA/CA-MRSA PVL

+/-) pneumonia, which increase mortality/morbidity. In an influenza epidemic/pandemic, the diagnosis of individual cases is obvious. With sporadic cases, or at the beginning of an influenza epidemic, some findings are helpful in differentiating influenza from influenza-like illnesses (Table 4.5).

The clinical diagnosis of influenza is suggested by its severity and characteristic signs/symptoms of influenza. The diagnosis of influenza may be confirmed by demonstrating influenza in respiratory secretions by DNA probe, PCR, or DIA/EIA during the first 2-days of illness. Influenza virus may be cultured from nasal aspirates, sputum or throat swabs. Influenza viruses are grown in cell culture or embryonic eggs. Rapid culture results may be obtained by using shell vial cell cultures/immunofluorescent antibody detection after 24 hours. Influenza may also be diagnosed serologically demonstrating an increase in influenza titers between acute and convalescent sera (convalescent titers should be obtained 3-4 weeks after acute titers). ELISA/CF assays may be used to determine antibody class or HA/NA typing. Diagnosis of avian influenza A (H_5N_1) resembles influenza A but is accompanied by diffuse infiltrates on chest x-ray and mild increases in serum transaminases. Diagnosis is by culture of respiratory secretions, hemoagglutinin specific RT-PCR for avian influenza A (H_5N_1).

Pitfalls: The main clinical problem is to differentiate viral influenza that requires therapy from ILIs (only supportive therapy available). Influenza A is unlikely if a patient presents with an ILI but with a subacute onset, temperature < 102°F, mild/moderate myalgias (particularly if not severe and over the back with pain), no retro-orbital eye pain, mild non-productive cough/coryza, and no conjunctival suffusion or severe prostration. Influenza should be accompanied by leukopenia and more specifically lymphopenia (relative > absolute). The presence of leukocytosis should suggest an alternate diagnosis in the absence of a superimposed bacterial pneumonia. In general, bacterial pneumonias are accompanied by pleuritic chest pain but viral pneumonias are not. In the absence of a superimposed bacterial pneumonia, the "pleuritic chest pain" that accompanies viral influenza is due to direct intercostal muscle invasion by the influenza virus (mimics the pleuritic chest pain of bacterial pneumonia). The chest x-ray in early primary influenza pneumonia has minimal/no infiltrates but later rapidly develop bilateral diffuse infiltrates. Segmental/lobar infiltrates in a patient with influenza indicates superimposed bacterial pneumonia. Influenza with bacterial pneumonia occurring at the outset is usually due to S. aureus (MSSA/CA-MRSA PVL-positive or negative). Superimposed bacterial pneumonia presenting after a week interval of improvement following influenza is usually due to S. pneumoniae/H. influenzae, not S. aureus. Viral influenza B being less severe than influenza A more closely resembles a ILIs in most cases. SARS is most likely to be confused with viral influenza A. SARS has a sudden onset accompanied by hypoxemia/↑ A-a gradient with diffuse infiltrates (usually without superimposed bacterial pneumonia as with influenza). Avian influenza A (H_5N_1) hemagglutinins are not detected by hemagglutinins inhibition serological tests for influenza A, therefore, a negative hemagglutinin inhibition serology for influenza A does not rule out avian influenza.

Therapeutic Considerations: Mild to moderate influenza A/B may be treated with neuraminidase inhibitors (oseltamivir (Tamiflu)/zanamivir (Relenza), which reduce symptoms by ~ 2 days. Treatment should be started as early as possible, and no later than 2 days of onset for optimal therapeutic effect. For severe influenza pneumonia, treat with oseltamivir (Tamiflu)/zanamivir (Relenza) plus either amantadine or amantadine. Unless amantadine resistant, amantadine and rimantadine are effective against the adherence of the influenza virus to cells and prevent cell to cell transmission. Amantadine/rimantadine also increases peripheral airway dilatation/oxygenation, which is vital in severe influenza pneumonia. If influenza presents together with bacterial pneumonia, S. aureus (MSSA/CA-MRSA PVL +/–) is likely. Anti-HA-MRSA antibiotics are also effective against CA-MRSA (PVL +/–). Late onset of bacterial pneumonia following viral influenza due to H. influenzae/S. pneumoniae should be treated with the same agents used for CAP (beta-lactams, respiratory quinolones, etc.).

Prognosis: Prognosis is good for mild to moderate influenza. Prognosis is poor if complicated by bacterial pneumonia (S. aureus, particularly if due to CA-MRSA PVL-positive strains) and guarded if later complicated by post-influenza CAP due to S. pneumoniae/H. influenzae. Severe influenza A is most often fatal because of profound hypoxemia. Severe influenza pneumonia may be fatal even in young adults. Influenza pneumonia may also be severe/fatal in debilitated/elderly adults, those with severe cardiopulmonary disease, or immunocompromised hosts. In non-fatal cases, full recovery usually occurs in 1-2 weeks. Myositis/rhabdomyolysis may occur, particularly in children. Influenza may be complicated by encephalitis, Reye's syndrome, or myocarditis. Post-influenza asthenia may persist for months.

Avian Influenza (Influenza virus, type A (H_5N_1)

Clinical Presentation: Influenza following close contact with infected poultry. Recent outbreaks in humans in Asia. Human-to-human transmission reported. Often fulminant respiratory illness rapidly followed by ARDS/death

Diagnostic Considerations: Often acute onset of severe influenza illness ± diarrhea with leukopenia, lymphopenia, and mildly ↑ serum transaminases. Diagnosis by hemagglutin-specific RT-PCR for avian influenza or culture of respiratory secretions

Pitfalls: Although avian influenza is caused influenza A virus, the hemagglutinin inhibition serological test used to diagnose influenza A is insensitive to avian hemagglutinin, resulting in negative testing

Therapeutic Considerations: Antivirals must be given early to be effective. Avian influenza strains may be resistant to oseltamivir and amantadine/rimantadine; high-dose oseltamivir may be more effective. Even if resistant, amantadine/rimantadine should be given to possibly increase peripheral airway dilatation/oxygenation

Prognosis: Often fulminant infection with ARDS/death

Staphylococcus aureus Pneumonia

Epidemiology: S. aureus (MSSA/MRSA) are gram-positive cocci in clusters and rarely a cause of CAP in normal adults. In virtually all cases, S. aureus CAP occurs only with viral influenza. S. aureus CAP may complicate avian influenza, but not HSV-1, RSV, or CMV.

Clinical Presentation: S. aureus CAP is not uncommon in children < 3 months of age, where it is characterized by cavitary lung lesions, pneumatoceles, pneumothorax, and lung abscesses. Among hospitalized patients, MSSA/MRSA commonly colonize respiratory secretions as a result of the many antimicrobials given to hospitalized/ICU patients. S. aureus pneumonia is an easily recognized clinical syndrome characterized by its acute presentation and severe course. Patients are acutely ill, develop high spiking fevers, and rapidly become cyanotic/hypoxic. In adults, the chest x-ray reveals multiple thick-walled cavitary lesions, which rapidly develop within 72 hours. Blood cultures are often positive for S. aureus (excluding contaminants from venipuncture). S. aureus CAP occurs *concurrently* with influenza pneumonia; in contrast, post-viral influenza pneumonia is usually due to S. pneumoniae or H.

influenzae and develops after an interval of improvement (~ 1 week) following influenza.

Diagnostic Considerations: S. aureus (MSSA, CO-MRSA, CA-MRSA) CAP occurs with influenza/influenza-like illness (ILI) and is characterized by the rapid ($\leq$ 72 hours) development of multiple cavitary lesions on chest x-ray. In CAP patients with an oxygen diffusion defect ($\uparrow$ A-a gradient), underlying viral influenza/SARS should be suspected to explain the profound hypoxemia. As with gram-negative necrotizing pneumonias, elastin fibers may be found in stained lower respiratory secretions. The diagnosis of S. aureus CAP is made by demonstrating gram-positive cocci in clusters in purulent sputum, positive blood cultures (3/4 or 4/4 with S. aureus), rapidly cavitating (< 72 hours) infiltrates on chest x-ray, and rapid clinical deterioration in a patient with influenza/ILI.

Pitfalls: Severe hypoxemia ($\downarrow$ pO_2/$\uparrow$ A-a gradient) should suggest an underlying viral pneumonia (influenza, SARS). With influenza or SARS, concurrent S. aureus CAP is likely if gram-positive cocci in clusters are found in purulent sputum, lung biopsy, cavitary aspirates, or blood cultures (excluding skin contaminants). Purulent sputum with MSSA/MRSA in a clinically stable intubated patient on a ventilator without rapidly cavitating infiltrates suggests S. aureus colonization or tracheobronchitis, not S. aureus nosocomial pneumonia.

Therapeutic Considerations: Although S. aureus CAP is virtually only with viral influenza, if suspected, empiric therapy should be active against both CA-MSSA and CO-MRSA. Daptomycin should not be used for staphylococcal pneumonias as it is inactivated by lung surfactant. In spite of early/appropriate anti-staphylococcal therapy, S. aureus CAP is a rapidly progressive/necrotizing pneumonia that may destroy multiple lung lobes. Therapy is continued for $\geq$ 2 weeks.

Prognosis: Prognosis is related to the extent of lung destruction, the severity of underlying influenza pneumonia, and the degree/duration of hypoxemia. CA-MRSA (PVL-negative) CAP with influenza resembles MSSA in severity. CA-MRSA (PVL-positive) CAP with influenza causes a fulminant/necrotizing pneumonia.

Severe Acute Respiratory Syndrome (SARS)

Clinical Presentation: Influenza-like illness with fever, dry cough, myalgias,, diarrhea in some. Patients are short of breath/hypoxic. Auscultation of the lungs resembles viral influenza (i.e., quiet, no rales). Biphasic infection: fever decreases after few days, patient improves, then fever recurs in a few days. Chest x-ray shows bilateral interstitial (upper/lower lobe) infiltrates. WBC and platelet counts are usually normal or slightly decreased. Relative lymphopenia is present early. Mild increases in SGOT/SGPT, LDH, CPK are common.

Diagnostic Considerations: Diagnosis by viral isolation or specific SARS serology. Important to exclude influenza A, Legionnaires' disease and tularemic pneumonia.

Pitfalls: Most likely to be confused with viral influenza A—both present with fever, myalgias, hypoxia. Chest x-ray in SARS has discrete infiltrates (influenza does not unless superimposed CAP) that are often ovoid. Commonly complicated by ARDS.

Therapeutic Considerations: Most patients are severely hypoxemic and require oxygen/ventilatory support. In a preliminary study, some patients benefitted from corticosteroids (pulse-dosed methylprednisolone 500 mg [IV] q24h x 3 days followed by taper/step down with prednisone [PO] to complete 20 days) plus Interferon alfacon-1 (9 mcg [SQ] q24h x at least 2 days, increased to 15 mcg/d if no response) x 8-13 days. Ribavirin of no benefit.

Prognosis: Related to underlying cardiopulmonary/immune status and severity/duration of hypoxemia. Frequently fatal.

Table 4.5. Winthrop-University Hospital Infectious Disease Division's Point System for Diagnosing Severe Influenza A in Adults

Presentation	Clinical Features	Point Score
Symptoms		
Onset	Acute	+5
Prostration	Acute/severe	+5
Generalized muscle soreness	Severe	+5
Pain neck/back	Severe	+5
Signs		
Fever (>102°F)	Present	+2
Dry cough	Present	−4
Coryza	Present	+1
Conjuctival suffusion	Otherwise unexplained	+5
Hemoptysis	Otherwise unexplained	+5
Blood-tinged/purulent sputum	Present	+3
Localized rales†	Present	−3
Cyanosis†	Otherwise unexplained	+5
Vascular collapse	Shock	+5
Laboratory Tests		
Leukocytosis	Present	−4
Leukopenia	Otherwise unexplained	+3
Lymphopenia	Otherwise unexplained	+3
Thrombocytopenia	Otherwise unexplained	+3
Chest x-ray	Minimal or no infiltrates (very early)	+3
	Focal segmental infiltrate*	−5
	Bilateral diffuse interstitial infiltrates (≤ 1 day)	+5
	Severe hypoxemia/(A-a gradient > 30)	+5
	Mild/no hypoxemia	−5
	Pleural effusion	−5

	Likelihood of Influenza A	
Total Points	> 20	Influenza A very likely
	10-20	Mild/moderate influenza A likely
	< 10	Influenza A unlikely; influenza B or influenza-like viral illness likely

* If influenza present, suggests S. aureus

Aspiration Pneumonia

Subset	Usual Pathogens*	Preferred IV Therapy	Alternate IV Therapy	PO Therapy or IV-to-PO Switch
Aspiration	Oral anaerobes S. pneumoniae H. influenzae M. catarrhalis	Levofloxacin 500 mg (IV) q24h x 2 weeks **or** Moxifloxacin 400 mg (IV) q24h x 2 weeks **or** Ceftriaxone 1 gm (IV) q24h x 2 weeks	Doxycycline 200 mg (IV) q12h x 3 days, then 100 mg (IV) q12h x 11 days	Levofloxacin 500 mg (PO) q24h x 2 weeks **or** Moxifloxacin 400 mg (PO) q24h x 2 weeks **or** Gemifloxacin 320 mg (PO) q24h x 2 weeks **or** Amoxicillin/clavulanic acid XR 2 tablets (PO) q12h x 2 weeks **or** Doxycycline 200 mg (PO) q12h x 3 days, then 100 mg (PO) q12h x 11 days** **or** Clarithromycin XL 1 gm (PO) q24h x 2 weeks

Duration of therapy represents total time IV, PO, or IV + PO
*   *Compromised hosts may require longer courses of therapy*
** *Loading dose is not needed PO if given IV with the same drug*

Epidemiology: Aspiration pneumonia accounts for 10% of community-acquired pneumonias and is a common cause of nosocomial pneumonia. Predisposing conditions include decreased consciousness (head trauma, stroke, medications, seizure disorder, general anesthesia, chronic alcoholism, drug overdose), neurological dysfunction (myasthenia gravis, pseudobulbar palsy, Parkinson's disease), esophageal obstruction (stricture, neoplasm, diverticula) or dysmotility, tracheoesophageal fistula, GERD, dental procedures, gastrointestinal/pulmonary instrumentation (bronchoscopy, upper GI endoscopy, endotracheal/NG tubes, tracheostomy), general debilitation, and recumbent position. Community-acquired bacterial aspiration pneumonia is usually caused by aspiration of normal anaerobic oropharyngeal flora and is typically polymicrobial. It is often localized to a single lobe but can be massive and involve both lungs in patients in the supine position.

Clinical Presentation: Aspiration pneumonia may also follow aspiration of gastric bacteria. Compared to the acute/dramatic presentation of chemical pneumonitis following aspiration of gastric acid, the clinical presentation of bacterial aspiration pneumonia is usually subacute/insidious (Table 4.6), with low-grade fevers (< 102°F without chills), cough, and purulent sputum. The chest x-ray shows an infiltrate in the dependent segment of the lung:

basilar infiltrates when aspiration occurs in the upright position, and infiltrates in the posterior segments of the upper lobes or the apical segments of the lower lobes when aspiration occurs in the supine position. Infiltrates usually progress slowly and often cavitate after $\geq$ 7 days. Nosocomial aspiration pneumonia is caused by aspiration of aerobic gram-negative bacilli colonizing the oropharynx/stomach in patients that have been hospitalized $\geq$ 7 days.

Diagnostic Considerations: Bacterial aspiration pneumonia is a clinical diagnosis that should be suspected in patients who are observed aspirating, or are predisposed to aspiration and develop unexplained infiltrates, especially in the basilar segments of the lower lobes (aspiration in the upright position), or in the posterior segments of the upper lobes or the apical segments of the lower lobes (aspiration in the supine position). The insidious/indolent nature of the clinical presentation (low-grade fever, cough, sputum production) is a clue to the diagnosis. Sputum Gram stain/culture are of no value in making the diagnosis, blood cultures are usually negative, and the WBC count is variably elevated. Aspiration pneumonia may be complicated by putrid empyema or lung abscess.

Pitfalls: The diagnosis of bacterial aspiration pneumonia is usually straightforward in patients with disorders that predispose to aspiration. Cavitation on the chest x-ray occurring $\geq$ 7 days distinguishes bacterial aspiration pneumonia from other causes of acute cavitary pneumonias, which cavitate sooner. Aspiration CAP is caused by anaerobic oropharyngeal flora, and sputum Gram stain/culture are of no value (normal flora). In hospital-acquired bacterial aspiration pneumonia, institutional aerobic gram-negative bacillary flora displace the usual normal anaerobic oropharyngeal flora after one week of hospitalization, and anaerobes are not important nosocomial pneumonia pathogens.

Therapeutic Considerations: Aspiration CAP should be treated with the same antibiotics used to treat typical CAP, as the oropharyngeal flora above the diaphragm, which are predominantly anaerobic (Peptostreptococci, "oral pigmented" Bacteroides [e.g., B. melaninogenicus], Veillonella, etc), are highly sensitive to beta-lactams, macrolides, tetracyclines, quinolones, etc. Specific anti-anaerobic therapy (clindamycin, metronidazole), which is required for anaerobic infections below the diaphragm (e.g., B. fragilis), is not required for aspiration CAP. In contrast to aspiration CAP, aspiration pneumonia occurring in hospitalized patients should be treated the same as nosocomial pneumonia (Chapter 7), as the predominant aspirated flora are gram-negative bacilli from the hospital microbial environment (e.g., P. aeruginosa, others), not anaerobes. Repeat aspiration pneumonia is due to a continuance of the same predisposing factors for aspiration rather than therapeutic failure. Aspiration pneumonia complicated by empyema requires antimicrobial therapy plus chest tube drainage. Aspiration pneumonia complicated by lung abscess requires prolonged (usually months) antimicrobial therapy until the lung abscess resolves.

Prognosis: The prognosis in bacterial aspiration pneumonia depends on the extent of the aspiration, the severity of the disorder predisposing to aspiration, and the functional capacity of the lungs. Prognosis is worst in patients with massive aspiration pneumonia or with aspiration pneumonia complicated by empyema/lung abscess.

Table 4.6. Classification of Aspiration Pneumonia

Inoculum	Pulmonary Sequelae	Clinical Features	Therapy
Acid	Chemical pneumonitis	Acute dyspnea, tachypnea, tachycardia, hypoxemia; ± cyanosis, bronchospasm, fever. Sputum is pink, frothy. Chest x-ray shows infiltrates in one or both lower lobes	Positive-pressure breathing, IV fluids, tracheal suction
Oropharyngeal bacteria	Bacterial infection	Usually insidious onset of cough, fever, purulent sputum. Chest x-ray shows infiltrate in dependent pulmonary segment/lobe ± cavitation	Antibiotics
Inert fluids	Mechanical obstruction, reflex airway closure	Acute dyspnea, cyanosis ± apnea; pulmonary edema	Tracheal suction; intermittent positive-pressure breathing with oxygen and isoproterenol
Particulate matter	Mechanical obstruction	Dependent on level of obstruction, ranging from acute apnea and rapid death to chronic cough ± recurrent infection	Removal of particulate matter, antibiotics for superimposed infection

In: Bartlett JG. Aspiration Pneumonia. Gorbach SL, Bartlett JG, Blacklow NR (eds). Infectious Diseases, 2nd edition. W.B. Saunders, Philadelphia, PA, 1998.

Typical/Atypical Tuberculosis

Subset	Usual Pathogens	Therapy
Tuberculosis (TB)	M. tuberculosis	INH 300 mg (PO) q24h x 6 months **plus** Rifampin 600 mg (PO) q24h x 6 months **plus** PZA 25 mg/kg (PO) q24h x 2 months **plus** EMB 15 mg/kg (PO) q24h (until susceptibilities known)[††]
Atypical tuberculosis	Mycobacterium avium-intracellulare (MAI)	<u>Treat for 6 months after sputum negative for MAI:</u> Ethambutol 15 mg/kg (PO) q24h **plus either** Clarithromycin 500 mg (PO) q12h **or** Azithromycin 500 mg (PO) q24h <u>May also choose to add:</u> Quinolone (PO)* q24h
	M. kansasii	<u>Preferred therapy</u> Rifampin 600 mg (PO) q24h **plus** INH 300 mg (PO) q24h **plus** pyridoxine 50 mg (PO) q24h **plus** EMB 15 mg/kg (PO) q24h. Treat x 18 months with 12 months of negative sputum <u>Alternate therapy</u> Clarithromycin 500 mg (PO) q12h **plus** INH 900 mg (PO) q24h **plus** pyridoxine 50 mg (PO) q24h **plus** EMB 25 mg/kg (PO) q24h **plus** sulfamethoxazole 1 gm (PO) q8h. Treat x 18 months with 12 months of negative sputum <u>For severe cases</u>, add streptomycin 0.5-1 gm (IM) 3x/week during first 3 months of preferred/alternate therapy

Duration of therapy represents total time IV, PO, or IV + PO
*   *Levofloxacin 500 mg or moxifloxacin 400 mg*
†† *If isolate is sensitive, discontinue EMB and continue as above, to complete 6 months. If INH-resistant, continue EMB, rifampin, and PZA to complete 6 months. If any other resistance is present, obtain infectious disease or pulmonary consult*

Tuberculous (TB) Pneumonia

Clinical Presentation: Community-acquired pneumonia with single/multiple infiltrates
Diagnostic Considerations: Diagnosis by sputum AFB smear/culture. Respiratory isolation important. Lower lobe effusion common in lower lobe primary TB. Reactivation TB is usually bilateral/apical ± old, healed Ghon complex; cavitation/fibrosis are common, but pleural effusion is absent
Pitfalls: Primary TB may present as CAP; reactivation TB presents as chronic pneumonia (Table 8.1)
Therapeutic Considerations: 1-2 weeks of therapy is usually required to eliminate AFBs from sputum
Prognosis: Related to underlying health status

Mycobacterium avium-intracellulare (MAI) Pneumonia

Clinical Presentation: Community-acquired pneumonia in normal hosts or immuno-suppressed/HIV patient with focal single/multiple infiltrates indistinguishable from TB
Diagnostic Considerations: Diagnosis by AFB culture. In HIV, MAI may disseminate,

resembling miliary TB. Diagnosis by culture of blood, liver, or bone marrow

Pitfalls: TB and MAI are indistinguishable on acid-fast smear; must differentiate TB from MAI by AFB culture, as therapy for MAI differs from TB

Therapeutic Considerations: MAI in normal hosts is readily treatable, but MAI in HIV patients requires life-long suppressive therapy after initial treatment

Prognosis: Related to degree of immunosuppression/CD_4 count

Mycobacterium kansasii Pneumonia

Clinical Presentation: Subacute CAP resembling TB/MAI that can occur in clusters/outbreaks

Diagnostic Considerations: Chest x-ray infiltrates/lung disease plus M. kansasii in a single sputum specimen. M. kansasii can cause disseminated infection, like TB, and is diagnosed by culturing M. kansasii from the blood, liver, or bone marrow

Pitfalls: M. kansasii in sputum with a normal chest x-ray does not indicate infection. Common colonizer of respiratory secretions in chronic bronchiectasis.

Therapeutic Considerations: M. kansasii is more readily treatable than TB. Use the alternate regimen for rifampin-resistant strains.

Prognosis: Good in normal hosts. May be rapidly progressive/fatal without treatment in HIV patients.

Miscellaneous Pneumonia Subsets

Subset	Usual Pathogens*	IV Therapy		PO Therapy or IV-to-PO Switch
Chronic alcoholics	K. pneumoniae S. pneumoniae H. influenzae M. catarrhalis	Ceftriaxone 1 gm (IV) q24h x 2 weeks	Quinolone[‡] (IV) q24h x 2 weeks	Quinolone[‡] (PO) q24hx 2 weeks
Bronchiectasis, cystic fibrosis	S. maltophilia B. cepacia	Cefepime 2 gm (IV) q8h[¶] **or** Meropenem 2 gm (IV) q8h[¶] **or** Minocycline 100 mg (IV) q12h[¶] **or** TMP-SMX 2.5 mg/kg (IV) q6h[¶]	Quinolone[‡] (IV) q24h[¶]	TMP-SMX 1 SS tablet (PO) q6h[¶] **or** Quinolone[‡] (PO) q24h[¶] **or** Minocycline mg (PO) q12h[¶]
	P . aeruginosa	See next page		
	MDR (multi-drug resistant) P. aeruginosa	See next page		

Miscellaneous Pneumonia Subsets

Subset	Usual Pathogens*	IV Therapy		PO Therapy or IV-to-PO Switch
Bronchiectasis, cystic fibrosis (cont'd)	P. aeruginosa	Meropenem 2 gm (IV) q8h¶	Levofloxacin 750 mg (IV) q24h¶ **or** Ciprofloxacin 750 mg (IV) q12h¶ **or** Cefepime 2 gm (IV) q8h¶ ± amikacin 1 gm (IV) q24h¶	Levofloxacin 750 mg (PO) q24h¶ **or** Ciprofloxacin XR 1 gm (PO) q24h¶
	MDR (multi-drug resistant) P. aeruginosa	Colistin 80 mg or 1.7 mg/kg (IV) q8h¶ **with or without** Rifampin 600 mg (IV/PO) q24h¶	Polymyxin B 1-1.25 mg/kg (IV) q12h¶†	Colistin **or** Polymyxin B 80 mg q8h (via nebulizer aerosol)¶†§¥
Other pathogens	Blastomyces, Histoplasma, Coccidioides, Paracoccidioides, Actinomyces, Nocardia, Pseudallescheria boydii, Sporothrix, Mucor (Chapter 8)			

Duration of therapy represents total time IV, PO, or IV + PO. Most patients on IV therapy able to take PO meds should be switched to PO therapy soon after clinical improvement
*   *Compromised hosts may require longer courses of therapy*
¶   *Treat until cured*
‡   *Levofloxacin 500 mg or moxifloxacin 400 mg or gatifloxacin 400 mg*
†   *1 mg colistin = 12,500 IU; 1 mg polymyxin B = 10,000 IU*
§   *Use 160 mg q8h for recurrent infection*
¥   *Nebulized/aerosolized antibiotics predispose to MDR strains*

Pneumonia in Chronic Alcoholics (also see K. pneumoniae, p. 54)

Clinical Presentation: Onset is acute with fever, chills, cough. Pleuritic chest pain and dyspnea are common. Sputum may be blood-tinged. Chest x-ray shows a lobar infiltrate ± consolidation with cavitation after 3-5 days

Diagnostic Considerations: Klebsiella pneumoniae pneumonia usually occurs only in chronic alcoholics and is characterized by blood-flecked "currant jelly" sputum and cavitation (typically in 3-5 days)

Pitfalls: Suspect Klebsiella with "pneumococcal" pneumonia that cavitates. Empyema is more common than pleural effusion.

Therapeutic Considerations: Monotherapy with newer anti-Klebsiella agents is as effective as "double-drug" therapy with older agents.

Prognosis: Related to degree of hepatic/splenic dysfunction.

Bronchiectasis/Cystic Fibrosis

Clinical Presentation: Onset is acute/subacute with fever ± chills, new infiltrate on chest x-ray, ↑ sputum volume/viscosity, and ↓ pulmonary function

Diagnostic Considerations: Cystic fibrosis/bronchiectasis is characterized by viscous secretions ± low grade fevers; less commonly may present as lung abscess. Onset of pneumonia/lung abscess heralded by cough/decrease in pulmonary function

Pitfalls: Sputum colonization is common with S. maltophilia or B. cepacia, which may or may not be pathogens

Therapeutic Considerations: Important to select antibiotics with low resistance potential and good penetration into respiratory secretions (e.g., quinolones, meropenem)

Prognosis: Related to extent of underlying lung disease/severity of infection

Pseudomonas aeruginosa Pneumonia

Epidemiology: Pseudomonas aeruginosa is an aerobic gram-negative bacillus that causes a necrotizing hospital-acquired pneumonia. It is not a cause of CAP in normal hosts, but may cause CAP in patients with cystic fibrosis/chronic bronchiectasis. High-risk groups predisposed to P. aeruginosa infection include IV drug abusers (bacteremia, tricuspid valve ABE ± septic pulmonary emboli) and patients with febrile neutropenia (bacteremia). HIV patients, organ transplants, and those on immunosuppressive/chronic steroid therapy are not predisposed to P. aeruginosa bacteremia/CAP, although some terminal HIV patients develop P. aeruginosa bacteremia. Despite being a common colonizer of respiratory secretions in intubated patients on ventilators, it is an uncommon albeit highly virulent cause of nosocomial pneumonia.

Clinical Presentation: P. aeruginosa CAP occurs only in patients with underlying suppurative lung disease (i.e., bronchiectasis/cystic fibrosis) and is usually secondary to inhalation/aspiration and localized to a lung segment/lobe.

Diagnostic Considerations: The diagnosis of P. aeruginosa CAP should be considered in patients with bronchiectasis/cystic fibrosis who develop otherwise unexplained clinical deterioration and new pulmonary infiltrates. On chest x-ray, P. aeruginosa CAP secondary to inhalation/aspiration is localized to a segment or lobe of the lung. Blood cultures are rarely positive. Patients with bronchiectasis/cystic fibrosis who develop increased copious/purulent respiratory secretions without pulmonary infiltrates or with no change in their pulmonary infiltrates typically have P. aeruginosa tracheobronchitis, but not P. aeruginosa pneumonia.

Pitfalls: The respiratory secretions of most patients with bronchiectasis/cystic fibrosis are colonized by non-fermentative aerobic gram-negative bacilli (P. aeruginosa). The recovery of P. aeruginosa from respiratory secretions in clinically stable patients with little or no change in their pulmonary infiltrates indicates colonization with P. aeruginosa, not P. aeruginosa CAP. The recovery of a "pathogen" in respiratory secretions does not prove its pathogenic role if not accompanied by characteristic clinical manifestations. Organisms presumptively identified as "Pseudomonas" may in fact be other non-fermentative gram-negative bacilli resembling P. aeruginosa (B. cepacia, S. maltophilia). In patients with cystic fibrosis/chronic bronchiectasis, P. aeruginosa, B. cepacia, S. maltophilia are common colonizers of respiratory secretions and may cause tracheobronchitis/pneumonia.

Therapeutic Considerations: Because P. aeruginosa is the most virulent potential pulmonary pathogen in patients with chronic bronchiectasis/cystic fibrosis, empiric coverage should be directed primarily against this organism. Initial empiric coverage using monotherapy with a highly active anti-P. aeruginosa antibiotic with low-resistance potential and the ability to achieve therapeutic concentrations in viscid secretions (e.g., meropenem) is the preferred approach. Empiric coverage with two anti-pseudomonal agents may be used but has no advantage over well-selected monotherapy. Empiric therapy is usually continued for 2 weeks, although a longer duration of therapy may be required.

Prognosis: The prognosis for P. aeruginosa CAP in patients with cystic fibrosis/chronic bronchiectasis is guarded and may be fatal. Successful antibiotic therapy restores residual pulmonary function.

REFERENCES AND SUGGESTED READINGS

Alvarez-Lerma F, Torres A. Severe community-acquired pneumonia. Curr Opin Crit Care 10:369-374, 2004.

Apisarnthanarak A, Mundy LM. Etiology of community-acquired pneumonia. Clin Chest Med 26:47-55, 2005.

Aronsky D, Dean NC. How should we make the admission decision in community-acquired pneumonia? Med Clin North Am 85:1397-411, 2001.

Bartlett JG. Diagnostic test for etiologic agents of community-acquired pneumonia. Infect Dis Clin North Am 18:791-807, 2004.

Beyrer K, Lai S, Dreesman J, et al. Legionnaires' disease outbreak associated with a cruise liner, August 2003: epidemiological and microbiological findings. Epidemiol Infect 135:802-10, 2007.

Blasi F, Tarsia P. Value of short-course antimicrobial therapy in community-acquired pneumonia. Int J Antimicrob Agents 26; Suppl 3:S148-55, 2005.

Blasi F, Tarsia P, Cosentini R, et al. Therapeutic potential of the new quinolones in the treatment of lower respiratory tract infections. Expert Opin Investig Drugs 12:1165-77, 2003.

Bochud PY, Moser F, Erard P, et al. Community-acquired pneumonia. A perspective outpatient study. Medicine (Baltimore) 80:75-87, 2001.

Bruns AH, Oosterheert JJ, Prokop M, et al. Patterns of resolution of chest radiograph abnormalities in adults hospitalized with severe community-acquired pneumonia. Clin Infect Dis 45:983-91, 2007.

Buising KL, Thursky KA, Black JF, et al. A prospective comparison of severity scores for identifying patients with severe community-acquired pneumonia: reconsidering what is meant by severe pneumonia. Thorax 61:419-424, 2006.

Carratala J, Martin-Herrero JE, Mykietiuk A, et al. Clinical experience in the management of community-acquired pneumonia: lessons from the use of fluoroquinolones. Clin Microbiol Infect 12; Suppl 3:2-11, 2006.

Chapman TM, Perry CM. Cefepime: a review of its use in the management of hospitalized patients with pneumonia. Am J Respir Med 2:75-107, 2003.

Cunha BA. Clinical relevance of penicillin-resistant Streptococcus pneumoniae. Semin Respir Infect 17:204-14, 2002.

Cunha BA. Community-acquired pneumonia. Diagnostic and therapeutic approach. Med Clin North Am 85:43-77, 2001.

Cunha BA. Empiric therapy of community-acquired pneumonia: guidelines for the perplexed? Chest 125:1913-9, 2004.

Cunha BA. Levofloxacin in the treatment of community-acquired pneumonia due to penicillin resistant s. pneumoniae. Penetration 5:39-46, 2005.

Cunha BA. Penicillin resistance in pneumococcal pneumonia. Antibiotics with low resistance potential are effective and pose less risk. Postgrad Med 113:42-4, 47-8, 52-4, 2003.

Cunha BA. Pneumonia in the elderly. Clin Microbiol Infect 7:581-8, 2001.

Cunha BA. Antibiotic pharmacokinetic considerations in pulmonary infections, Volume II. Gerding D, (eds). Seminars in Respiratory Infections, 1991.

Cunha BA. The atypical pneumonias: clinical diagnosis and importance. Clin Microbiol and Infect Dis 12:12-24, 2006.

Cutler, SJ, Bouzid M, Cutler RR. Q fever. J of Infect 54:313-318, 2007.

Dattwyler RJ. Community-acquired pneumonia in the age of bio-terrorism. Allergy Asthma Proc 26:191-194, 2005.

den Boer JW, Yzerman EP, Jansen R, et al. Legionnaires' disease and gardening. Clin Microbiol Infect 13:88-91, 2007.

Dunbar LM, Wunderink RG, Habib MP, et al. High-dose, short-course levofloxacin for community-acquired pneumonia: a new treatment paradigm. Clin Infect Dis 37:752-760, 2003.

File TM Jr. A new dosing paradigm: high-dose, short-course fluoroquinolone therapy for community-acquired pneumonia. Clin Cornerstone Suppl 3:S21-8, 2003.

File TM Jr. Clinical efficacy of newer agents in short-duration therapy for community-acquired pneumonia. Clin Infect Dis 1;39(Suppl 3):S159-64, 2004.

File TM Jr. Community-acquired pneumonia. Lancet 13;362:1991-2001, 2003.

File TM Jr. The epidemiology of respiratory tract infections. Semin Respir Infect 15:184-94, 2000.

File TM Jr., Garau J, Blasi F, et al. Guidelines for empiric antimicrobial prescribing in community-acquired pneumonia. Chest 125:1888-901, 2004.

File TM Jr., Niederman MS. Antimicrobial therapy of community-acquired pneumonia. Infect Dis Clin North Am 18:993-1016, 2004.

File TM Jr. Streptococcus pneumoniae and community-acquired pneumonia: a cause for concern. Am J Med 117; (Suppl 3A):39S-50S, 2004.

Fish DN. Levofloxacin: update and perspectives on one of the original respiratory quinolones. Expert Rev Anti Infect Ther 1:371-87, 2003.

Garau J. Role of beta-lactam agents in the treatment of community-acquired pneumonia. Eur J Clin Microbiol Infect Dis 24:83-99, 2005.

Gillet Y, Vanhems P, Lina G, et al. Factors predicting mortality in necrotizing community-acquired pneumonia caused by Staphylococcus aureus containing Panton-Valentine leukocidin. Clin Infect Dis 45:315-21, 2007.

Grau S, Antonio JM, Ribes E, et al. Impact of rifampicin addition to clarithromycin in Legionella pneumophila pneumonia. Int J Antimicrob Agents 28:249-252, 2006.

Hedlund J, Stralin K, Ortqvist A, et al. Swedish guidelines for the management of community-acquired pneumonia in immunocompetent adults. Scand J Infect Dis 37: 791-805, 2005.

Houck PM, Bratzler DW. Administration of first hospital antibiotics for community-acquired pneumonia: does timeliness affect outcomes? Curr Opin Infect Dis 18:151-156, 2005.

Hsu MC, Lin TM, Huang CT, Liao MH, Li SY.Chlamydia pneumoniae respiratory infections in Taiwan.Microbiol Immunol 51:539-42, 2007.

Kamath AV, Myint PK. Recognizing and managing severe community-acquired pneumonia. Br J Hosp Med (Lond). 67: M76-78, 2006.

Keam SJ, Croom KF, Keating GM. Gatifloxacin: a review of its use in the treatment of bacterial infections in the US. Drugs 65:695-724, 2005.

Kunimoto D, Long R. Tuberculosis still overlooked as a cause of community-acquired pneumonia—how not to miss it. Respir Care Clin N Am 11:25-34, 2005.

Leal FE, Cavazzana CL, de Andrade HF, et al. Toxoplasma gondii pneumonia in immunocompetent subjects: case report and review. Clin Infect Dis 44:e62-6, 2007.

Lee I, Kim TS, Yoon HK. Mycoplasma pneumoniae pneumonia: CT features in 16 patients. Eur Radiol 16:719-25, 2006.

Leung-Shea C, Danaher PJ. Q fever in members of the United States armed forces returning from Iraq. Clin Infect Dis 43:e77-82, 2006.

Loeb M. Epidemiology of community- and nursing home-acquired pneumonia in older adults. Expert Rev Anti Infect Ther 3:263-270, 2005.

Loeb M. Pneumonia in the elderly. Curr Oppin Infect Dis 17:127-30, 2004.

Mandell LA, Bartlett JG, Dowell SF, File TM, et al. Update of practice guidelines for the management of community-acquired pneumonia in immunocompetent adults. Clin Infect Dis 37:1405-1433, 2003.

Mandell LA. Epidemiology and etiology of community-acquired pneumonia. Infect Dis Clin North Am 18:761-776, 2004.

Mandell LA. Update of community-acquired pneumonia. New pathogens and new concepts in treatment. Postgrad Med 118:35-36, 2005.

Marrie TJ. Empiric treatment of ambulatory community-acquired pneumonia: always include treatment of atypical agents. Infect Dis Clin North Am 18:829-41, 2004.

Mason CM, Nelson S. Pulmonary host defenses and factors predisposing to lung infection. Clin Chest Med 26:11-7, 2005.

McCormack PL, Keating GM. Amoxicillin/clavulanic acid 2000 mg/125 mg extended release (XR): a review of its use in the treatment of respiratory tract infections in adults. Drugs 65:121-36, 2005.

McDonough EA, Metzgar D, Hansen CJ, et al. A cluster of Legionella-associated pneumonia cases in a population of military recruits. J Clin Microbiol 45:2075-7, 2007.

Miedzinski L. Community acquired pneumonia: new facets of an old disease–Hantavirus pulmonary syndrome. Respir Care Clin N Am 11:45-58, 2005.

Mulvey JM, Padowitz A, Lindley-Jones M. Mycoplasma pneumoniae associated with Stevens Johnson syndrome. Anaesth Intensive Care 35:414-7, 2007.

Nagappan V, Deresinski S. Posaconazole: A broad-spectrum triazole antifungal agent. Clin Infect Dis 45:1610-1617, 2007.

Nambu A, Saito A, Araki T, et al. Chlamydia pneumoniae: comparison with findings of Mycoplasma pneumoniae and Streptococcus pneumoniae at thin-section CT. Radiol 238:330-8, 2006.

Nausheen S, Cunha BA. Q Fever in Community-Acquired Pneumonia in a Patient with Crohn's Disease on Immunosuppressive Therapy. Heart & Lung 36:300-303, 2007.

Oliveira AG. Current management of hospitalized community-acquired pneumonia in Portugal. Consensus statements of an expert panel. Rev Port Pneumol 11:243-282, 2005.

Paradisi F, Corti G, Cinelli R. Streptococcus pneumoniae as an agent of nosocomial infection: treatment in the era of penicillin-resistant strains. Clin Microbiol Infect 7(Suppl 4):34-42, 2001.

Parker NR, Barralet JH, Bell AM. Q fever. Lancet 367:679-88, 2006.

Plouffe JF. Importance of atypical pathogens of community-acquired pneumonia. Clin Infect Dis 31(Suppl 2):S35-9, 2000.

Quintiliani R. Clinical management of respiratory tract infections in the community: experience with telithromycin. Infection 29(Suppl):16-22, 2001.

Reinert RR. Clinical efficacy of ketolides in the treatment of respiratory tract infections. J Antimicrob Chemother 53:918-27, 2004.

Rzeszutek M, Wierbowski A, Hoban DJ, et al. A review of clinical failures associated with macrolide-resistant Streptococcus pneumoniae. Int J Antimicrob Agents 24:95-104, 2004.

Sakai F, Tokuda H, Goto H. Computed Tomographic

Features of Legionella pneumophila Pneumonia in 38 Cases. Comput Assist Tomogr 31:125-131, 2007.

Segreti J, House HR, Siegel RE. Principles of antibiotic treatment of community-acquired pneumonia in the outpatient setting. Am J Med 118; Suppl 7A:21S-28S, 2005.

Shefet D, Robenshtok E, Paul M, et al. Empirical atypical coverage for inpatients with community-acquired pneumonia: systematic review of randomized controlled trials. Arch Intern Med 165:1992-2000, 2005.

Simpson SH, Marrie TJ, Majumdar SR. Do guidelines guide pneumonia practice? A systematic review of interventions and barriers to best practice in the management of community-acquired pneumonia. Respir Care Clin N Am 11:1-13, 2005.

Skull SA, Andrews RM, Byrnes GB, et al. Pneumococcal polysaccharide vaccine may not prevent hospitalization for pneumonia in elderly individuals. Clin Infect Dis 44:617, 2007.

Sopena N, Force L, Pedro-Botet ML, et al. Sporadic and epidemic community legionellosis: two faces of the same illness. Eur Respir J 29:138-42, 2007.

Tan JS. Nonresponses and treatment failures with conventional empiric regimens in patients with community-acquired pneumonia. Infect Dis Clin North Am 18:883-897, 2004.

Tan JS, File TM Jr. Management of community-acquired pneumonia: a focus on conversion from hospital to the ambulatory setting. Am J Respir Med 2:385-94, 2003.

Traver RD, Teague SD, Heitkamp DE, et al. Legionnaires' disease in long-term care facilities: overview and proposed solutions. J Am Geriatr Soc 43:497-512, 2005.

Traver RD, Teague SD, Heitkamp DE, et al. Radiology of community-acquired pneumonia. Radiol Clin North Am 43: 497-512, 2005.

Tseng MH, Wei BH, Lin WJ, et al. Fatal sepsis and necrotizing pneumonia in a child due to community-acquired methicillin-resistant *Staphylococcus aureus*: case report and literature revue. Scand J Infect Dis 2005;37:504-507, 2005.

Tubach F, Ravaud P, Salmon-Céron D, et al. Emergence of Legionella pneumophila pneumonia in patients receiving tumor necrosis factor-alpha antagonists. Clin Infect Dis 43:e95-100, 2006.

Weiss K, Tillotson GS. The controversy of combination vs monotherapy in the treatment of hospitalized community-acquired pneumonia. Chest 128: 940-6, 2005.

Wellington K, Noble S. Telithromycin. Drugs 64:1683-94;1695-6, 2004.

Wellington K, Curran MP. Cefditoren pivoxil: a review of its use in the treatment of bacterial infections. Drugs 64:2597-618.

Weyers CM, Leeper KV. Noresolving pneumonia. Clin Chest Med 26:143-58, 2005.

Woodhead M. Community-acquired pneumonia: severity of illness evaluation. Infect Dis Clin North Am 18:791-807, 2004.

Zhanel GG, Johanson C, Embil JM, et al. Ertapenem: review of a new carbapenem. Expert Rev Anti Infect Ther 3:23-39, 2005.

GUIDELINES

Bartlett JG, Dowell SF, Mandell LA, et al. Practice guidelines for the management of CAP. Am Rev Resp Care 172:655-656, 2005.

Madhi SA, Albrich W. WHO guidelines for treatment of severe pneumonia. Lancet 370:386-7, 2007.

Mandell LA, Wunderink RG, Anzueto A, et al. Infectious Diseases Society of America/American Thoracic Society consensus guidelines on the management of community-acquired pneumonia in adults. Clin Infect Dis 44:S27-S72, 2007.

Wheat LJ, Freifeld AG, Kleiman MB. Clinical practice guidelines for the management of patients with histoplasmosis: 2007 update by the Infectious Diseases Society of America. Clin Infect Dis 45:807-25, 2007.

TEXTBOOKS

Cunha BA. Antibiotic Essentials, 7th Edition. Physicians' Press, Royal Oak, MI, 2008.

Cunha BA. Infectious Diseases in Critical Care Medicine. Informa Healthcare, New York, 2007.

Gorbach SL, Bartlett JG, Blacklow NR (eds). Infectious Diseases, 3rd Edition. Philadelphia, Lippincott, Williams & Wilkins, 2004.

Mandell GL, Bennett JE, Dolin R (eds). Mandell, Douglas and Bennett's Principles and Practice of Infectious Disease, 6th Edition. Philadelphia, Elsevier, 2005.

Marrie TJ. Community-acquired Pneumonia. Kluwer Academic Publishers, New York, NY. 2001.

Chapter 5

Bioterrorist Agents and Pneumonia

Burke A. Cunha, MD
Dennis J. Cleri, MD

Bioterrorist Agents and Pneumonia[¶]

Subset	Pathogen	IV/IM Therapy	IV-to-PO Switch
Anthrax (inhalation)	Bacillus anthracis	Quinolone* (IV) x 2 weeks **or** Doxycycline 200 mg (IV) q12h x 3 days, then 100 mg (IV) q12h x 11 days[‡] **or** Penicillin G 4 MU (IV) q4h ± clindamycin 600 mg (IV) q8h x 2 weeks	Quinolone* (PO) x 2 weeks **or** Doxycycline 200 mg (PO) q12h x 3 days, then 100 mg (PO) q12h x 11 days (loading dose not needed PO if given IV)
Tularemic pneumonia	Francisella tularensis	Streptomycin 1 gm (IM) q12h x 10 days **or** Gentamicin 5 mg/kg (IM or IV) q24h x 10 days **or** Doxycycline 200 mg (IV) q12h x 3 days, then 100 mg (IV) q12h x 7 days[‡] **or** Chloramphenicol 500 mg (IV) q6h x 10 days **or** Quinolone* (IV) x 10 days	Doxycycline 200 mg (PO) q12h x 3 days, then 100 mg (PO) q12h x 7 days (loading dose not needed PO if given IV) **or** Quinolone* (PO) x 10 days
Pneumonic plague	Yersinia pestis	Treat the same as tularemia pneumonia (above)	

Duration of therapy represents total treatment time. Most patients on IV therapy able to take PO meds should be switched to PO therapy after clinical improvement

*   *Ciprofloxacin 400 mg (IV) q12h or 500 mg (PO) q12h or levofloxacin 500 mg (IV or PO) q24h*

‡   *Patients who remain critically ill after doxycycline 200 mg (IV) q12h x 3 days should continue receiving 200 mg (IV) q12h for the full course of therapy. For patients who have improved after 3 days, the dose may be decreased to 100 mg (IV or PO) q12h to complete the course of therapy*

¶   *Additional information can be obtained at www.bt.cdc.gov. For post-exposure prophylaxis, see Chapter 13*

Anthrax (Bacillus anthracis)

Clinical Presentation: Bioterrorist anthrax usually presents as cutaneous or inhalational anthrax. Cutaneous anthrax has the same clinical presentation as naturally-acquired anthrax: Lesions begin as painless, sometimes mildly pruritic papules, usually on the upper extremities, neck, or face, and evolve into a vesicular lesion which may be surrounded by satellite lesions. A "gelatinous halo" surrounds the vesicle as it evolves into an ulcer, and a black eschar eventually develops over the ulcer. Inhalational anthrax is a biphasic illness. Initially, there is a viral illness-like prodrome with fever, chills, and myalgias with chest discomfort 3-5 days after inhaling anthrax spores. Bacteremia is common. Patients often improve somewhat over the next 1-2 days, only to rapidly deteriorate and become critically ill with high fevers, dyspnea, cyanosis, crushing substernal chest pain, and shock

Diagnostic Considerations: Inhalation anthrax is suspected in patients with fevers, chest pain, and mediastinal widening accompanied by bilateral pleural effusions on chest x-ray. If chest x-ray findings are equivocal, then a chest CT/MRI is recommended to demonstrate mediastinal lymph node enlargement. Inhalational anthrax presents as a hemorrhagic mediastinitis, not community-acquired pneumonia. The diagnosis is clinical but supported by Gram stain of hemorrhagic pleural fluid demonstrating gram-positive bacilli. Patients with inhalational anthrax often have positive blood cultures and may have associated anthrax meningitis. If meningitis is present, the CSF is hemorrhagic and CSF Gram stain shows encapsulated gram-positive bacilli, which, when cultured, are non-hemolytic on blood agar

Pitfalls: Inhalation anthrax most closely resembles tularemic pneumonia; both have bloody pleural effusions and a widened mediastinum on chest x-ray, but tularemia is not accompanied by substernal chest pain. Be alert to the possibility of smallpox following outbreaks of other bioterrorist agents such as anthrax, as the genome of smallpox is easily modified and can be incorporated into bacteria

Therapeutic Considerations: B. anthracis is highly susceptible to nearly all antibiotics; in the U.S. bioterrorist experience, no strains were resistant to antibiotics. Traditionally, penicillin has been used to treat natural anthrax, but because of concern for resistant bioterrorist strains, doxycycline or quinolones are preferred. There is no need for double therapy or synergy for susceptible strains. However, clindamycin, which by itself is active against B. anthracis, has been used in combination with other agents because of its potential anti-exotoxin activity. Although the 2001 inhalational anthrax experience was limited to a few patients, some patients seemed to respond somewhat better when clindamycin 600 mg (IV) q8h or 300 mg (PO) q8h plus rifampin 300 mg (PO) q12h was added to either a quinolone or doxycycline

Prognosis: With inhalational anthrax, prognosis is related to the inhaled dose of the organism, underlying host status, and rapidity of initiating antimicrobial therapy. Inhalational anthrax remains a highly lethal infectious disease, but with early intervention/supportive care, some patients survive. Patients with associated anthrax meningitis have a poor prognosis

Tularemic Pneumonia (Francisella tularensis)

Clinical Presentation: Fever, chills, myalgias, headache, dyspnea and a nonproductive cough may occur, but encephalopathy is absent. Chest x-ray resembles other causes of community-acquired pneumonia, but tularemic pneumonia is usually accompanied by hilar adenopathy and pleural effusion, which is serosanguineous or frankly bloody. Cavitation sometimes occurs.

Relative bradycardia is not present and serum transaminases are not elevated

Diagnostic Considerations: Tularemic pneumonia can resemble other atypical pneumonias, but in a patient presenting with community-acquired pneumonia, the presence of hilar adenopathy with pleural effusions should suggest the diagnosis. F. tularensis may be seen in the Gram stain of the sputum or bloody pleural effusion fluid as a small, bipolar staining, gram-negative bacillus. Diagnosis is confirmed serologically or by culture of the organism from respiratory fluid/blood

Pitfalls: Gram-negative bacilli in the sputum may resemble Y. pestis but are not bipolar staining. Chest x-ray may resemble inhalational anthrax (hilar adenopathy/mediastinal widening). Both tularemic pneumonia and inhalational anthrax may be accompanied by bloody pleural effusions. In contrast to inhalational anthrax (which may be accompanied by anthrax meningitis), CNS involvement is not a feature of tularemic pneumonia

Therapeutic Considerations: Streptomycin is the antibiotic traditionally used to treat tularemia. Gentamicin may be substituted for streptomycin if it is not available. Doxycycline, chloramphenicol, or a quinolone are also effective

Prognosis: Depends on inoculum size and health of host. Mortality rates for severe untreated infection can be as high as 30%, although early treatment is associated with mortality rates < 1%

Pneumonic Plague (Yersina pestis)

Clinical Presentation: Bioterrorist plague presents as pneumonic plague and has the potential for person-to-person spread. After an incubation period of 1-4 days, the patient presents with acute onset of fever, chills, headache, myalgias and dizziness, followed by pulmonary manifestations including cough, chest pain, dyspnea. Hemoptysis may occur, and increasing respiratory distress and circulatory collapse are common. Compared to community-acquired pneumonia, patients presenting with plague pneumonia are critically ill. Sputum is pink and frothy and contains abundant bipolar staining gram-negative bacilli. Chest x-ray is not diagnostic

Diagnostic Considerations: Yersinia pestis may be demonstrated in sputum Gram stain (bipolar staining gram-negative bacilli) and may be recovered from blood cultures. Laboratory confirmation requires isolation of Y. pestis from body fluid or tissue culture. Consider the diagnosis in any critically ill patient with pneumonia and bipolar staining gram-negative bacilli in the sputum

Pitfalls: Plague pneumonia can resemble tularemic pneumonia, but there are several distinguishing features. Unlike plague, tularemic pneumonia is usually associated with hilar enlargement and pleural effusion. Although gram-negative bacilli may be present in the sputum of patients with tularemia, the organisms are not bipolar staining

Therapeutic Considerations: Streptomycin is the preferred drug for pneumonic plague. Doxycycline or a quinolone are also effective

Prognosis: Depends on inoculum size, health of the host, and the rapidity of treatment. Left untreated, mortality rates exceed 50%. ARDS, DIC, and other manifestations of gram-negative sepsis are more common when treatment is delayed

REFERENCES AND SUGGESTED READINGS

Albrink WX, Brooks SM, Biron RE, et al. Human inhalation anthrax. Am J Pathol 36:457-471, 1960.

Barakat LA, Quentzel HL, Jeringan JA, et al. Fatal inhalational anthrax in a 94-year-old Connecticut woman. JAMA 287:863-868, 2002.

Brachman PS. Inhalation anthrax. Ann NY Acad Sci 353:83-93, 1980.

Campbell GL, Hughes JM. Plague in India: a new warning from an old nemesis. Ann Intern Med 122:151-153, 1995.

Chol E. Tularemia and Q fever. Med Clin North Am 86:393-416, 2002.

Cleri DJ, Vernaleo JR, Lombardi LJ. Plague pneumonia disease caused by Yersina Pestis. Semin Respir Infect 12:12-23, 1997.

Cunha BA. Zoonotic anthrax: A clinical perspective (Part I). Infect Dis Pract 25:69-76, 2001.

Crook LD, Tempest B. Plague. A clinical review of 27 cases. Arch Intern Med 152:1253-1256, 1992.

Cunha BA. Bioterrorist anthrax: a clinician's perspective (part II). Infectious Disease Practice 26:81-85, 2002.

Cunha BA. Bioterrorism in the emergency room: Anthrax, tularemia, plague, ebola and smallpox. Clinical Microbiology & Infection 8:489-503, 2002.

Dienst FT Jr. Tularemia, a perusal of 339 cases. J La State Med Soc 115:114-127, 1963.

Doganay M, Aydin N. Antimicrobial susceptibility of Bacillus anthracis. Scand J Infect Dis 23:333-335, 1991.

Doll JM, Zeitz OS, Ettestad P. Cat-transmitted fatal pneumonic plague in a person who traveled from Colorado to Arizona. Am J Trop Med Hyg 51:109-114, 1994.

Ellis J, Oyston PC, Green M, et al. Tularemia. Clin Microbial Rev 15:631-46, 2002.

Enderlin G, Morales L, Jacobs RE, et al. Streptomycin and alternative agents for the treatment of tularemia: a review of the literature. Clin Infect Dis 19:42-47.

Friedlander AM. Anthrax: clinical features, pathogenesis, and potential biological warfare threat. Curr Clin Top Infect Dis 20:335-49, 2000.

Friedlander AM Weldos SL, Pitt ML. Postexposure prophylaxis against experimental inhalation anthrax. J Infect Dis 167-1239-1243, 1993.

Fetai L, Alrahji AA, Hart, B, et al. Radiologic manifestations of potential bioterrorist agents of infection. AJR Am J Roentgenol 180:565-75, 2003.

Gallagher-Smith M, Kim J, Al-Bawardy R. Et al. Francisella tularensis: possible agent in bioterrorism. Clin Lab Sci 17:35-9, 2004.

Gill MV, Cunha BA. Tularemia pneumonia. Semin Respir Infect 12:61-67, 1997.

Gold H. Anthrax: a report of one hundred seventeen cases. Arch Intern Med 96:387-396, 1955.

Henderson RJ. Plague. Trop Dis Bull 66:653-659, 1969.

Hull HF, Montes JM, Mann JM. Septicemia plague in New Mexico. J Infect Dis 155:113-118, 1987.

Inglesby TV, Henderson DA, Bartlett JG, et al. Anthrax as a biological weapon. JAMA 281:1735-1745, 1999.

Khardori N, Kanchanapoom T. Overview of biological terrorism: Potential agents and preparedness. Clin Microbiol News 27:1-9, 2005.

Krishna G, Chitkara RK. Pneumonic plague. Semin Respir Infect 18:159-67, 2003.

Mason WL, Eigelsbach HAT, Little SF, et al. Treatment of tularemia, including pulmonary tularemia, with gentamicin. Am Rev Respir Dis 121:39-45, 1980.

Mayer TA, Bersoff-Matcha S, Murphy C, et al. Clinical presentation in inhalational anthrax following bioterrorism exposure: report of 2 surviving patients. JAMA 286:2549-2553, 2001.

Mettler FA, Mann JM. Radiographic manifestations of plague in New Mexico, 1975-1980. A review of 42 proved cases. Radiology 139:61-565, 1981.

Mina B, Dym JP, Kuepper R, et al. Fatal inhalational anthrax with unknown source of exposure in a 61-year-old woman in New York City. JAMA 287:858-862, 2002.

Mock M, Fouet A. Anthrax. Annu Rev Microbial 55:647-71, 2001.

Stuart BM, Pullen RL. Tularemic pneumonia. Am J Med 210:223-236, 1945.

Tarnvick A, Berglund L. Tularaemia. Eur Respir 21:361-71, 2003.

Whitby M, Ruff TA, Street AC, et al. Biological agents as weapons 2: anthrax and plague. Med J Aust 17;176:605-8, 2002.

Wortmann G. Pulmonary manifestations of other agents: brucella, Q fever, tularemia and smallpox. Respir Care Cllin N Am 10:99-109, 2004.

TEXTBOOKS

Beran GW. Handbook of Zoonoses,. Section A: Bacterial, Rickettsial, Chlamydial, and Mycotic, 2nd Edition CRC Press, Boca Raton, 1994.

Christine AB. Infectious Disease: Epidemiology and Clinical practice. Anthrax. Vol 2. Churchill Livingstone, New York, 2001.

Gorbach SL, Bartlett JG, Blacklow NR (eds). Infectious Diseases, 3rd Edition. Philadelphia, Lippincott, Williams & Wilkins, 2004.

Mandell GL, Bennet JE, Dolin R. Mandell, Douglas, and Bennett's Principles and Practice of Infectious Diseases, 6th Edition. Elsevier, 2005.

Schlossberg D. Medical Interventions for Bioterrorism and Emerging Infections. Newtown, PA, Handbooks in Health Care Co., 2004.

Weinberg AN, Weber DJ (eds). Animal-associated human infections. Infect Dis Clin North Am. 1991.

Chapter 6

Nursing Home-Acquired Pneumonia (NHAP)

Burke A. Cunha, MD

Nursing Home-Acquired Pneumonia (NHAP)

Subset	Usual Pathogens*	Preferred IV Therapy	PO Therapy or IV-to-PO Switch
NHAP	H. influenzae S. pneumoniae M. catarrhalis MDR gram negative bacilli	Ertapenem 1 gm (IV) q24h x 2 weeks **or** Cefepime 2 gm (IV) q12h x 2 weeks	Levofloxacin 500 mg (IV) q24h x 2 weeks **or** Moxifloxacin 400 (IV) q24h x 2 weeks **or** Piperacillin/tazobactam 3.375 gm (IV) q6h x 2 weeks	Levofloxacin 500 mg (PO) q24h x 2 weeks **or** Moxifloxacin 400 mg (PO) q24h x 2 weeks **or** Doxycycline 200 mg (PO) q12h x 3 days, then 100 mg (PO) q12h x 11 days[†]

Duration of therapy represents total time IV, PO, or IV + PO
* *Compromised hosts may require longer courses of therapy*
† Loading dose is not needed PO if given IV with the same drug

A. **Epidemiology:** Nursing home residents are predisposed to NHAP due to the high frequency of strokes, swallowing disorders, tube feedings, and sedative use among elderly individuals in chronic care facilities. NHAP accounts for 10-15% of all pneumonia admissions in the United States and is most often caused by S. pneumoniae, aerobic gram-negative bacilli, or aspiration pneumonia pathogens, the latter accounting for one-third of NHAP. NHAP may resemble community-acquired (CAP) or nosocomial (hospital-acquired) pneumonia (NP) with respect to pathogen distribution, and may occur sporadically or as part of a nursing home outbreak

B. **Clinical Presentation:** NHAP in relatively healthy, active nursing home residents often presents similar to CAP in younger patients, with fever, chills, pulmonary symptoms (cough, dyspnea, sputum production, pleuritic chest pain), and one or more infiltrates/opacities on chest x-ray. In contrast, frail debilitated residents may present with malaise, anorexia, confusion, or diarrhea rather than with prominent pulmonary symptoms. Tachypnea may be the first manifestation of NHAP and precede the actual clinical diagnosis by 1-2 days

C. **Diagnostic Considerations:** Nursing home residents with suspected pneumonia are often transferred to an acute care facility. As with NP, respiratory secretions of nursing home patients are frequently colonized with bacteria and do not correlate well with the etiology of NHAP

D. **Pitfalls:** Many nursing home residents admitted for suspected NHAP have conditions that can mimic pneumonia, including decompensated emphysema, AECB, pulmonary embolism, heart failure, MI, pulmonary hemorrhage, or pulmonary drug reactions. NHAP often presents as malaise or confusion rather than with prominent pulmonary symptoms, and fever may be minimal/absent, due to coexisting renal insufficiency or other medical conditions. Many nursing home residents are unable to produce adequate sputum for

Gram stain/culture. K. pneumoniae is uncommon in this population, even in alcoholics

E. **Therapeutic Considerations:** It is important or rule out noninfectious mimics of NHAP (see pitfalls, above) so that appropriate therapy may be initiated. If noninfectious causes are ruled out and NHAP is likely, antibiotic therapy should be started as soon as possible. Some cases of NHAP can be treated effectively with IV/PO antibiotics in the nursing home if appropriate laboratory/support services are available, thus avoiding transfer to a hospital. Reasonable candidates for treatment in the nursing home generally should have a respiratory rate < 30/min, O_2 saturation $\geq$ 92% on room air, pulse < 90/min, temperature 36.5°C – 38.1°C, unchanged blood pressure, no feeding tube or impaired consciousness, and adequate medical/nursing care. Antimicrobial therapy during outbreaks of NHAP include coverage of atypical pathogens, as most outbreaks are due to C. pneumoniae, M. pneumoniae, or Legionella. (Outbreaks due to influenza are common in winter months, and pulmonary TB is also a diagnostic consideration in NHAP outbreaks.) Non-outbreak NHAP may be treated the same as for CAP and based on local pathogen epidemiology. For NHAP due to multidrug-resistant (MDR) aerobic gram-negative bacilli, treatment is the same as for NP. Appropriate antibiotic therapy is usually administered for approximately 2 weeks and may be given IV, IV-to-PO switch, or PO

F. **Prognosis:** Mortality rates are high (up to 30% in-hospital and 50% at 1 year) due to multiple medical comorbidities and impaired cardiopulmonary reserve in the elderly

G. **Prevention:** Steps to minimize the risk of aspiration are described in Chapter 7. Use of influenza, pneumococcal, and TB prophylaxis are described in Chapter 13

REFERENCES AND SUGGESTED READINGS

Buehrens PE. Effectiveness of oral antibiotic treatment in nursing-home acquired pneumonia. J Am Geriatr Soc 43:144-4, 1995.

Crossley KB, Thrun JR. Nursing home-acquired pneumonia. Semin Respir Infect 4:64-72, 1989.

Cunha BA. Pneumonia in the elderly. Clin Microbiol Infect 7:581-8, 2001.

Cunha BA. Pneumonia in the elderly. Drugs Today (Barc)36:785-91, 2000.

Cunha BA. Pneumonia in the elderly. J of Respir Infect 22:195-233, 2001.

Degelau J, Guay D, Straub K, et al Effectiveness of oral antibiotic treatment in nursing home-acquired pneumonia. J Am Geriatr Soc 43:245-51, 1995.

El Solh AA, Pietrantoni C, Bhat A, et al. Indicators of potentially drug-resistant bacteria in severe nursing home-acquired pneumonia. Clin Infect Dis 39:474-480, 2004.

Fernandez-Sabe N, Carratala J, Roson B, et al. Community-acquired pneumonia in very elderly patients: causative organisms, clinical characteristics, and outcomes. Medicine (Baltimore)82:159-69, 2003.

Garb JL, Brown RB, Garb JR, et al. Differences in etiology of pneumonias in nursing home and community patients. JAMA 10;240:2169-72, 1978.

Hutt E, Reznickova N, Morgenstern N, et al. Improving care for nursing home-acquired pneumonia in a managed care environment. Am J Manag Care 10:681-686, 2004.

Janssens JP, Krause KH. Pneumonia in the very old. Lancet Infect Dis 4:112-24, 2004.

Lim WS, Macfarlane JT. A prospective comparison of nursing home acquired pneumonia with community acquired pneumonia. Eur Respir J 18:362-8, 2001.

Loeb M. Epidemiology of community- and nursing home-acquired pneumonia in older adults. Expert Rev Anti Infect Ther 3:263-70, 2005.

Loeb M. Pneumonia in the elderly. Curr Opin Infect Dis 17:127-30, 2004.

Madariaga MG, Thomas A, Cannady PB Jr. Risk factors for nursing home-acquired pneumonia. Clin Infect Dis 37:148-9, 2003.

Marrie TJ, Blanchard W. A comparison of nursing home-acquired pneumonia patients with patients with community-acquired and nursing home patients without pneumonia. J Am Geriatr Soc 45:50-5, 1997.

Marrie TJ. Community-acquired pneumonia in the elderly. Clin Infect Dis 31:1066-78, 2000.

Marrie TJ, Durant H, Kwan C. Nursing home-acquired pneumonia. A case-control study. J Am Geriatr Soc 34:697-702, 1986.

Mathei C, Nicales L, Suetens C, et al. Infections in residents of nursing homes. Infect Dis Clin North Am 21:761-772, 2007.

Medina-Walpole AM, Datz PR. Nursing home-acquired pneumonia. J Am Geriatr Soc 47:1005-15, 1999.

Minnaganti VR, Patel PJ, Cunha BA. Nursing Home Acquired Pneumonia (NHAP): Community Acquired or Nosocomial? Infect Dis Pract 24:20-23, 2000.

Muder RR, Aghababian RV, Loeb MB, et al. Nursing home-acquired pneumonia: an emergency department treatment algorithm. Curr Med Opin 20:1309-20, 2004.

Muder RR, Brennen C, Swenson DL, et al. Pneumonia in a long-term care facility. A prospective study of outcome. Arch Intern Med 11;156:2365-70, 1996.

Mylotte JM. Nursing home-acquired pneumonia. Clin Geriatr Med 23:553-65, 2007.

Nakashima K, Tanaka T, Kramer MH, et al. Outbreak of Chlamydia pneumoniae infection in a Japanese nursing home, 1999-2000. Infect Control Hosp Epidemiol 27:1171-7, 2006.

Naughton BJ, Mylotte JM, Ramadan F, et al. Antibiotic use, hospital admissions, and mortality before and after implementing guidelines for nursing home-acquired pneumonia. J Am Geriatr Soc 49:1020-4, 2001.

Naughton BJ, Mylotte JM, Tayara A. Outcome of nursing home-acquired pneumonia: derivation and application of a practical model to predict 30 day mortality. J Am Geriatr Soc 48:1292-9, 2000.

Paladino JA. Eubanks DA. Adelman MH. Schentag JJ. Once-daily cefepime versus ceftriaxone for nursing home-acquired pneumonia. J Am Geriatr Soc 55:651-7, 2007.

Phares CR, Russell E, Thigpen MC, et al. Legionnaires' disease among residents of a long-term care facility: the sentinel event in a community outbreak. Am J Infect Control 5:319-23, 2007.

Quagliarello V, Ginter S, Han L, et al. Modifiable risk factors for nursing home-acquired pneumonia. Clin Infect Dis 1;40:1-6, 2005.

Seenivansan MH, Yu, VL, Muder RR. Legionnaires' disease in long-term care facilities: overview and proposed solutions. J Am Geriatr Soc 53:875-80, 2005.

Stout JE, Brennen C, Muder RR. Legionnaires' disease in a newly constructed long-term care facility. J Am Geriatr Soc 48:1589-92, 2000.

Sund-Levander M, Ortqvist A, Grodzinsky E, et al. Morbidity, mortality and clinical presentation of nursing home-acquired pneumonia in a Swedish population. Secand J Infect Dis 35:306-10, 2003.

Trivalle C. Treatment guideline for nursing home-acquired pneumonia. J Am Geriatr Soc 48:1347-8, 2000.

Troy CJ, Peeling RW, Ellis AG, et al. Chlamydia pneumoniae as a new source of infectious outbreaks in nursing homes. JAMA. 277:1214-1218, 1997.

Yoshikawa TT. Treatment of nursing home-acquired pneumonia. J Am Geriatr Soc 39:1040-1, 1991.

Yoshikawa TT, Norman DC. Approach to fever and infection in the nursing home. J Am Geriatr Soc 44:74-82, 1996.

Zimmer JG, Hall WJ. Nursing home-acquired pneumonia: avoiding the hospital. J Am Geriatr Soc 45:380-1, 1997.

GUIDELINES

ATS Board of Directors, Infectious Disease Society of America. Guidelines for the management of adults with hospital-acquired, ventilator-associated, and healthcare-associated pneumonia. Am J Respir Crit Care Med 171:388-416, 2005.

Mandell LA, Wunderink RG, Anzueto A, et al. Infectious Diseases Society of America/American Thoracic Society consensus guidelines on the management of community-acquired pneumonia in adults. Clin Infect Dis 44(S2):S27-S72, 2007.

TEXTBOOKS

Gorbach SL, Bartlett JG, Blacklow NR (eds). Infectious Diseases, 3rd Edition. Philadelphia, Lippincott, Williams & Wilkins, 2004.

Karetzky M, Cunha BA, Brandstetter RD. The Pneumonias. New York, Springer-Verlag, 1993.

Levison ME. The Pneumonias: Clinical Approaches in Infectious Diseases of the Lower Respiratory Tract. Littleton, MA, John Wright, PSG Inc., 1984.

Mandell GL, Bennet JE, Dolin R. Mandell, Douglas, and Bennett's Principles and Practice of Infectious Diseases, 6th Edition. Elsevier, 2005.

Chapter 7
Nosocomial (Hospital-Acquired) Pneumonia

Burke A. Cunha, MD

Nosocomial (Hospital-Acquired) Pneumonia

Subset	Usual Pathogens	Preferred IV Therapy	IV-to-PO Switch
Empiric therapy	P. aeruginosa E. coli K. pneumoniae S. marcescens	Meropenem 1 gm (IV) q8h x 1-2 weeks **or** Levofloxacin 750 mg (IV) q24h x 1-2 weeks **or** Piperacillin/tazobactam 4.5 gm (IV) q6h *plus* amikacin 1 gm (IV) q24h x 1-2 weeks **or** Cefepime 2 gm (IV) q8h x 1-2 weeks	Levofloxacin 750 mg (PO) q24h x 1-2 weeks **or** Ciprofloxacin 750 mg (PO) q12h x 1-2 weeks
Specific therapy	P. aeruginosa	Meropenem 1 gm (IV) q8h x 2 weeks **or** Levofloxacin 750 mg (IV) q24h x 2 weeks **or** Ciprofloxacin 400 mg (IV) q8h x 2 weeks **or** Piperacillin/tazobactam 4.5 gm (IV) q6h *plus* amikacin 1 gm (IV) q24h x 2 weeks	Levofloxacin 750 mg (PO) q24h x 2 weeks **or** Ciprofloxacin 750 mg (PO) q12h x 2 weeks
	MDR P. aeruginosa MDR Klebsiella MDR Acineto-bacter	Colistin 1.7 mg/kg (IV) q8h x 2 weeks **or** Polymyxin B 1-1.25 mg/kg (IV) q12h x 2 weeks	Not applicable
	S. aureus[‡] (HA-MRSA)	Linezolid 600 mg (IV) q12h x 2 weeks **or** Vancomycin 1 gm (IV) q12h x 2 weeks	Linezolid 600 mg (PO) q12h x 2 weeks **or** Minocycline 100 mg (PO) q12h x 2 weeks
	S. aureus[‡] (MSSA)	Nafcillin 2 gm (IV) q4h x 2 weeks **or** Clindamycin 600 mg (IV) q8h x 2 weeks **or** Linezolid 600 mg (IV) q12h x 2 weeks	Linezolid 600 mg (PO) q12h x 2 weeks **or** Clindamycin 300 mg (PO) q8h x 2 weeks **or** Cephalexin 1 gm (PO) q6h x 2 weeks
	HSV	Acyclovir 10 mg/kg (IV) q8h x 2 weeks	

HA = hospital-acquired; MDR = multidrug resistant; MSSA/MRSA = methicillin-sensitive/resistant S. aureus. Duration of therapy represents total time IV or IV + PO. Most patients on IV therapy able to take PO meds should be switched to PO therapy after clinical improvement

‡ *If lab report identifies gram-positive cocci in clusters, treat initially for MRSA. If later identified as MSSA, treat as MSSA or continue MRSA therapy*

A. Epidemiology. Nosocomial (hospital-acquired) pneumonia (NP) is defined as pneumonia that develops ≥ 48 hours after hospital admission. NP occurs in 5-15 cases per 1000 hospital admissions; the rate is 6-20–fold higher in mechanically-ventilated patients. It is useful to classify NP into ventilator-associated pneumonia (VAP) and non-ventilator-associated pneumonia (Table 7.1), as this distinction has implications for microbiology, evaluation, and treatment. VAP refers to pneumonia that develops ≥ 48-72 hours after endotracheal intubation. VAP occurs in 10-25% of intubated patients, with an incidence of 3% per day during days 1-5 of ventilation, 2% per day during days 6-10 of ventilation, and 1% per day thereafter. Early-onset NP, defined as pneumonia that develops within the first 5 days of hospitalization, is usually caused by incubating CAP pathogens and typically carries a better prognosis. In contrast, late-onset NP (≥ 5 days) is often caused by gram-negative aerobic bacilli, which may be multidrug-resistant, and is associated with high mortality and morbidity rates. The overall mortality rate for NP is 33-50%.

B. Etiology. Most cases of NP are caused by aerobic gram-negative bacilli (e.g., P. aeruginosa, K. pneumoniae) (Table 7.2). Gram-positive cocci (e.g., S. aureus [MSSA/MRSA]) are common colonizers of respiratory secretions in ventilated patients, but uncommonly cause NP. Rates of Legionella vary between hospitals, and Legionnaires' disease occurs most commonly with serogroup 1. Nosocomial Legionella outbreaks have been associated with colonized water supply or ongoing construction. Anaerobes are not important pathogens in NP. Except for HSV-1 pneumonia, nosocomial viral and fungal infections are uncommon causes of NP in immunocompetent patients. Many patients with NP are at increased risk for colonization and infection with multidrug-resistant (MDR) pathogens (see below).

    1. Necrotizing Pulmonary Pathogens. Necrotizing pneumonia with rapid (within 72 hours) cavitation implies a rapidly destructive process within the lung parenchyma and is the hallmark of S. aureus and P. aeruginosa pneumonias. After chest x-ray appearance and tissue biopsy, the next best indirect method for establishing the diagnosis of necrotizing pneumonia is to demonstrate elastin fibers (stained by potassium hydroxide) in respiratory tract secretion specimens.

Table 7.1. Nosocomial Pneumonia Terminology

Condition	Comments
Pneumonia ≥ 5 days after hospitalization	Represents true nosocomial pneumonia (NP). Subdivision into ventilator-associated pneumonia (VAP) and non-ventilator-associated pneumonia has implications for microbiology, diagnosis, and therapy. NP occurs in 5-15 cases per 1000 hospital admissions. VAP occurs in 10-25% of intubated patients
Pneumonia < 5 days after hospitalization	Represents incubating community-acquired pneumonia

a. **Klebsiella pneumoniae** (also see p. 54 for detailed pathogen characteristics). Klebsiella pneumoniae causes a necrotizing pneumonia with cavitation at 3-5 days. Absent microbiological data, cavitation rates may suggest K. pneumoniae (necrosis/cavitation at 3-5 days) versus S. aureus or P. aeruginosa (necrosis/cavitation < 3 days).

b. **Pseudomonas aeruginosa** (also see p. 77 for detailed pathogen characteristics). P. aeruginosa commonly colonizes respiratory tract secretions and may cause nosocomial pneumonia. Nevertheless, P. aeruginosa adheres to respiratory tract cells more avidly than other aerobic gram-negative bacilli, and its ability to invade the lung and produce a necrotizing pneumonia surpasses K. pneumoniae in its destructive capability. Although P. aeruginosa is not the most common cause of nosocomial pneumonia, it is the most virulent pulmonary pathogen, and coverage for suspected nosocomial pneumonia should be directed primarily against P. aeruginosa.

2. **Nonpathogens in Nosocomial Pneumonia.** Certain organisms are nonpathogens and represent the gram-negative nonfermentative bacillary flora of the hospital environment. Most of these organisms breed in an aqueous environment (e.g., respiratory secretions, irrigating solutions, sinks) and rapidly colonize the patient's respiratory secretions while in the hospital. (There are no good studies indicating that such organisms actually cause nosocomial pneumonia, and studies citing these organisms are based only on cultures of respiratory tract secretions.) Organisms that can be dismissed from therapeutic consideration if only obtained from respiratory secretions include Enterobacter, Citrobacter, Flavobacterium, and non-aeruginosa pseudomonads (i.e., Burkholderia [formally Pseudomonas] maltophilia). Burkholderia and Stenotrophomonas are potentially pathogenic, but only in patients with extensive bronchiectasis or cystic fibrosis. Anaerobic organisms aspirated along with aerobic bacillary flora in hospitalized patients are also an insignificant cause of nosocomial pneumonia.

3. **Outbreaks of Nosocomial Pneumonia.** Acinetobacter and Legionella cause nosocomial pneumonias in outbreaks. Acinetobacter outbreaks are associated with contaminated respiratory support equipment (Acinetobacter may be transferred between patients from contaminated respiratory secretions on the hands of medical personnel.) Nevertheless, most Acinetobacter recovered from specimens of respiratory secretions represent colonization, and Acinetobacter pneumonia outbreaks are uncommon. Legionella as a cause of nosocomial pneumonia also usually occurs in outbreaks, and the source of Legionella is usually contaminated water. Legionella in hospital outbreaks has been cultured from a variety of sources, including ice cubes and shower heads.

Table 7.2. Microbiology of Nosocomial Pneumonia (NP)

Pathogens	Comments
Common Pathogens	
S. pneumoniae (early) H. influenzae (early) P. aeruginosa (late) K. pneumoniae (late) E. coli (late)	Many cases diagnosed as NP probably are not NP
Uncommon Pathogens	
Serratia	The only upper lobe NP; ± "pseudohemoptysis"
Acinetobacter	Acinetobacter is a common colonizer of respiratory tract secretions in the ICU, usually in association with use of respiratory support equipment
Legionella	Legionella NP usually occurs only in outbreaks or clusters
S. aureus (MSSA/HA-MRSA)	S. aureus (MSSA/HA-MRSA) is a common colonizer of respiratory tract secretions in the ICU, but is an uncommon cause lung biopsy proven NP
Common Respiratory Secretion Colonizers (Rare Pathogens)	
Enterobacter Stenotrophomonas (Pseudomonas) maltophilia Burkholderia (Pseudomonas) cepacia Oropharyngeal anaerobes (non-B-fragilis)	These organisms are rarely, if ever, proven causes of NP. The recovery of a potential pathogen from respiratory secretions does not prove it is the cause of NP

4. **HSV-1 Pneumonia**. Suspect HSV-1 pneumonia in an intubated patient in the ICU with persistent fevers, leukocytosis, and pulmonary infiltrates with at least two weeks of antibiotic therapy, otherwise unexplained hypoxemia/increased A-a gradient, and "failure to wean." Cultures of respiratory secretions from such patients are usually negative for HSV-1. Results of other testing are shown in Table 7.3. Most often, the diagnosis of HSV-1 is suggested/confirmed by the cytology report, which indicates the presence of Cowdry type A inclusion bodies and cytopathic effects of HSV-1 (Table 7.4). The cytology in HSV pneumonitis demonstrates active viral infection of cells in the lower respiratory tract and not merely colonization of respiratory oropharyngeal secretions. The cytopathic effects of HSV-1 are diagnostic and need not be accompanied by positive HSV viral cultures, HSV vesicles in the distal airways, or positive HSV-1 serology. Patients with HSV pneumonia who have not received specific anti-HSV-1 therapy usually improve very slowly over a prolonged period of time, and

are eventually extubated. Therapy with acyclovir results in prompt (within 3-5 days) improvement of the patient's hypoxemia. The prognosis for HSV NP treated early with acyclovir is good.

C. Multidrug Resistant (MDR) Pathogens. Patients with late-onset NP are more likely to be infected with MDR pathogens and have higher mortality rates than patients with early-onset NP. The prevalence of MDR pathogens varies according to antibiotic selection/usage and type of ICU, highlighting the need for local surveillance data. Risk factors for MDR pathogens in NP are shown in Table 7.5.

D. Pathogenesis. Sources of pathogens for NP include the environment (air, water, equipment, fomites), respiratory care equipment, and transfer of microorganisms between patients and staff or other patients (common). The primary routes of bacterial entry into the lower respiratory tract include inhalation or direct inoculation of pathogens into the lower airway, hematogenous spread from infected intravenous catheters, or bacterial translocation from the gastrointestinal tract lumen. Infected biofilm on/in the endotracheal tube with subsequent involvement of the distal airways may be important in the pathogenesis of VAP.

Table 7.3. Clinical Characteristics of HSV-1 Pneumonia

Symptoms	• Failure to wean off respirator (in patients without advanced preexisting lung disease)
Signs	• Low grade fever • Unexplained hypoxemia with normal/near-normal chest x-ray • No HSV vesicles in respiratory passages
Laboratory tests	• Leukocytosis (± left shift) • ↓ pO_2/↑ A-a gradient (> 30) • Serology: negative HSV-1 IgM ± ↑ IgG titers, or HSV-1 ↑ IgM ± ↑ IgG titers • Chest x-ray: normal or diffuse "ground glass" opacities • Gallium/Indium scan: bilateral symmetrical diffuse uptake • Spiral chest CT: diffuse "ground glass" opacities • Bronchoscopy: ± HSV-1 virus cultured from respiratory secretions • Cytology: HSV-1 intranuclear (Cowdry type A) inclusion bodies

Adapted from: Cunha BA. Herpes Simplex Virus-1 (HSV-1) Pneumonia. Infectious Disease Practice 29:375-378, 2005.

Table 7.4. Cytopathic Features of HSV and CMV Inclusion Bodies in BAL Cytologic Specimens

Cytopathic Effects	HSV	CMV
Cell size	• Normal	• Cellular "gigantism"
Nucleus	• "Ground glass" appearing nuclei • "Owl's eye" intranuclear inclusion bodies • Nuclear chromatin displaced to edge of cell nucleus	• "Kidney bean" shaped intranuclear inclusions • Enlarged nucleus surrounded by clear halo (mimics "Owl's eye" inclusion bodies) take up ~ ½ of enlarged nucleus
Cytoplasm	• No cytoplasmic inclusions	• Multiple/diffuse cytoplasmic inclusions
Cellular polymorphism	• Absent	• Present

BAL = bronchoalveolar lavage

E. Clinical Presentation. NP presents as a pulmonary infiltrate compatible with a bacterial pneumonia occurring ≥ 7 days of hospitalization ± fever/leukocytosis. Criterion for severe NP are shown in Table 7.6.

F. Diagnostic Considerations. The presumptive diagnosis of nosocomial pneumonia is suggested by the presence of a pulmonary infiltrate compatible with a bacterial pneumonia occurring in a patient who has been hospitalized for ≥ 48-72 hours. Infiltrates on chest x-ray are not diagnostic of nosocomial pneumonia, even when accompanied by fever and leukocytosis, and it is important to rule out noninfectious mimics (Table 7.7). Leukocytosis and fever are nonspecific/nondiagnostic of NP, and definitive diagnosis requires lung biopsy culture. Except for S. aureus (MSSA/MRSA), there are no other common NP gram-positive pathogens.

G. Therapeutic Consideration. The initial approach to therapy is based on selecting optimal anti-P. aeruginosa coverage, which is also effective against all other common aerobic gram-negative bacillary pathogens that cause NP. Pneumonia occurring < 5 days of hospitalization often represents incubating CAP due to S. pneumoniae (including drug-resistant strains) or H. influenzae. Empiric therapy should cover "early" and "late" NP pathogens. Monotherapy is as effective as combination therapy for non-P. aeruginosa NP, but double-drug therapy is recommended for confirmed P. aeruginosa pneumonia. After 2 weeks of appropriate antibiotic therapy, nonprogressive/stable pulmonary infiltrates with fever and leukocytosis are usually due to a noninfectious cause rather than persistent infection or antibiotic resistance; the general approach to these cases is shown in Figure 7.1.

H. Pitfalls. Do not cover non-pulmonary pathogens cultured from respiratory secretions in ventilated patients (e.g., Enterobacter, B. cepacia, S. maltophilia, Citrobacter, Flavobacterium, Enterococci); these organisms rarely if ever cause VAP. S. aureus

(MSSA/HA-MRSA) cultured from BAL fluid is not diagnostic of S. aureus NP; semi-quantitative BAL/protected brush specimens reflect airway colonization, not lung pathogens. Tissue (lung) culture is needed for definitive diagnosis of P. aeruginosa/S. aureus NP.

I. **Prevention.** Recommendations to reduce the risk of NP are shown in Table 7.8.

Table 7.5. Risk Factors For Multidrug-Resistant (MDR) Pathogens in NP*

- "High-resistance potential" antimicrobial therapy before/during hospitalization (e.g., ceftazidime)
- Prolonged hospitalization
- High incidence of antibiotic resistance in the CCU/ICU
- Presence of risk factors for MDR pathogens in NP
  - Residence in a nursing home or extended care facility
  - Home infusion therapy (including antibiotics)
  - Chronic dialysis within 30 days
  - Home wound care
- Immunosuppressive disease/therapy

* Major pathogens include P. aeruginosa, Acinetobacter, Enterobacteriaceae (ESBL-producing)
Adapted from: American Thoracic Society. Guidelines for Management of Adults with Hospital-acquired, Ventilator-associated, and Healthcare-associated Pneumonia. Am J Respir Crit Care Med 171:388-416, 2005.

Table 7.6. Presumptive Diagnosis of Severe Nosocomial Pneumonia*

- Admission to the CCU/ICU
- Respiratory failure (need for mechanical ventilation or need for > 35% oxygen to maintain arterial oxygen saturation > 90%)
- Otherwise unexplained rapidly progressing multilobar pneumonia ± cavitation
- Otherwise unexplained hypotension or end-organ dysfunction (shock, vasopressors > 4 hours, urine output < 20 mL/h or total urine output < 80 mL in 4 hours [unless another explanation is available], acute renal failure requiring dialysis)

* Excluding non-infectious mimics of NP (e.g., pulmonary embolism/infarct, acute myocardial infarction, ARDS, decompensated emphysema, exacerbation of heart failure, pulmonary hemorrhage).
Adapted from: American Thoracic Society. Guidelines for Management of Adults with Hospital-acquired, Ventilator-associated, and Healthcare-associated Pneumonia. Am J Respir Crit Care Med 171:388-416, 2005.

Table 7.7. Chest X-Ray Mimics of Nosocomial Pneumonia*

- Interstitial lung disease
- Primary or metastatic lung carcinoma
- Pulmonary emboli/infarction
- Pulmonary drug reactions
- Pulmonary hemorrhage
- Collagen vascular disease affecting the lungs (SLE, RA)
- Acute respiratory distress syndrome (ARDS)
- Bronchiolitis obliterans with organizing pneumonia (BOOP)
- Heart failure

* Also see chest x-ray atlas (Chapter 11)

Table 7.8. Prevention of Nosocomial Pneumonia

Factor	Preventative Measures
General prophylaxis	• Emphasize staff education, compliance with hand washing, isolation to reduce patient-to-patient transmission of MDR organisms (colonization more problematic than infection) • Obtain CCU/ICU isolates to differentiate colonization from infection and to identify/quantify endemic MDR pathogens
Intubation and mechanical ventilation	• Avoid mechanical ventilation and use noninvasive ventilation whenever possible • Orotracheal intubation and orogastric tubes are preferred over nasotracheal intubation and nasogastric tubes • Continuous aspiration of subglottic secretions in ventilated patients, if available • Maintain endotracheal tube cuff pressure > 20 cm H_2O to prevent leakage of bacterial pathogens around the cuff into the lower respiratory tract • Contaminated condensate should be carefully emptied from ventilator circuits and condensate should be prevented from entering either the endotracheal tube or inline medication nebulizers • Minimize duration of intubation and mechanical ventilation
Aspiration, body position, enteral feeding	• Keep patients in the semirecumbent position (30-45°) rather than supine to prevent aspiration, especially when receiving enteral feeding • Enteral nutrition is preferred over parenteral nutrition (reduces central IV catheter complications; prevents reflux villous atrophy of the intestinal mucosa that may increase the risk of bacterial translocation)
Modulation of colonization	• Daily interruption or lightening of sedation to avoid constant heavy sedation and try to avoid paralytic agents, both of which can depress cough and thereby increase the risk of NP
Stress bleeding prophylaxis, hyperglycemia	• If needed, stress bleeding prophylaxis with either H_2 antagonists or sucralfate is acceptable • Intensive insulin therapy is recommended to maintain serum glucose levels of 80-110 mg/dL in CCU/ICU patients to reduce nosocomial blood stream infections, duration of mechanical ventilation, ICU stay, and morbidity/mortality

MDR = multidrug-resistant
Adapted from: American Thoracic Society. Guidelines for Management of Adults with Hospital-acquired, Ventilator-associated, and Healthcare-associated Pneumonia. Am J Respir Crit Care Med 171:388-416, 2005.

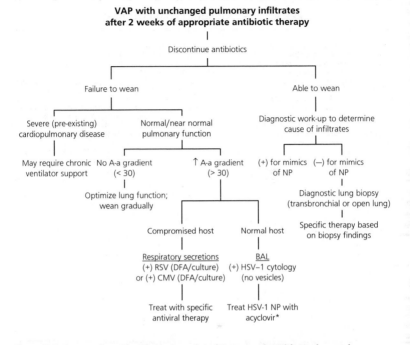

**VAP with unchanged pulmonary infiltrates
after 2 weeks of appropriate antibiotic therapy**

Discontinue antibiotics

Failure to wean

Severe (pre-existing)
cardiopulmonary disease

May require chronic
ventilator support

Normal/near normal
pulmonary function

No A-a gradient
(< 30)

Optimize lung function;
wean gradually

↑ A-a gradient
(> 30)

Compromised host

Respiratory secretions
(+) RSV (DFA/culture)
or (+) CMV (DFA/culture)

Treat with specific
antiviral therapy

Normal host

BAL
(+) HSV–1 cytology
(no vesicles)

Treat HSV-1 NP with
acyclovir*

Able to wean

Diagnostic work-up to determine
cause of infiltrates

(+) for mimics
of NP

(—) for mimics
of NP

Diagnostic lung biopsy
(transbronchial or open lung)

Specific therapy based
on biopsy findings

**Figure 7.1. Approach to Ventilator-Associated Pneumonia With Unchanged
Pulmonary Infiltrates After 2 Weeks of Appropriate Anti-P. aeruginosa Therapy**

* Expected response to acyclovir therapy: ↓ FIO_2/↑ PO_2, and ↓ A-a gradient within 72 hours; rapidly able to wean within 1 week

REFERENCES AND SUGGESTED READINGS

Alvarez-Lerma F, Grau S, Alvarez-Beltran M. Levofloxacin in the treatment of ventilator-associated pneumonia. Clin Microbiol Infect 12 (Suppl 3):81-92, 2006.

Bartlett JG, O'Keffe P, Tally F, et al. Bacteriology of hospital-acquired pneumonia. Arch Intern Med. 146:868-871, 1986.

Baughman RP. Microbiologic diagnosis of ventilator-associated pneumonia. Clin Chest Med 26:81-86, 2005.

Borade PS, Lee DK. Antibiotic resistance and nosocomial pneumonia. Respir Med 99:1462, 2005.

Branson RD. The ventilator circuit and ventilator-associated pneumonia. Respir Care 50:774-785, 2005.

Chapman TM, Perry CM. Cefepime: a review of its use in the management of hospitalized patients with pneumonia. Am J Respir Med. 2:75-107, 2003.

Chastre J, Fagon JY, Bornet-Lesco M, et al. Evaluation of bronchoscopic techniques for the diagnosis of nosocomial pneumonia. Am J Respir Crit Care Med. 152:231, 1995.

Chastre J, Fagon JY. Invasive diagnostic testing should be routinely used to manage ventilated patients with suspected pneumonia. Am J Respir Crit Care Med. 150:570-574, 1994.

Chua Tde J, File TM Jr. Ventilator-associated pneumonia: gearing towards shorter-course therapy. Curr Opin Infect Dis 19:185-8, 2006.

Crnich CJ, Safdar N, Maki DG. The role of intensive care unit environment in the pathogenesis and prevention of ventilator-associated pneumonia. Respir Care 50:813-838, 2005.

Cunha BA. Antibiotic selection is crucial for optimal monotherapy of ventilator associated pneumonia. Crit Care Med 35:1992-1994, 2007.

Cunha BA. Fever in the intensive care unit. Intensive Care 25:648-651, 1999.

Cunha BA. Herpes Simplex-1 (HSV-1) Pneumonia. Infect Dis Pract 29:375-378, 2005.

Cunha BA. Monotherapy for nosocomial pneumonias. Antibiotics for the Clinician 2:34-37, 1998.

Cunha BA. Nosocomial pneumonia. Med Clin North Am. 85:79-114, 2001.

Cunha BA, Eisenstein LE, Dillard T, et al. Herpes Simplex Virus (HSV) pneumonia in heart transplant: diagnosis and therapy. Heart & Lung 36:72-78, 2007.

Cunha BA. S. aureus nosocomial pneumonia: clinical aspects. Infect Dis Pract 31:557-560, 2007.

Daubin C, Vincent S, Vabret A, et al. Nosocomial viral ventilator-associated pneumonia in the intensive care unit: a prospective cohort study. Intensive Care Med 31:1116-22, 2005.

Depuydt P, Myny D, Blot S. Nosocomial pneumonia: aetiology, diagnosis and treatment. Curr Opin Pulm Med 12:192-197, 2006.

Depuydt P, Blot SI, Benoit DD, et al. Antimicrobial resistance in nosocomial bloodstream infection associated with pneumonia and the value of systemic surveillance cultures in an adult intensive care unit. Crit Care Med 34:653-659, 2006.

Eisenstein L, Cunha BA. Herpes simples virus Type I (HSV-I) pneumonia presenting as failure to wean. Heart Lung. 32:65-66, 2003.

Flanders SA, Collard HR, Saint S. Nosocomial pneumonia: state of the science. Am J Infect Control 34:84-93, 2006.

Franzetti F, Grassini A, Piazza M, et al. Nosocomial bacterial pneumonia in HIV-infected patients: risk factors for adverse outcome and implications for rational empiric antibiotic therapy. Infection 34:9-16, 2006.

Fritsche TR, Sader HS, Stilwell MG, et al. Antimicrobial activity of tigecycline tested against organisms causing community-acquired respiratory tract infection and nosocomial pneumonia. Diagn Microbiol Infect Dis 52:187-193, 2005.

Hijazi M, Al-Ansari M. Therapy for ventilator-associated pneumonia: what works, what doesn't. Respir Care Clin N Am 10:341-358, 2004.

Hurley JC. Inapparent outbreaks of ventilator-associated pneumonia: an ecologic analysis of prevention and cohort studies. Infect Control Hosp Epidemiol 26:374-390, 2005.

Klainer AS, Oud L, Randazzo, et al. Herpes simplex virus involvement of the lower respiratory tract following surgery. Chest 106:8S-14S, 34S-35S, 1994.

Garbino J, Gerbase MW, Wunderli W, et al. Respiratory viruses and severe lower respiratory tract complications in Hospitalized patients. Chest 125:1033-39, 2004.

Herout V, Vortel V, Vondrackova A. Herpes simplex involvement of the respiratory tract. Am J Clin Pathol 46:411-19, 1966.

Levy PY, Teysseire N, Etienne J, et al. A Nosocomial Outbreak of Legionella pneumophila Caused by Contaminated Transesophageal Echocardiography Probes. Concise Communications 24:619-622, 2004.

Mayhall CG. In pursuit of ventilator-associated pneumonia prevention: the right path. Clin Infect Dis 45:712-4, 2007.

Mubareka S, Rubinstein E. Aerosolized colistin for the treatment of nosocomial pneumonia due to multidrug-resistant gram-negative bacteria in patients without cystic fibrosis. Crit Care 9:29-30, 2005.

Park DR. Antimicrobial treatment of ventilator-associated pneumonia. Respir Care 50:932-952, 2005.

Park DR. The microbiology of ventilator-associated pneumonia. Respir Care 50:742-763, 2005.

Pierce AD, Sanford JP. Aerobic gram-negative bacillary pneumonia. A Rev Respir Dis. 110:647-658, 1974.

Pennington JE, Reynolds HY, Carbone PP. Pseudomonas pneumonia: a retrospective study of 36 cases. Am J Med. 55:155-60, 1973.

Porzecanski I, Bowton DL. Diagnosis and treatment of ventilator-associated pneumonia. Chest 130:597-604, 2006.

Randazzo JP, Bisaccia E, Klainer AS. Herpes simplex virus respiratory tract infection. Infect Dis Pract 20:43-55, 1996.

Robert R, Grollier G, Dore P, et al. Nosocomial pneumonia with isolation of anaerobic bacteria in ICU patients: therapeutic considerations and outcome. J Crit Care 14:114-119, 1999.

Rose HD, Heckman MG, Unger JD. Pseudomonas aeruginosa pneumonia in adults. Am Rev Respir Dis. 107:416-422, 1973.

Safdar N, Dezfulian C, Collard HR, et al. Clinical and economic consequences of ventilator-associated pneumonia: a systematic review. Crit Care Med 33:2184-93, 2005.

Shales DM, Lederman M, Chmielewski R, et al. Sputum elastin fibers and the diagnosis of necrotizing pneumonia. Chest. 85:763-766, 1984.

Shaw MJ. Ventilator-associated pneumonia. Curr Opin Pulm Med 11:236-241, 2005.

Shorr AF, Susla GB, Kollef MH. Quinolones for treatment of nosocomial pneumonia: a meta analysis. Clin Infect Dis 40: Suppl 2: S115-22.

Sun HK, Kuti JL, Nicolau DP. Pharmacodynamics of antimicrobials for the empirical treatment of nosocomial pneumonia: a report from the OPTIMA Program. Crit Care Med 33:2222-7, 2005.

Sung-Levander M, Ortqvist A, Grodzinsky E, et al. Morbidity, mortality, and clinical presentation of nursing home-acquired pneumonia in a Swedish population. Scand J Infect Dis. 35:306-310, 2003.

Tillotson JR, Lerner Am. Characteristics of nonbacteremic Pseudomonas pneumonia. Ann Intern Med. 68:295-307, 1968.

Tillotson JR, Lerner Am. Pneumonia caused by gram-negative bacilli. Medicine (Baltimore). 45:65-76, 1966.

Vincent JL. Ventilator-associated pneumonia. J Hos Infect. 57:272-280, 2004.

Vitkauskiene A, Scheuss S, Sakalauskas R, et al. Pseudomonas aeruginosa strains from nosocomial pneumonia are more serum resistant than P. aeruginosa strains from noninfectious respiratory colonization processes. Infection 33:356-361, 2005.

Wenzel RP. Hospital-acquired pneumonia: Overview of the current state of the art for prevention and control. Eur J Clin Microbial Infect Dis. 8:56-60, 1989.

Wunderink RG. Nosocomial pneumonia, including ventilator-associated pneumonia. Proc Am Thorac Soc 2:440-444, 2005.

Wunderink RG, Woldenburg LS, Zeiss J, et al. The radiologic diagnosis of autopsy proven ventilator-associated pneumonia. Chest. 101:458-463, 1992.

GUIDELINES

American Thoracic Society Guidelines for the Management of Adults with Hospital-Acquired, Ventilator-Associated, and Healthcare-Associated Pneumonia. Am J Respir Crit Care Med 171;388-416, 2005.

Guidelines for Preventing Health-Care-Associated Pneumonia, 2003. MMWR;Vol 53, No RR3;1, March 26, 2004.

Mandell LA, Wunderink RG, Anzueto A, et al. Infectious Diseases Society of America/American Thoracic Society consensus guidelines on the management of community-acquired pneumonia in adults. Clin Infect Dis 44(S2):S27-S72, 2007.

TEXTBOOKS

Burgener FA, Kormano M. Differential Diagnosis in Conventional Radiology, 2nd Edition. Stuttgart, Georg Thieme Verlag, 1991.

Chapman S, Nakielny R. Aids to Radiological Differential Diagnosis, 2nd Edition. London, Bailliere Tindall, 1990.

Conn RB, Borer WZ, Snyder JW. Current Diagnosis 9. Philadelphia, W. B. Saunders Company, 1997.

Crapo JD, Glassroth J, Karlinsky JB, King TE. Baum's Textbook of Pulmonary Diseases, 7th Edition. Philadelphia, Lippincott Williams & Wilkins, 2004.

Cunha BA. Nosocomial Pneumonias. In Kassirer J (ed). Current Therapy in Infectious Diseases. 4th Edition. The C.V. Mosby Co., St Louis, Missouri, 1997.

Cunha BA. Nosocomial Pneumonias. In Schlossberg D (ed). Current Therapy of Infectious Diseases, 3rd Edition. Cambridge University Press, Cambridge, 2007.

Eisenberg RL. Clinical Imaging. An Atlas of Differential Diagnosis, 2nd Edition. Gaithersburg, Aspen Publishers, Inc., 1992.

Gorbach SL, Bartlett JG, Blacklow NR (eds). Infectious Diseases, 3rd Edition. Philadelphia, Lippincott, Williams & Wilkins, 2004.

Jarvis WR (ed). Nosocomial Pneumonia. Marcel Dekker, New York, NY, 2000.

Karetzky M, Cunha BA, Brandstetter R. The Pneumonias. New York, Springer-Verlag, 1993.

Kasper L, Braunwald E, Fauci AS, Hauser SL, Longo DL, Jameson JL. Harrison's Principles of Internal Medicine, 16th Edition. New York, The McGraw Hill Companies, 2004.

Levison ME. The Pneumonias: Clinical Approaches to Infectious Diseases of the Lower Respiratory Tract. Boston, John Wright, PSG Inc., 1984.

Lillington GA, Jamplis RW. A Diagnostic Approach to Chest Diseases, 2nd Edition. Baltimore, The Williams & Wilkins Company, 1977.

Murray JF, Nadel JA. Textbook of Respiratory Medicine, 3rd Edition. Philadelphia, W.B. Saunders Company, 2000.

Mandell GL, Bennett JE, Dolin R (eds). Mandell, Douglas and Bennett's Principles and Practice of Infectious Disease, 6th Edition. Philadelphia, Elsevier, 2005.

Penington JE (ed). Pseudomonas aeruginosa Infections and Treatment. Marcel Dekker, New York, NY, 1995.

Pennington JE (ed). Respiratory Infections: Diagnosis and Management, 2nd Edition. Raven Press, New York, NY, 1994.

Teplick JE, Haskin ME. Roentgenologic Diagnosis, 3rd Edition. Philadelphia, W. B. Saunders Company, 1976.

Wright FW. Radiology of the Chest and Related Conditions. London, Taylor & Francis, 2002.

Chapter 8

Chronic Pneumonias: Parasites, Fungi, Unusual Organisms

Burke A. Cunha, MD • John H. Rex, MD
Kenneth F. Wagner, DO • James H. McGuire, MD
David Schlossberg, MD

Parasites, Fungi, Unusual Organisms in Lungs

Pulmonary Infiltrates/Mass Lesions

Subset	Pathogens	Preferred Therapy	Alternate Therapy
Pulmonary blastomycosis	Blastomyces dermatitidis	Itraconazole 200 mg (PO)* q12h until cured <u>Severely ill</u> Amphotericin B deoxycholate 0.7-1 mg/kg (IV) q24h until 1-2 grams given	Fluconazole 400-800 mg (PO) q24h until cured
Pulmonary histoplasmosis	Histoplasma capsulatum	<u>Immunocompetent</u> Itraconazole 200 mg (PO)* q24h until cured <u>Immunocompromised or severely ill</u> Amphotericin B deoxycholate 1 mg/kg (IV) q24h x 7 days[†] or 0.8 mg/kg q48h until 2-2.5 grams given	<u>Immunocompetent</u> Itraconazole 200 mg (IV) q12h x 7-14 days, then 200 mg (PO) q12h until cured **or** Fluconazole 1600 mg (PO) x 1 dose, then 800 mg (PO) q24h until cured <u>Immunocompromised or severely ill</u> Itraconazole 200 mg (IV) q12h x 7-14 days, then 200 mg (PO) q12h until cured
Pulmonary paracoccidioidomycosis (South American blastomycosis)	Paracoccidioides brasiliensis	Itraconazole 200 mg (PO) q24h x 6 months **or** Ketoconazole 400 mg (PO) q24h x 18 months	Amphotericin B 0.5 mg/kg (IV) q24h until 1.5-2.5 grams given
Pulmonary actinomycosis	Actinomyces israelii	Amoxicillin 1 gm (PO) q8h x 6 months **or** Doxycycline 100 mg (PO) q12h x 6 months	Clindamycin 300 mg (PO) q8h x 6 months **or** Chloramphenicol 500 mg (PO) q6h x 6 months

Pulmonary Infiltrates/Mass Lesions (cont'd)

Subset	Pathogens	Preferred Therapy	Alternate Therapy
Pulmonary aspergillosis *BPA*	Aspergillus	Systemic oral steroids	Itraconazole 200 mg (PO) q12h x 8 months
Acute invasive pneumonia	Aspergillus	Voriconazole (see "usual dose," p. 345) x 6-18 months **or** Amphotericin B deoxycholate 1-1.5 mg/kg (IV) q24h until 2-3 gm total dose given (duration of therapy poorly defined)	Itraconazole 200 mg (IV) q12h x 2 days, then itraconazole 200 mg (PO) solution q12h x 6-18 months **or** Caspofungin 70 mg (IV) x 1 dose, then 50 mg (IV) q24h x 6-18 months **or** Amphotericin B lipid formulation (p. 279) (IV) q24h x 6-18 months
Chronic pneumonia	Aspergillus	Posaconazole 400 mg (PO) q12h until cured **or** Voriconazole (see "usual dose," p. 345) until cured¶ **or** Itraconazole 200 mg (IV) q12h x 2 days, then 200 mg (IV) q24h x 1-2 weeks, then 200 mg (PO) solution q12h until cured¶	Lipid-associated amphotericin B (p. 279) (IV) q24h until cured **or** Amphotericin B deoxycholate 1-1.5 mg/kg (IV) q24h until 2-3 grams given **or** Caspofungin 70 mg (IV) x 1 dose, then 50 mg (IV) q24h x 1-2 weeks, then itraconazole 200 mg (PO) solution q12h until cured
Pulmonary sporotrichosis	Sporothrix schenckii	Lipid-associated formulation of amphotericin B (p. 279) (IV) q24h x 3 weeks **or** Amphotericin B deoxycholate 0.5 mg/kg (IV) q24h until 1-2 grams given	Itraconazole 200 mg (PO)* q12h until cured
Pulmonary coccidioido-mycosis	Coccidioides immitis	Itraconazole 200 mg (PO)* q12h until cured **or** Fluconazole 800 mg (IV or PO) x 1 dose, then 400 mg (PO) q24h until cured	Amphotericin B deoxycholate 1 mg/kg (IV) q24h x 7 days†

Pulmonary Infiltrates/Mass Lesions (cont'd)

Subset	Pathogens	Preferred Therapy	Alternate Therapy
Pulmonary nocardiosis	Nocardia asteroides	TMP-SMX 5-10 mg/kg/d (TMP) in 2-4 doses (IV) x 3-6 weeks, then 1 DS tablet (PO) q12h until cured	Minocycline 100 mg (PO) q12h until cured
Pulmonary cryptococcosis	Cryptococcus neoformans	Fluconazole 800 mg (IV or PO) x 1 dose, then 400 mg (PO) q24h until cured	Amphotericin B deoxycholate 0.5 mg/kg (IV) q24h until 1-2 grams given **or** Lipid-associated formulation of amphotericin B (p. 279) (IV) q24h x 3 weeks
Pulmonary zygomycosis (mucormycosis)	Rhizopus Mucor Absidia	Lipid-associated formulation of amphotericin B (p. 279) (IV) q24h x 1-2 weeks[†] or x 3 weeks **or** Amphotericin B deoxycholate 1-1.5 mg/kg (IV) q24h x 1-2 weeks[†] or until 2-3 grams given	Itraconazole 200 mg (PO)* q12h until cured
Pulmonary pseudall-escheriasis	Pseudallescheria boydii Scedosporium apiospermum	Voriconazole (see "usual dose," p. 345) until cured	Itraconazole 200 mg (PO)* q12h until cured

BPA = bronchopulmonary aspergillosis
* Initiate therapy with itraconazole 200 mg (IV) q12h x 7-14 days
† Follow with itraconazole 200 mg (PO) solution q12h until cured
¶ Significant drug interactions are possible when voriconazole or itraconazole is administered with usual immunosuppressive agents (e.g., tacrolimus). Review all concomitant medications for potential interactions

Pulmonary Blastomycosis (Blastomyces dermatitidis)

Clinical Presentation: Highly variable. May present as a chronic/non-resolving pneumonia with fever/cough and characteristic "right-sided perihilar infiltrate" ± small pleural effusion (Table 8.1)

Diagnostic Considerations: May be recovered from sputum or demonstrated in lung tissue specimens (Table 8.2). Usual sites of dissemination include skin, bones and prostate, not CNS or adrenals

Pitfalls: Dissemination to extra-pulmonary sites may occur years after pneumonia

Prognosis: Related to severity/extent of infection. One-third of cases are self-limited and do not require treatment

Pulmonary Histoplasmosis (Histoplasma capsulatum)

Clinical Presentation: Acute primary infection presents as self-limiting flu-like illness with fever, headache, nonproductive cough, chills, and chest pain. Minority of patients become overtly ill with complicated respiratory or progressive pulmonary infection. Can cause arthralgias, E. nodosum, E. multiforme, or pericarditis. May occur in outbreak. Chronic infection presents as chronic pneumonia resembling TB or chronic disseminated infection (Tables 8.2, 8.3)

Diagnostic Considerations: May be recovered from sputum or demonstrated in lung tissue specimens (Table 8.2). Worldwide distribution, but most common in Central/South Central United States. Acute disseminated histoplasmosis suggests HIV/AIDS. Acute histoplasmosis with immunodiffusion (ID) assay M band precipitins; chronic histoplasmosis with ID assay H band precipitins or CF ≥ 1:32. Peripheral eosinophilia (acute > chronic histoplasmosis) vs. TB (no eosinophilia)

Pitfalls: Pleural effusion is uncommon. Do not treat old/inactive/minimal histoplasmosis, histoplasmosis pulmonary calcification, or histoplasmosis fibrosing mediastinitis. Mimics TB

Prognosis: Related to severity/extent of infection. No treatment is needed for self-limiting acute histoplasmosis presenting as flu-like illness. HIV/AIDS patients should receive life-long suppressive therapy with itraconazole

Pulmonary Paracoccidioidomycosis (South American Blastomycosis)

Clinical Presentation: Typically presents as a chronic pneumonia syndrome with productive cough, blood-tinged sputum, dyspnea, and chest pain. May also develop fever, malaise, weight loss, mucosal ulcerations in/around mouth and nose, dysphagia, changes in voice, cutaneous lesions on face/limbs, or cervical adenopathy. Can disseminate to prostate, epididymis, kidneys, or adrenals

Diagnostic Considerations: Characteristic "pilot wheel" shaped yeast in sputum. Diagnosis by culture and stain (Gomori) of organism from clinical specimen. Found only in Latin American. One-third of cases have only pulmonary involvement. Skin test is non-specific/non-diagnostic

Pitfalls: No distinguishing radiologic features. No clinical adrenal insufficiency, in contrast to TB or histoplasmosis. Hilar adenopathy/pleural effusions are uncommon

Prognosis: Related to severity/extent of infection. HIV/AIDS require life-long suppression with TMP-SMX 1 DS tablet (PO) q24h or itraconazole 200 mg (PO) solution q24h

Pulmonary Actinomycosis (Actinomyces israelii)

Clinical Presentation: Indolent, slowly progressive infiltrates involving the pulmonary parenchyma ± pleural space. Presents with fever, chest pain, weight loss. Cough/hemoptysis are less common. Chest wall sinuses frequently develop. Chest x-ray shows adjacent dense

infiltrate. "Sulfur granules" are common in sinus drainage fluid
Diagnostic Considerations: Diagnosis by stain/culture of drainage from sinuses or lung/bone biopsy specimens. Actinomyces are non-acid fast and anaerobic
Pitfalls: No CNS lesions, but bone erosion is common with chest lesions. Prior antibiotic therapy may interfere with isolation of organism
Prognosis: Excellent when treated until lesions resolve. Use IV regimen in critically ill patients, then switch to oral regimen

Bronchopulmonary Aspergillosis (BPA / ABPA)
Clinical Presentation: Migratory pulmonary infiltrates in chronic asthmatics. Eosinophilia is common, and sputum shows Charcot-Leyden crystals/brown flecks containing Aspergillus
Diagnostic Considerations: Diagnosis by Aspergillus in sputum and high-titers of Aspergillus precipitins in serum. BPA is an allergic reaction in chronic asthmatics, *not* an infectious disease. Pulmonary infiltrates with peripheral eosinophilia in chronic asthmatics suggests the diagnosis
Pitfalls: Correct diagnosis is important since therapy is steroids, not antifungals
Prognosis: Related to severity/duration of asthma and promptness of steroid therapy

Acute Invasive Aspergillus Pneumonia
Clinical Presentation: Pleuritic chest pain, hemoptysis, cough in a patient with advanced HIV disease
Diagnostic Considerations: Diagnosis by bronchoscopy with biopsy/culture. Open lung biopsy (usually video-assisted thorascopic surgery) is sometimes required. Radiographic appearance includes cavitation, nodules, sometimes focal consolidation. Dissemination to CNS may occur, and manifests as focal neurological deficits
Pitfalls: Positive sputum culture for Aspergillus in advanced HIV disease should heighten awareness of possible infection
Therapeutic Considerations: Decrease/discontinue corticosteroids, if possible. Consider granulocyte-colony stimulating factor (G-CSF) if neutropenic
Prognosis: Poor unless immune deficits can be corrected

Chronic Aspergillus Pneumonia
Clinical Presentation: Occurs in patients with AIDS, chronic granulomatous disease, alcoholism, diabetes, and those receiving steroids for chronic pulmonary disease. Usual features include chronic productive cough ± hemoptysis, low-grade fever, weight loss, and malaise. Chronic Aspergillus pneumonia resembles TB, histoplasmosis, melioidosis
Diagnostic Considerations: Diagnosis by lung biopsy demonstrating septate hyphae invading lung parenchyma. Aspergillus may be in sputum, but is not diagnostic of Aspergillus pneumonia
Pitfalls: May extend into chest wall, vertebral column, or brachial plexus
Prognosis: Related to severity/extent of infection

Pulmonary Sporotrichosis (Sporothrix schenckii)
Clinical Presentation: Usually presents as productive cough, low-grade fever, and weight loss. Chest x-ray shows cavitary thin-walled lesions with associated infiltrate. Hemoptysis is unusual. Differential diagnosis includes other thin-walled cavitary lung lesions (e.g., histoplasmosis, coccidioidomycosis, atypical TB, paragonimiasis)
Diagnostic Considerations: Diagnosis by lung biopsy demonstrating invasive lung disease, not broncho-alveolar lavage. Usually a history of puncture/traumatic wound involving an extremity. May be associated with septic arthritis/osteomyelitis

Pitfalls: Sporotrichosis in lungs implies disseminated disease. May need repeated attempts at culture
Prognosis: Related to extent of infection/degree of immunosuppression

Pulmonary Coccidioidomycosis (Coccidioides immitis)

Clinical Presentation: Usually presents as a solitary, peripheral, thin-walled cavitary lesion in early or later stage of primary infection. May present as a solitary pulmonary nodule. E. nodosum and bilateral hilar adenopathy are common (in contrast to sporotrichosis). Hemoptysis is unusual
Diagnostic Considerations: Diagnosis by biopsy/Coccidioides serology (Table 8.2). Increased incidence of dissemination in Filipinos, Blacks, and American Indians. May be associated with chronic meningitis/osteomyelitis, peripheral eosinophilia. CF IgG titer $\geq 1:32$ diagnostic of active disease
Pitfalls: Dissemination is preceded by $\rightrightarrows$ Coccidioides titers/disappearance of E. nodosum
Prognosis: Related to extent of infection/degree of immunosuppression

Pulmonary Nocardiosis (Nocardia asteroides)

Clinical Presentation: Usually presents as a dense lower lobe lung mass ± cavitation. May have associated mass lesions in CNS. Chest wall sinuses are more common with Actinomycosis
Diagnostic Considerations: Diagnosis by demonstrating organisms by stain/culture of lung specimens. Nocardia are weakly acid-fast and aerobic
Pitfalls: Use IV regimens in critically ill patients. HIV/AIDS patients require life-long suppressive therapy with TMP-SMX or minocycline
Prognosis: Related to extent of infection/degree of immunosuppression

Pulmonary Cryptococcosis (Cryptococcus neoformans)

Clinical Presentation: Individual focus of infection is usually inapparent/minimal when patient presents with disseminated cryptococcal infection. Pneumonia is typically a minor part of disseminated disease; CNS manifestations usually predominate (e.g., headache, subtle cognitive changes, occasional meningeal signs, focal neurological deficits)
Diagnostic Considerations: Diagnosis by demonstrating organisms in sputum/lung specimens
Pitfalls: Clinical presentation of isolated cryptococcal pneumonia is rare. HIV/AIDS patients require life-long suppressive therapy with fluconazole
Prognosis: Related to extent of dissemination/degree of immunosuppression

Pulmonary Zygomycosis (Mucormycosis) (Rhizopus/Mucor/Absidia)

Clinical Presentation: Progressive pneumonia with fever, dyspnea, and cough unresponsive to antibiotic therapy. Usually seen only in compromised hosts. Chest x-ray is not characteristic, but shows infiltrate with consolidation in > 50% of patients. Cavitation occurs in 40% as neutropenia resolves
Diagnostic Considerations: Diagnosis by demonstrating organisms in lung biopsy. Pleural effusion is not a feature of pulmonary mucormycosis
Pitfalls: Causes rhinocerebral mucormycosis in diabetics, pneumonia in leukopenic compromised hosts
Prognosis: Related to degree of immunosuppression and underlying disease

Pulmonary Pseudallescheriasis (P. boydii/S. apiospermum)

Clinical Presentation: Progressive pulmonary infiltrates indistinguishable from Aspergillosis or Mucor. Usually seen only in compromised hosts (e.g., prolonged neutropenia, high-dose steroids, bone marrow or solid organ transplants, AIDS). Manifests as cough, fever, pleuritic pain, and often hemoptysis. No characteristic chest x-ray appearance

Diagnostic Considerations: Diagnosis by demonstrating organism in lung biopsy. Hemoptysis is common in patients with cavitary lesions. CNS involvement is rare

Pitfalls: One of few invasive fungi unresponsive to amphotericin B deoxycholate. Cause of sinusitis in diabetics, and pneumonia in leukopenic compromised hosts

Prognosis: Related to severity/extent of infection and degree of immunosuppression. Cavitary lesions causing hemoptysis often require surgical excision. Disseminated infection is often fatal

Table 8.1. Features of Chronic Granulomatous Pneumonias

Findings	Histoplasmosis	Tuberculosis	Blastomycosis
Laboratory tests			
Pancytopenia	a	a	–
Hypergammaglobulinemia	–	–	–
Leukemoid reaction	–	±	–
Chest x-ray			
Miliary calcifications	±	±	–
Hilar adenopathy	+	–	–
Pleural effusion	–	±	–
Abdominal x-ray			
Hepatic/splenic calcifications	+	±	–
Organ involvement			
Meningitis	a	a	–
Oropharyngeal ulcers	a	–	–
Pulmonary infiltrates	+	+	±
Addison's disease	a	a	–
Granulomatous hepatitis	+	+	±
Splenomegaly	a	a	±
Generalized adenopathy	a	a	–
Bone/joint lesions	a	+	+
Glomerulonephritis	–	–	–
Epididymoorchitis	–	+	+
Granulomatous prostatitis	a	–	+
Skin ulcers	a	–	+
Erythema nodosum	+	+	–

+ usually present; ± may be present; – usually absent; a = present only in disseminated histoplasmosis/miliary TB
Also see chest x-ray atlas (Chapter 11)
Adapted from: Cunha BA. Histoplasmosis. Infect Dis Pract 9:1-8, 1986.

Table 8.2. Characteristics of Selected Opportunistic and Pathogenic Fungi

Fungus	Culture Characteristics	Morphology		Additional Tests
		Culture	Tissue	
Histoplasma capsulatum	Colonies slow-growing, white or buff-brown, suede-like to cottony with pale yellow-brown reverse (25°C). Yeast-phase colonies smooth, white, pasty (37°C)	Thin, branching, septate hyphae that produce tuberculate macroconidia and microconidia (25°); small round to oval budding yeast-like cells (37°C)	Small, narrow-based budding yeasts (2-4 μm); often clustered due to growth within mononuclear phagocytes	Conversion from mold yeast phase; exoantigen test; nucleic acid probe test
Coccidioides immitis	Colonies initially moist and glabrous, rapidly becoming suede like to downy, grayish white with a tan to brown reverse	Single-celled, hyaline, rectangular to barrel-shaped, alternate arthroconidia, 2-4 x 3-6 μm, separated by disjunctor cell	Spherical, thick-walled, endosporulating spherules, 20-200 μm; mature spherules contain small, 2-5 μm endospores; arthroconidia and hyphae may form in cavitary lesions	Exoantigen and nucleic acid probe tests
Blastomyces dermatitidis	Colonies may grow rapidly with fluffy white mycelium or slowly as glabrous, tan, nonsporulation colonies (25°C). Yeast phase colonies wrinkled, folded, glabrous (37°C)	Hyaline, ovoid to pyriform, one-celled, smooth conidia, borne on short lateral or terminal hyphal branches (25°C). Large (8-15 μm), thick-walled, budding yeast (37°C)	Spherical, multinucleated yeasts, 8-15 μm, with thick walls and single, broadbased buds	Conversion from mold yeast; exoantigen and nucleic acid probe test

Adapted from: Anaissie EJ, McGinnis MR, Pfaller MA (eds). Clinical Mycology. New York, Churchill Livingstone, 2003. Dismukes WE, Pappas PG, Sobel JD (eds). Clinical Mycology. Oxford, Oxford University Press, 2003. Bottone EJ. An Atlas of the Clinical Microbiology of Infectious Diseases, Volume 2. Viral, fungal, and parasitic agents. Taylor and Francis, 2006.
Also see chest x-ray atlas (Chapter 11)

Table 8.3. Organ Involvement in Histoplasmosis

Organ System	Manifestations
Hematologic	Thrombocytopenia, anemia, leukopenia, pancytopenia, splenomegaly, generalized adenopathy, eosinophilia
Dermatologic	Erythema nodosum, skin ulcers
Gastrointestinal	Granulomatous hepatitis, intestinal ulceration
Pulmonary	"Thick-walled" cavities, apical infiltrates, coin lesions, hilar adenopathy, "buckshot" calcifications, miliary calcifications, "marching cavities," mediastinal fibrosis, obstruction of pulmonary/artery vein*, obstruction of superior vena cava*
Cardiac	Endocarditis, pericarditis
HEENT	Nose ulcers, lip ulcers, gum ulcers, mouth ulcers, tongue ulcers, laryngeal ulcers
Neurologic	Chronic meningitis
Other	Addison's disease

* Secondary to lymph node compression/mediastinal fibrosis
Adapted from: Cunha BA. Histoplasmosis. Infect Dis Pract 9:1-8, 1986.

Pulmonary Cystic Lesions/Masses

Subset	Pathogens	Preferred Therapy	Alternate Therapy
Alveolar echinococcosis	Echinococcus multilocularis	<u>Operable cases</u> Wide surgical resection plus albendazole 400 mg* (PO) q12h or mebendazole 50 mg/kg (PO) q24h until cured	<u>Inoperable cases</u> Albendazole 400 mg* (PO) q12h x 1 month, then repeat therapy after 2 weeks x 3 cycles (i.e., 4 total months of albendazole)
Pulmonary amebiasis	Entamoeba histolytica	Metronidazole 750 mg (PO) q8h x 10 days	Tinidazole 800 mg (PO) q8h x 5 days
Pulmonary paragonimiasis (lung fluke)	Paragonimus westermani	Praziquantel 25 mg/kg (PO) q8h x 2 days	Bithionol 50 mg/kg (PO) q48h x 4 weeks (14 doses)

* If < 60 kg, give albendazole 7.5 mg/kg

Alveolar Echinococcosis (Echinococcus multilocularis)
Clinical Presentation: Slowly growing cysts remain asymptomatic for 5-20 years, until space-occupying effect elicits symptoms. Rupture or leak into bronchial tree can cause cough, chest pain, and hemoptysis
Diagnostic Considerations: Diagnosis is suggested by typical "Swiss cheese calcification"

findings on chest x-ray, and confirmed by specific E. multilocularis serology (which does not cross react with E. granulosus). Most common in Northern forest areas of Europe, Asia, North America, and Arctic. Acquired by ingestion of viable parasite eggs in food. Tapeworm-infected canines/cats or wild rodents are common vectors. Less common than infection with E. granulosus
Pitfalls: Do not confuse central cavitary lesions with squamous cell carcinoma
Prognosis: Related to size/location of cysts

Pulmonary Amebiasis (Entamoeba histolytica)
Clinical Presentation: Cough, pelvic pain, fever, and right lung/pleural mass mimicking pneumonia or lung abscess. Bronchopleural fistulas may occur. Sputum has "liver-like" taste if cyst ruptures into bronchus. Bacterial co-infection is rare. Amebic lung lesions are associated with hepatic liver abscesses, and invariably involve the right lobe of lung/diaphragm
Diagnostic Considerations: Diagnosis by aspiration of lungs cysts, which may be massive. Amebic serology is sensitive and specific. Worldwide distribution. Acquired by ingesting amebic cysts. Key to diagnosis is concomitant liver involvement; liver abscess presents years after initial diarrheal episode
Pitfalls: Lung involvement is rarely the sole manifestation of amebic infection, and is usually due to direct extension of amebic liver abscess (10-20% of amebic liver abscesses penetrate through the diaphragm and into the lungs). Follow metronidazole with paromomycin 500 mg (PO) q8h x 7 days to eliminate intestinal focus
Prognosis: Related to severity/extent of cysts

Pulmonary Paragonimiasis (Paragonimus westermani) Lung Fluke
Clinical Presentation: Mild infection; may be asymptomatic. Acute phase of infection is accompanied by abdominal pain, diarrhea and urticaria, followed by pleuritic chest pain. Chronic symptoms occur within 6 months after exposure, with dyspnea/dry cough leading to productive cough ± hemoptysis. Complications include pleural effusion, lung abscess, bronchiectasis, cough, and night sweats. Eosinophilia may be evident acutely
Diagnostic Considerations: Oriental lung fluke acquired by ingestion of freshwater crayfish/crabs. After penetration of the gut/peritoneal cavity, the fluke migrates through the diaphragm/pleural space and invades lung parenchyma. Incubation period is 2-20 days. Diagnosis by demonstrating operculated eggs in sputum, pleural fluid, or feces. Multiple sputum samples are needed to demonstrate P. westermani eggs. Charcot-Leyden crystals are seen in sputum, and eosinophils are present in pleural effusion. Characteristic chest x-ray findings of ring-shaped/crescent infiltrates with "thin-walled" cavities are evident in ~ 60%. Endemic in Asia, Africa, and Latin America. Chest x-ray findings take months to resolve
Pitfalls: May have extrapulmonary (ectopic) organ involvement (e.g., cerebral, subcutaneous, abdominal). Up to 20% have normal chest x-rays
Prognosis: Related to degree of lung damage (e.g., bronchiectasis) and extrapulmonary organ involvement, especially CNS

Pulmonary Coin Lesions

Subset	Pathogens	Preferred Therapy	Alternate Therapy
Dog heartworm	Dirofilaria immitis	No therapy necessary	
Aspergilloma	Aspergillus	No therapy if asymptomatic. Surgery for massive hemoptysis	Itraconazole 200 mg (PO) solution q24h x 3-6 months **or** Voriconazole (see "usual dose," p. 345) x 3-6 months

Dog Heartworm (Dirofilaria immitis)
Clinical Presentation: Asymptomatic "coin lesion" after bite of infected mosquito transmits parasite from dogs to humans. Differential diagnosis includes granulomas and malignancy
Diagnostic Considerations: Diagnosis by specific serology or pathological demonstration of organism in granuloma, usually when a coin lesion is biopsied to rule out malignancy. Worldwide distribution. Acquired from pet dogs. Dirofilariasis causes dog heartworm in carrier, but presents as a solitary lung nodule in humans
Pitfalls: Often confused with malignancy
Prognosis: Excellent

Pulmonary Aspergilloma
Clinical Presentation: Coin lesion(s) ± productive cough, hemoptysis, wheezing. May be asymptomatic. Usually occurs in pre-existing cavitary lung lesions, especially TB with cavity > 2 cm
Diagnostic Considerations: Diagnosis by chest x-ray appearance of fungus ball in cavity and Aspergillus precipitins/biopsy. May present with "crescent sign" on chest x-ray (white fungus ball silhouetted against black crescent of the cavity)
Pitfalls: Role of itraconazole or voriconazole as therapy is unclear
Prognosis: Related to degree of hemoptysis

REFERENCES AND SUGGESTED READINGS

Johnson DH, Cunha BA. Rhodococcus equi pneumonia. Seminars in respiratory infections 13:57-60, 1997.

Klein NC, Cunha BA. Pasteurella multocida pneumonia. Seminars in respiratory infections 13:54-56, 1997.

GUIDELINES

Galgiani JN, Ampel NM, Blair JE, et al. Coccidioidomycosis. Clin Infect Dis 41:1217-23, 2005.

TEXTBOOKS

Anaissie EJ, McGinnis MR, Pfaller MA (eds). Clinical Mycology. New York, Churchill Livingstone, 2003.

Brandstetter RD. Pulmonary Medicine. Oradell, NJ, Medical Economics Books, 1989.

Burgener FA, Kormano M. Differential Diagnosis in Conventional Radiology, 2nd Edition. Stuttgart, Georg Thieme Verlag, 1991.

Chapman S, Nakielny R. Aids to Radiological Differential Diagnosis, 2nd Edition. London, Bailliere Tindall, 1990.

Conn RB, Borer WZ, Snyder JW. Current Diagnosis 9. Philadelphia, W. B. Saunders Company, 1997.

Cook GC, Zumla A (eds). Manson's Tropical Diseases, 21st Edition. London, Elsevier Science Limited, 2003.

Crapo JD, Glassroth J, Karlinsky JB, King TE. Baum's Textbook of Pulmonary Diseases, 7th Edition. Philadelphia, Lippincott Williams & Wilkins, 2004.

de Hoog GS, Guarro J, Gene J, Figueras MJ. Atlas of Clinical Fungi, 2nd Edition. Utrecht, NL, Centraalbureau voor Schimmelcultures, 2000.

Despommier DD, Gwadz RW, Hotez PJ, Knirsch CA. Parasitic Diseases, 4th Edition. New York, Apple Trees Productions, LLC., 2000.

Dismukes WE, Pappas PG, Sobel JD (eds). Clinical Mycology. Oxford, Oxford University Press, 2003.

Eisenberg RL. Clinical Imaging. An Atlas of Differential Diagnosis, 2nd ed. Gaithersburg, Aspen Publishers, 1992.

Garcia LS. Diagnostic Medial Parasitology (4th ed). Washington, D.C., ASM Press, 2001.

Gillespie SH, Pearson RD (eds). Principles and Practice of Clinical Parasitology. Chichester, UK, John Wiley & Sons, LTD, 2001.

Gorbach SL, Bartlett JG, Blacklow NR. Infectious Diseases, 3rd Edition. Philadelphia, Lippincott Williams & Wilkins, 2004.

Gutierrez Y. Diagnostic Pathology of Parasitic Infections with Clinical Correlations, 2nd Edition. New York, Oxford University Press, 2000.

Karetzky M, Cunha BA, Brandstetter. The Pneumonias. New York, Springer-Verlag, 1993.

Kasper L, Braunwald E, Fauci AS, Hauser SL, Longo DL, Jameson JL. Harrison's Principles of Internal Medicine, 16th Edition. New York, The McGraw Hill Companies, 2004.

Levison ME. The Pneumonias: Clinical Approaches to Infectious Diseases of the Lower Respiratory Tract. Boston, John Wright, PSG Inc., 1984.

Lillington GA, Jamplis RW. A Diagnostic Approach to Chest Diseases, 2nd Edition. Baltimore, The Williams & Wilkins Company, 1977.

Madkour MM (ed). Tuberculosis. Berlin, Spring-Verlag, 2003.

Mandell GL, Bennet JE, Dolin R. Mandell, Douglas, and Bennett's Principles and Practice of Infectious Diseases, 6th Edition. Elsevier, 2005.

Murray JF, Nadel JA. Textbook of Respiratory Medicine, 3rd Edition. Philadelphia, W.B. Saunders Company, 2000.

Rom WN, Garay SM (eds). Tuberculosis. Ed 2, Philadelphia, Lippincott Williams & Wilkins, 2004.

Schlossberg D (ed). Tuberculosis and Nontuberculosis Mycobacterial Infections, 4th Edition. Philadelphia, WB Saunders Company, 1999.

Sharma OP (ed). Lung Disease in the Tropics. New York, Marcel Dekker, 1991.

Strickland GT. Hunter's Tropical Medicine and Emerging Infectious Diseases, 8th Edition. Philadelphia, W.B. Saunders Company, 2000.

Teplick JE, Haskin ME. Roentgenologic Diagnosis, 3rd Edition. Philadelphia, W. B. Saunders Company, 1976.

Walzer PD, Cushion MT (eds). Pneumocystis Pneumonia, 3rd Edition. New York, Marcel Dekker, 2005.

Wingard JR, Anaissie EJ (eds). Fungal Infections in the Compromised Patient. Boca Raton, FL, Taylor & Francis Group, 2005.

Chapter 9

Pneumonias in the Immunocompromised Host

Paul E. Sax, MD
Burke A. Cunha, MD
David Schlossberg, MD

RESPIRATORY TRACT OPPORTUNISTIC INFECTIONS IN HIV

Infection with Human Immunodeficiency Virus (HIV-1) leads to a chronic and without treatment usually fatal infection characterized by progressive immunodeficiency, a long clinical latency period, and opportunistic infections. The hallmark of HIV disease is infection and viral replication within T-lymphocytes expressing the CD4 antigen (helper-inducer lymphocytes), a critical component of normal cell-mediated immunity. Qualitative defects in CD4 responsiveness and progressive depletion in CD4 cell counts increase the risk for opportunistic infections such as Pneumocystis (carinii) jiroveci pneumonia. HIV infection can also disrupt blood monocyte, tissue macrophage, and B-lymphocyte (humoral immunity) function, predisposing to infection with encapsulated bacteria (e.g., invasive pneumococcal infection is 100-fold higher in HIV patients than in normal hosts). More than 1 million people in the United States and 40 million people worldwide are infected with HIV. Without treatment, the average time from acquisition of HIV to an AIDS-defining opportunistic infection is about 10 years; survival then averages 1-2 years. There is tremendous individual variability in these time intervals, with some patients progressing from acute HIV infection to death within 1-2 years, and others not manifesting HIV-related immunosuppression for more than 20 years after HIV acquisition. Antiretroviral therapy and prophylaxis against opportunistic infections have markedly improved the overall prognosis of HIV disease.

Patients with HIV disease are at risk for infectious complications not otherwise seen in immunocompetent patients. Such opportunistic infections occur in proportion to the severity of immune system dysfunction (reflected by CD4 cell count depletion). While community acquired infections (e.g., pneumococcal pneumonia) can occur at any CD4 cell count, "classic" HIV-related opportunistic infections (PCP, toxoplasmosis, cryptococcus, disseminated M. avium-intracellulare, CMV) do not occur until CD4 cell counts are dramatically reduced. Specifically, it is rare to encounter PCP in HIV patients with CD4 > $200/mm^3$, and CMV and disseminated MAI occur at median CD4 cell counts < $50/mm^3$. Recommendations for the prophylaxis and treatment of respiratory tract opportunistic infections in HIV are shown in Table 9.1 and pp. 119-123, respectively. The U.S. Public Health Service/Infectious Diseases Society of America guidelines are periodically updated at www.hivatis.org/trtgdlns.html#Opportunistic

Table 9.1. Prophylaxis of Respiratory Tract Opportunistic Infections in HIV

Infection	Indications and Prophylaxis	Comments
P. (carinii) jiroveci pneumonia (PCP)	Indications: CD4 < 200/mm³, oral thrush, constitutional symptoms, or previous history of PCP Preferred prophylaxis: TMP-SMX 1 DS tablet (PO) q24h or 1 SS tablet (PO) q24h. 1 DS tablet (PO) 3x/week is also effective, but daily dosing may be slightly more effective based on 1 comparative study Alternate prophylaxis: Dapsone 100 mg (PO) q24h (preferred as second-line by most; more effective than aerosolized pentamidine when CD4 < 100/mm³) **or** Atovaquone 1500 mg (PO) q24h (comparably effective to dapsone and aerosolized pentamidine; more GI toxicity vs. dapsone, but less rash) **or** Aerosolized pentamidine 300 mg via Respirgard II nebulizer once monthly (exclude active pulmonary TB first to avoid nosocomial transmission)	Without prophylaxis, 80% of AIDS patients develop PCP, and 60-70% relapse within one year after the first episode. Prophylaxis with TMP-SMX also reduces the risk for toxoplasmosis and possibly bacterial infections. Among patients with prior non-life-threatening reactions to TMP-SMX, 55% can be successfully rechallenged with 1 SS tablet daily, and 80% can be rechallenged with gradual dose escalation using TMP-SMX elixir. Macrolide-regimens for MAC (azithromycin, clarithromycin) add to efficacy of PCP prophylaxis. Primary and secondary prophylaxis may be discontinued if CD4 cell counts increase to > 200 cells/mm³ for 3 months or longer in response to antiretroviral therapy (i.e., immune reconstitution). Prophylaxis should be resumed if the CD4 cell count decreases to < 200/mm³
Tuberculosis (M. tuberculosis)	Indications: PPD induration ≥ 5 mm or history of positive PPD without prior treatment, or close contact with active case of TB. Must exclude active disease (chest x-ray). Indicated at any CD4 cell count Preferred prophylaxis: INH 300 mg (PO) q24h x 9 months + pyridoxine 50 mg (PO) q24h x 9 months Alternate prophylaxis: Rifampin 600 mg (PO) q24h x 2 months + pyrazinamide 20 mg/kg (PO) q24h x 2 months. Rifampin should not be give to patients receiving amprenavir, indinavir, lopinavir +amprenavir, indinavir, lopinavir + ritonavir, nelfinavir, saquinavir, or delavirdine	Consider prophylaxis for skin test negative patients when the probability of prior TB exposure is > 10% (e.g., patients from developing countries, IV drug abusers in some cities, prisoners). However, a trial testing this strategy in the U.S. did not find a benefit for empiric prophylaxis. INH prophylaxis delayed progression to AIDS and prolonged life in Haitian cohort with positive PPD treated x 6 months. Rifampin plus pyrazinamide x 2 months was effective in a multinational clinical trial (but the combination may ↑ hepatotoxicity). Rifabutin may be substituted for rifampin in rifampin-containing regimens (see p. 122 for dosing)

Table 9.1. Prophylaxis of Respiratory Tract Opportunistic Infections in HIV

Infection	Indications and Prophylaxis	Comments
M. avium-intracellulare (MAI)	<u>Indications:</u> CD4 < 50/mm^3 <u>Preferred prophylaxis:</u> Azithromycin 1200 mg (PO) once a week (fewest number of pills; fewest drug interactions; may add to efficacy of PCP prophylaxis) **or** Clarithromycin 500 mg (PO) q12h (more effective than rifabutin; associated with survival advantage; resistance detected in some breakthrough cases) <u>Alternate prophylaxis:</u> Rifabutin (less effective). See TB (p. 122) for dosing	Macrolide options (azithromycin, clarithromycin) preferable to rifabutin. Azithromycin is preferred for patients on protease inhibitors (fewer drug interactions). Primary prophylaxis may be discontinued if CD4 cell counts increase to > 100/mm^3 and HIV RNA suppresses for 3-6 months or longer in response to antiretroviral therapy. Secondary prophylaxis may be discontinued for CD4 cell counts that increase to > 100/mm^3 x 6 months or longer in response to antiretroviral therapy if patients have completed 12 months of MAI therapy and have no evidence of disease. Resume MAC prophylaxis for CD4 < 100/mm^3
Pneumococcus (S. pneumoniae)	<u>Indications:</u> CD4 > 200/mm^3 <u>Preferred prophylaxis:</u> Pneumococcal polysaccharide (23 valent) vaccine.* Re-vaccinate x 1 at 5 years	Incidence of invasive pneumococcal disease is > 100-fold higher in HIV patients. Re-immunize if initial vaccine is given when CD4 < 200/mm^3, but is now > 200/mm^3 due to antiretroviral therapy
Influenza	<u>Indications:</u> Generally recommended for all patients <u>Preferred prophylaxis:</u> Influenza vaccine (inactivated whole virus and split virus vaccine)*	Give annually (optimally October–January). Some experts do not give vaccine if CD4 is < 100/mm^3 (antibody response is poor). New intranasal live virus vaccine is contraindicated in immuno-suppressed patients

* Same dose as for normal hosts (see Chapter 13). If possible, give vaccines early in course of HIV infection, while immune system may still respond. Alternatively, to increase the likelihood of response in patients with advanced HIV disease, vaccines may be administered after 6-12 months of effective antiretroviral therapy. Vaccines should be given when patients are clinically stable, not acutely ill (e.g., give during a routine office visit, rather than during hospitalization for an opportunistic infection). Live vaccines (e.g., oral polio, oral typhoid, Yellow fever) are generally contraindicated, but measles vaccine is well-tolerated in children, and MMR vaccine is recommended for adults as described above

TREATMENT OF RESPIRATORY OPPORTUNISTIC INFECTIONS IN HIV

Antiretroviral therapy (ART) and specific antimicrobial prophylaxis regimens have led to a dramatic decline in HIV-related opportunistic infections. Today, opportunistic infections occur predominantly in patients not receiving ART (due to undiagnosed HIV infection or nonacceptance of therapy), or in the period after starting ART (due to lack of immune reconstitution or from eliciting a previously absent inflammatory host response). Despite high rates of virologic failure in clinical practice, the rate of opportunistic infections in patients compliant with ART remains low, presumably due to continued immunologic response despite virologic failure, a phenomenon that may be linked to impaired "fitness" (virulence) of resistant HIV strains. For patients on or off ART, the absolute CD4 cell count provides the best marker of risk for opportunistic infections. Diagnostic clues for community-acquired pneumonia based on chest x-ray and CD4 count are shown in Table 9.2.

Bacterial Pneumonia

Usual Pathogens	Preferred Therapy	Comments
S. pneumoniae (most common) H. influenzae P. aeruginosa S. aureus	**Combination therapy with** Ceftriaxone 1-2 gm (IV) q24h (or cefotaxime 1 gm [IV] q8h) *plus* azithromycin 500 mg q24h x 7-14 days **or monotherapy with** Levofloxacin 750 mg (PO/IV) q24h or moxifloxacin 400 mg (PO/IV) q24h x 7-14 days, depending on severity	For severe immunodeficiency (CD4 < 100/mm^3), neutropenia, or a prior history of pseudomonas infection, broaden coverage to include P. aeruginosa and other gram-negative bacilli by adding ceftazidime 1 gm (IV) q8h **or** cefepime 1 gm (IV) q12h **or** ciprofloxacin 750 mg (PO) q12h or 400 mg (IV) q8h

Clinical Presentation: HIV-infected patients with bacterial pneumonia present similar to those without HIV, with a relatively acute illness (over days) that is often associated with chills, rigors, pleuritic chest pain, and purulent sputum. Patients who have been ill over weeks to months are more likely have PCP, tuberculosis, or a fungal infection. Since bacterial pneumonia can occur at any CD4 cell count, this infection is frequently the presenting symptom of HIV disease, prompting initial HIV testing and diagnosis

Diagnostic Considerations: The most common pathogens are Streptococcus pneumoniae, followed by Haemophilus influenzae, Pseudomonas aeruginosa, and Staphylococcus aureus. The pathogens of atypical pneumonia (Legionella pneumophila, Mycoplasma pneumoniae, and Chlamydia pneumoniae) are rarely encountered, even with extensive laboratory investigation. A lobar infiltrate on chest radiography is a further predictor of bacterial pneumonia. Blood cultures should be obtained, as HIV patients have an increased rate of bacteremia compared to those without HIV

Pitfalls: Sputum gram stain and culture are generally only helpful if collected prior to starting antibiotics, and only if a single organism predominates. HIV patients with bacterial pneumonia may rarely have a more subacute opportunistic infection concurrently, such as PCP or TB

Therapeutic Considerations: Once improvement has occurred, a switch to oral therapy is generally safe. Patients with advanced HIV disease are at greater risk of bacteremic pneumonia due to gram-negative bacilli, and should be covered empirically for this condition

Prognosis: Response to therapy is generally prompt and overall prognosis is good

Invasive Pulmonary Aspergillosis

Pathogen	Preferred Therapy	Alternate Therapy
Aspergillus fumigatus (rarely other species)	Posaconazole 400 mg (PO) q12h until cured **or** Voriconazole 400 mg (IV or PO) q12h x 2 days, then 200 mg (IV or PO) q12h until cured (typically 6-18 months)	Amphotericin B deoxycholate 1 mg/kg (IV) q24h until 2-3 gm total dose given (optimal duration of therapy poorly defined) **or** Amphotericin B lipid formulations (Abelcet or Ambisome) 5 mg/kg/day (IV) until cured

Clinical Presentation: Pleuritic chest pain, hemoptysis, cough in a patient with advanced HIV disease. Additional risk factors include neutropenia and use of corticosteroids

Diagnostic Considerations: Diagnosis by bronchoscopy with biopsy/culture. Open lung biopsy (usually video-assisted thorascopic surgery) is sometimes required. Radiographic appearance includes cavitation, nodules, sometimes focal consolidation. Dissemination to CNS may occur, and manifests as focal neurological deficits

Pitfalls: Positive sputum culture for Aspergillus in advanced HIV disease should heighten awareness of possible infection

Therapeutic Considerations: Decrease/discontinue corticosteroids, if possible. If present, treat neutropenia with granulocyte-colony stimulating factor (G-CSF) to achieve absolute neutrophil count > 1000/mm^3. There are insufficient data to recommend chronic suppressive or maintenance therapy

Prognosis: Poor unless immune deficits can be corrected

Pneumocystis (carinii) jiroveci Pneumonia (PCP)

Subset	Preferred Therapy	Alternate Therapy
Mild or moderate disease (pO$_2$ > 70 mmHg, A-a gradient < 35)	TMP-SMX DS 2 tablets (PO) q8h x 21 days	Dapsone 100 mg (PO) q24h x 21 days plus TMP 5 mg/kg (PO) q8h x 21 days (less leukopenia/hepatitis vs. TMP-SMX) **or** Primaquine 30 mg (PO) q24h x 21 days plus clindamycin 300-450 mg (PO) q6h-q8h x 21 days **or** Atovaquone 750 mg (PO) q12h with food x 21 days **or** Trimetrexate 45 mg/m^2 or 1.2 mg/kg (IV) q24h x 21 days plus leucovorin 20 mg/m^2 or 0.5 mg/kg (IV or PO) q6h (leucovorin must be continued for 3 days after the last trimetrexate dose)
Severe disease (pO$_2$ < 70 mmHg, A-a gradient > 35)	TMP-SMX (5 mg/kg TMP) (IV) q6h x 21 days **plus** Prednisone 40 mg (PO) q12h on days 1-5, then 40 mg (PO) q24h on days 6-10, then 20 mg (PO) q24h on days 11-21. Methylprednisolone (IV) can be substituted at 75% of prednisone dose	Pentamidine 4 mg/kg (IV) q24h (infused over at least 60 minutes) x 21 days plus prednisone x 21 days. (Dose reduction of pentamidine to 3 mg/kg [IV] q24h may reduce toxicity)

Clinical Presentation: Fever, cough, dyspnea; often indolent presentation. Physical exam is usually normal. Chest x-ray is variable, but commonly shows a diffuse interstitial pattern. Elevated LDH and exercise desaturation are highly suggestive of PCP

Diagnostic Considerations: Diagnosis by immunofluorescent stain of induced sputum or bronchoscopy specimen. Check ABG if O$_2$ saturation is abnormal or respiratory rate is increased

Pitfalls: Slight worsening of symptoms is common after starting therapy, especially if not treated with steroids. Do not overlook superimposed bacterial pneumonia or other secondary infections, especially while on pentamidine. Patients receiving second-line agents for PCP prophylaxis—in particular aerosolized pentamidine—may present with atypical radiographic findings, including apical infiltrates, multiple small-walled cysts, pleural effusions, pneumothorax, or single/multiple nodules

Therapeutic Considerations: Outpatient therapy is possible for mild disease, but only when close follow-up is assured. Adverse reactions to TMP-SMX (rash, fever, GI symptoms, hepatitis, hyperkalemia, leukopenia, hemolytic anemia) occur in 25-50% of patients, many of whom will need a second-line regimen to complete therapy (e.g., trimethoprim-dapsone or atovaquone). Unless an adverse reaction to TMP-SMX is particularly severe (e.g., Stevens-Johnson syndrome or other life-threatening problem), TMP-SMX may be considered for PCP prophylaxis, since prophylaxis requires a much lower dose (only 10-15% of treatment dose). Patients being treated for severe PCP with TMP-SMX who do not improve after one week may be switched to pentamidine, although there are no prospective data to confirm this approach. In general, patients receiving antiretroviral therapy when PCP develops should have their treatment continued, since intermittent antiretroviral therapy can lead to drug resistance. For newly-diagnosed or antiretroviral-naive HIV patients, treatment of PCP may be completed before starting antiretroviral therapy. Steroids should be tapered (p. 121), not discontinued abruptly. Adjunctive steroids increase the risk of thrush/herpes simplex infection, but probably not CMV, TB, or disseminated fungal infection

Prognosis: Usually responds to treatment. Adverse prognostic factors include ↑ A-a gradient, hypoxemia, ↑ LDH

Pulmonary Tuberculosis (for isolates sensitive to INH and rifampin)

Pathogen	Patients NOT Receiving PI's or NNRTI's	Patients Receiving PI's or NNRTI's*
Mycobacterium tuberculosis (MTB)	Initial phase (8 weeks) INH 300 mg (PO) q24h **plus** rifampin† 600 mg (PO) q24h **plus** pyrazinamide (PZA) 25 mg/kg (PO) q24h **plus** ethambutol (EMB) 15-20 mg/kg (PO) q24h Continuation phase (18 weeks) INH 300 mg (PO) q24h **plus** rifampin† 600 mg (PO) q24h	Initial phase (8 weeks) INH 300 mg (PO) q24h **plus** rifabutin* **plus** PZA 25 mg/kg (PO) q24h **plus** EMB 15 mg/kg (PO) q24h x 8 weeks. Continuation phase (18 weeks) INH 300 mg (PO) q24h **plus** rifabutin*

*   Rifabutin dose: If PI is nelfinavir, indinavir, amprenavir or fosamprenavir, then rifabutin dose is 150 mg (PO) q24h. If PI is ritonavir, lopinavir/ritonavir or atazanavir, then rifabutin dose is 150 mg (PO) 2-3 times weekly. If NNRTI is efavirenz, then rifabutin dose is 450 mg (PO) q24h or 600 mg (PO) 2-3 times weekly. If NNRTI is nevirapine, then rifabutin dose is 300 mg (PO) q24h. Rifabutin is **contraindicated** in patients receiving delavirdine or hard-gel saquinavir. Patients receiving PI's AND NNRTI's: treat as above, except adjust rifabutin to 300 mg (PO) q24h.

†   For patients receiving triple NRTI regimens, substitute rifabutin 300 mg (PO) q24h for rifampin

Clinical Presentation: May present atypically. HIV patients with high (> 500/mm³) CD4 cell counts are more likely to have a typical pulmonary presentation, but patients with advanced HIV disease may have a diffuse interstitial pattern, hilar adenopathy, or a normal chest x-ray. Tuberculin skin testing (TST) is helpful if positive, but unreliable if negative due to anergy

Diagnostic Considerations: In many urban areas, TB is one of the most common HIV-related respiratory illnesses. In other areas, HIV-related TB occurs infrequently except in immigrants or patients arriving from highly TB endemic areas. Maintain a high Index of suspicion for TB in HIV patients with unexplained fevers/pulmonary infiltrates

Pitfalls: Extrapulmonary and pulmonary TB often coexist, especially in advanced HIV disease

Therapeutic Considerations: Treatment by directly observed therapy (DOT) is strongly recommended for all HIV patients. If patients have cavitary disease or either positive sputum cultures or lack of clinical response at 2 months, total duration of therapy should be increased up to 9 months. If hepatic transaminases are elevated (AST > 3 times normal) before treatment initiation, treatment options include: (1) standard therapy with frequent monitoring; (2) rifamycin (rifampin or rifabutin) + EMB + PZA for 6 months; or (3) INH + rifamycin + EMB for 2 months, then INH + rifamycin for 7 months. Once-weekly rifapentine is not recommended for HIV patients. Non-severe immune reconstitution inflammatory syndrome (IRIS) may be treated with nonsteroidal anti-inflammatory drugs (NSAIDs); severe cases should be treated with corticosteroids. In all cases of IRIS, antiretroviral therapy should be continued if possible. Monitor carefully for signs of rifabutin drug toxicity (arthralgias, uveitis, leukopenia)

Prognosis: Usually responds to treatment. Relapse rates are related to the degree of immunosuppression and local risk of re-exposure to TB

Table 9.2. Acute Community-Acquired Pneumonia in HIV: Diagnostic Clues Based on Chest X-Ray and CD4 Count

Chest X-Ray	CD4 Count	↑ A-a gradient[†]	Sputum AFB stain	Usual Pathogens
Focal pulmonary infiltrate	Normal/near normal	–	–	S. pneumoniae, H. influenzae, Legionella, Salmonella
		–	+	M. tuberculosis
	< 50/mm^3	–	+	MAI
Normal/near normal or diffuse pulmonary infiltrates	Normal/decreased	+	–	PCP, CMV, HSV
Multiple diffuse pulmonary infiltrates	< 50/mm^3	–	–	S. aureus, P. aeruginosa

† A-a gradient > 30
Adapted from: Cunha BA. Community-acquired pneumonia in patients with HIV. Drugs for Today. 31:739, 1998.

PNEUMONIAS IN ORGAN TRANSPLANTS

Patients with organ transplants are subject to the same pneumonia pathogens as in normal hosts. Although less common than typical bacterial pathogens, organ transplants are at increased risk of developing opportunistic infections related to the severity and type of immune defect (T-cell, B-cell, mixed). The immune defect may be caused by an underlying immune disorder and/or immunosuppressive drug therapy, and may be amplified by the presence of immunomodulating viruses, (e.g., CMV, HHV-6, EBV, HIV). Reactivation of latent infections, especially TB and HSV, accounts for the majority of opportunistic infections in transplant patients. Hospitalized transplant patients are also susceptible to outbreaks of Legionnaires' disease and aspergillosis. Most causes of nosocomial pneumonia in the days following transplantation are the same as for normal hosts who undergo surgery, and the type of pneumonia can often be predicted based on the post-transplant period (Tables 9.3, 9.4). Transplant patients harbor a variety of microorganisms that are variably suppressed as potential pathogens. These pathogens appear sequentially rather than simultaneously, so that only one potential transplant pathogen is clinically predominant at any given time. If the first pathogen is successfully treated or suppressed, subsequent pathogens will sequentially manifest themselves. Absent microbiological data, the rapidity of onset of pneumonia, the distribution of infiltrates on chest x-ray, and the presence or absence of an oxygen diffusion defect (↑ A-a gradient) in patients with diffuse pulmonary infiltrates can be used to establish a differential diagnosis (Tables 9.5, 9.6). Empiric therapy can often be administered for acute focal/segmental infiltrates. However, subacute or chronic infiltrates require a tissue diagnosis for specific therapy. Noninfectious mimics of pneumonia should be excluded (e.g., pulmonary drug reactions, pulmonary emboli, pulmonary hemorrhage).

Community-Acquired Pneumonia in Organ Transplants

Subset	Usual Pathogens*	Therapy
Focal/segmental infiltrates *Acute*	S. pneumoniae Legionella H. Influenzae	Treat the same as in normal hosts (Chapter 4)
Subacute	Aspergillus	Preferred Therapy Voriconazole (see "usual dose," p. 345) until cured¶ **or** Anidulafungin 200 mg (IV) x 1 dose, then 100 mg (IV) q24h until cured **or** Itraconazole 200 mg (IV) q12h x 2 days, then 200 mg (IV) q24h x 1-2 weeks, then 200 mg (PO) solution q12h until cured¶ **or** Posaconazole 400 mg (PO) q12h until cured **or** Caspofungin 70 mg (IV) x 1 dose, then 50 mg (IV) q24h x 1-2 weeks, then itraconazole 200 mg (PO) solution q12h until cured Alternate Therapy Lipid-associated amphotericin B (p. 279) (IV) q24h until cured **or** Amphotericin B deoxycholate 1 mg/kg (IV) q24h until 2-3 grams given
	M. tuberculosis	INH 300 mg (PO) q24h x 6 months **plus** Rifampin 600 mg (PO) q24h x 6 months **plus** PZA 25 mg/kg (PO) q24h x 2 months **plus** EMB 15 mg/kg (PO) q24h (until susceptibilities known)††
	C. neoformans	Preferred Therapy Fluconazole 800 mg (IV or PO) x 1 dose, then 400 mg (PO) q24h until cured Alternate Therapy Amphotericin B deoxycholate 0.5 mg/kg (IV) q24h until 1-2 grams given **or** Lipid-associated formulation of amphotericin B (p. 279) (IV) q24h x 3 weeks

Community-Acquired Pneumonia in Organ Transplants (cont'd)

Subset	Usual Pathogens*	Therapy
Diffuse infiltrates	S. stercoralis (hyperinfection syndrome)	<u>Preferred Therapy</u> Thiabendazole 25-50 mg/kg (PO) q12h (max. 3 gm/day) until cured <u>Alternate Therapy</u> Ivermectin 200 mcg/kg (PO) q24h until cured
	PCP, RSV, HHV-6	Treat PCP the same as in patients receiving chronic steroid therapy (see p. 130)
	CMV	Ganciclovir 5 mg/kg (IV) q12h until clinical improvement followed by valganciclovir 900 mg (PO) q12h until cured **plus** CMV immunoglobulin (CMV-IG) 500 mg/kg (IV) q48h x 2 weeks

*   Compromised hosts are predisposed to organisms listed, but may be infected by usual pathogens in normal hosts
¶   Significant drug interactions are possible when voriconazole or itraconazole is administered with usual immunosuppressive agents (e.g., tacrolimus). Review all concomitant medications for potential interactions

Focal or Segmental Pulmonary Infiltrates in Organ Transplants

Clinical Presentation: Acute or subacute community-acquired pneumonia (CAP) with respiratory symptoms and fever

Diagnostic Considerations: Bone marrow transplant (BMT)/solid organ transplant (SOT) patients with focal/segmental infiltrates are most commonly infected with the usual CAP pathogens affecting normal hosts (e.g., S. pneumoniae, H. influenzae, Legionella). The clinical presentation of CAP in organ transplants is indistinguishable from that in normal hosts. However, BMT/SOT patients presenting subacutely with focal/segmental infiltrates are usually infected with pulmonary pathogens with a slower clinical onset (e.g., Nocardia, Aspergillus). Empiric therapy will not cover all possible pathogens; tissue biopsy is necessary for definitive diagnosis and specific therapy. Preferred diagnostic modalities include transbronchial lung biopsy, percutaneous thin needle biopsy, or open lung biopsy, not BAL

Pitfalls: Patients presenting with subacute onset of CAP have a different pathogen distribution than those presenting with acute CAP. PCP/CMV does not present with focal/segmental infiltrates

Therapeutic Considerations: Bone marrow transplant (BMT)/Solid organ transplant (SOT) patients with acute onset of CAP are treated with the same antibiotics used to treat CAP in normal hosts. Empiric coverage is directed against both typical and atypical bacterial pathogens. If no improvement in clinical status after 72 hours, proceed to lung biopsy to identify non-bacterial pathogens (e.g., Nocardia, Aspergillus)

Prognosis: Best with acute focal/segmental infiltrates. Not as good with subacute or chronic focal/segmental infiltrates

Diffuse Pulmonary Infiltrates in Organ Transplants

Clinical Presentation: Insidious onset of interstitial pneumonia usually accompanied by low-grade fevers. Focal/segmental infiltrates are absent

Diagnostic Considerations: Bilateral diffuse infiltrates, which can be minimal or extensive, fall into two clinical categories: those with and without hypoxemia/↑ A-a gradient (> 30). Diffuse pulmonary infiltrates without hypoxemia suggest a noninfectious etiology (e.g., CHF, pulmonary drug reaction, pulmonary hemorrhage). The differential diagnosis of diffuse pulmonary infiltrates with hypoxemia includes PCP, CMV, HSV, RSV, others. For interstitial infiltrates with hypoxemia, the chest x-ray may be only minimally abnormal, but gallium/indium scans reveal intense bilateral, diffuse lung uptake, explaining the apparent discrepancy between clinical status and chest x-ray findings. RSV/HSV may be detected by specific monoclonal antibody tests of respiratory secretions. CMV/PCP require tissue biopsy for definitive diagnosis. A highly elevated LDH suggests the possibility of PCP. Transbronchial biopsy is preferable, but BAL may be used. The incidence of CMV pneumonia is highest in lung transplants. CMV has a predilection for infecting the transplanted organ. (T. gondii myocarditis is the most common opportunistic infection in the transplanted heart)

Pitfalls: Because infections in BMT/SOT are sequential, the majority of patients with PCP pneumonia may have underlying CMV as well. In BMT, CMV found alone on lung biopsy suggests it is the primary pathogen. Serological tests are unhelpful for CMV; a semiquantitative CMV antigenemic assay is preferred. Candida pneumonia does not exist as a separate entity but only as part of disseminated/invasive candidiasis

Therapeutic Considerations: Nocardia and Aspergillus should be treated aggressively until lesions resolve. Among the subacute diffuse pneumonias, PCP is readily treatable. Initiate treatment for CMV pneumonia with ganciclovir IV; after clinical improvement, complete therapy with valganciclovir (PO) until cured. If after treatment, there is an increase in CMV antigen levels, treat pre-emptively to prevent CMV pneumonia with valganciclovir 900 mg (PO) q24h until CMV antigen levels return to previous levels. Specific therapy exists for HSV and RSV but not adenovirus or HHV-6/7/8

Prognosis: Related to underlying immune status, promptness of therapy, and general health of host

Table 9.3. Post-Transplant Pneumonias

Period	Infections	Comments
Early period (< 1 month post-transplant)	Nosocomial pneumonia	Infections predominantly related to the surgical procedure
Middle period (1-6 months post-transplant)	Peak incidence of intracellular bacterial, viral, and fungal pathogens, including: • PCP • CMV • Aspergillus	Period of maximal immunosuppression to prevent transplant rejection. Peak effect of immunomodulating viruses (HHV-6, HBV/HCV, EBV, CMV) adds to net state of immunosuppression
Late period (≥ 6 months post-transplant) *Good graft function*	Same community-acquired respiratory infections as normal hosts	Transplant immunosuppressive therapy results in baseline immunosuppression
Poor graft function or rejection	Pathogens similar to middle post-transplant period, including: • PCP • CMV • Aspergillus	Intensive immunosuppressive therapy for rejection results in greater immunosuppression than organ transplants without rejection

Table 9.4. Infections in Heart Transplant Patients

Early transplant period (0-1 month)	Middle post-transplant period (1-6 months)	Late post-transplant period (> 6 months)
Surgical site infections Nosocomial infections (IV site, pneumonias, UTI's) HSV reactivation	CMV* HHV-6* PCP* HSV Histoplasmosis Coccidioidomycosis Cryptococcus Listeria Nocardia Toxoplasmosis Mycobacterial infections	Aspergillus* PCP Influenza Community-acquired pathogens CMV

* Most common pathogens

Table 9.5. Focal Pulmonary Infiltrates in Transplant Patients

Presentation	Nodular	Perihilar	Multifocal	Consolidation	Cavitation
Acute	Legionella	Heart failure PCP	Legionella Heart failure	Typical bacterial pneumonias Heart failure	Pseudomonas aeruginosa
Subacute or chronic	Aspergillus Nocardia Cryptococcus	RSV CMV	Aspergillus Nocardia TB	Aspergillus Nocardia Cryptococcus	Nocardia Aspergillus TB

Adapted from: Cunha BA. Pneumonias in the Compromised Host. Infect Dis Clin North Am. 2001;15:591-612.

Table 9.6. Diffuse Pulmonary Infiltrates in Transplant Patients

Presentation	Normal A-a gradient (< 30)	↑ A-a gradient (> 30)
Acute *Noninfectious*	Heart failure, pulmonary hemorrhage	ARDS
Infectious	Bacterial pneumonia, TB	PCP, CMV, HSV
Subacute/chronic *Noninfectious*	Drug-induced	BOOP, pulmonary fibrosis
Infectious	Nocardia, Aspergillus, Cryptococcus	RSV, HHV-6

Adapted from: Cunha BA. Pneumonias in the Compromised Host. Infect Dis Clin North Am. 2001;15:591-612.

PNEUMONIAS IN CHRONIC STEROID THERAPY

Corticosteroids are widely used as antiinflammatory agents for a variety of disorders, including rheumatological diseases, immune anemias, asthma, COPD, and interstitial lung disease. They are also important agents to prevent/treat transplant rejection. Steroid use results in lymphocytopenia with a selective depletion of circulating T-lymphocytes, which in turn results in impaired cell-mediated immunity. Consequently, patients receiving chronic high-dose steroids are at increased risk of pneumonias caused by intracellular bacterial, viral, and fungal pathogens, including TB, Legionella, Nocardia, Aspergillus, CMV, HSV, RSV, Strongyloides stercoralis, toxoplasmosis, and PCP. These patients may also develop reactivation fungal pneumonias caused by one of the endemic mycoses (e.g., Histoplasma, Coccidioides, Cryptococcus, Blastomyces). The clinical approach to pneumonias in patients receiving chronic steroid therapy is similar to that of the transplant patient (pp. 124-129). Absent microbiological data, the rapidity of onset of pneumonia and the distribution of infiltrates on chest x-ray can be used to generate a differential diagnosis (Table 9.7). Empiric therapy can often be administered for acute focal or segmental pneumonias. However, subacute or chronic infiltrates require a tissue diagnosis (tissue biopsy rather than respiratory secretion or BAL culture) for specific therapy. Noninfectious mimics of pneumonia should be excluded (e.g., pulmonary embolism, pulmonary hemorrhage/infarction).

Pneumonias in Chronic Steroid Therapy

Subset	Usual Pathogens*	Preferred IV Therapy	Alternate IV Therapy	IV-to-PO Switch
Chronic steroid therapy (If perihilar infiltrates/ hypoxemia, treat as PCP until lung biopsy)	Aspergillus	Posaconazole 400 mg (PO) q12h¶ **or** Voriconazole (see "usual dose," p. 345)¶ **or** Anidulafungin 200 mg (IV) x 1 dose, then 100 mg (IV) q24h¶ **or** Caspofungin 70 mg (IV) x 1 dose, then 50 mg (IV) q24h¶	Amphotericin B deoxycholate 1 mg/kg (IV) q24h until 2-3 grams **or** Lipid-associated formulation of amphotericin B (p. 279) (IV) q24h x 4-6 weeks **or** Itraconazole 200 mg (IV) q12h x 2 days, then 200 mg (IV) q24h¶	Voriconazole (see "usual dose," p. 345)¶ **or** Posaconazole 400 mg (PO) q12h¶ **or** Itraconazole 200 mg (IV) q12h x 2 days, then 200 mg (PO) solution q12h†¶
	P. (carinii) jiroveci (PCP)	TMP-SMX 5 mg/kg (IV) q6h x 3 weeks	Pentamidine 4 mg/kg (IV) q24h x 3 weeks	TMP-SMX 5 mg/kg (PO) q6h x 3 weeks

Duration of therapy represents total time IV, PO, or IV + PO. Most patients on IV therapy able to take PO meds should be switched to PO therapy soon after clinical improvement
* *Compromised hosts are predisposed to organisms listed, but may be infected by usual pathogens in normal hosts*
† *Loading dose is not needed PO if given IV with the same drug*
¶ *Treat until cured*

Pneumonia with Chronic Steroid Therapy
If fungal infection is suspected, obtain lung biopsy to confirm diagnosis/identify causative organism. Non-responsiveness to appropriate antibiotics should suggest fungal infection. Avoid empirically treating fungi; due to the required duration of therapy, it is advantageous to confirm the diagnosis by lung biopsy first. Prognosis related to degree of immunosuppression

Acute Aspergillus Pneumonia
Clinical Presentation: Chest x-ray shows progressive necrotizing pneumonia unresponsive to antibiotic therapy. No characteristic appearance on chest x-ray. Usually seen only in compromised hosts
Diagnostic Considerations: Diagnosis by lung biopsy (not broncho-alveolar lavage) demonstrating hyphae invading lung parenchyma/blood vessels. Usually occurs only in patients receiving chronic steroids or cancer chemotherapy, organ transplants, leukopenic compromised

hosts, or patients with chronic granulomatous disease
Pitfalls: Aspergillus pneumonia does not occur in normal hosts
Prognosis: Almost always fatal despite appropriate therapy

Pneumocystis (carinii) jiroveci pneumonia (PCP): *see p. 121*

Table 9.7. Pneumonia in Organ Transplants and Patients on Chronic Steroid Therapy: Diagnostic Clues Based on Chest X-Ray

Infiltrate	Causes
Focal/segmental *Acute*	Bacterial pneumonia, Legionella, pulmonary embolism/infarct, CHF
Subacute/chronic	Aspergillosis, Nocardia, cryptococcus, TB/MAI, reactivation of systemic mycoses (histoplasmosis, blastomycosis, etc.)
Bilateral/diffuse *Acute*	PCP, CHF, ARDS, pulmonary hemorrhage, influenza
Subacute/chronic	RSV, CMV, HHV-6, miliary TB, drug-induced pneumonitis, radiation pneumonitis, leukagglutinin reaction, oxygen toxicity, lymphangitic spread (malignancy), bronchiolitis obliterans organizing pneumonia (BOOP), sarcoidosis, idiopathic pulmonary fibrosis

REFERENCES AND SUGGESTED READINGS

Abernathy-Carver KJ, Fan LL, Boguniewicz M, et al. Legionella and Pneumocystis pneumonia in asthmatic children on high doses of systemic steroids. Pediatr Pulmonol. 18:135-138, 1994.

Alsiua AE, Krisiunas L, Rosenburg RJ, et al. Value of 111-indium leukocyte scanning in febrile organ transplant patients. Clin Transplant. 5:368-372, 1991.

Arya B, Hussian S, Hariharan S. Rhodococcus equi pneumonia in a renal transplant patient: a case report and review of literature. Clin Transplant. 18:748-752, 2004.

Balthesen M, Messerie M, Reddehase MJ. Lungs are a major organ site of cytomegalovirus latency and recurrence. J Virol. 67:5360-5366, 1993.

Bozzette SA, Finkelstein DM, Spector SA, et al. A randomized trial of three antipneumocystis agents in patients with advanced human immunodeficiency virus infection. NIAID AIDS Clinical Trials Group. N Engl J Med 332:693, 1995.

Bozzette SA, Sattler FR, Chiu J, et al. A controlled trial of early adjunctive treatment with corticosteroids for Pneumocystis carinii pneumonia in the acquired immunodeficiency syndrome. California Collaborative Treatment Group. N Engl J Med 323:1451, 1990.

Brosgart CL, Louis TA, Hillman DW, et al. A randomized, placebo-controlled trial of the safety and efficacy of oral ganciclovir for prophylaxis of cytomegalovirus disease in HIV-infected individuals. AIDS 12:269-277, 1998.

Chakinala MM, Trulock EP. Pneumonia in the solid organ transplant patient. Clin Chest Med. 26:113-121, 2005.

Clift RA, Buckner CD, Fever A, et al. Infectious complications of marrow transplantation. Transplant Proc. 6:389-393, 1974.

Colonna JO II, Winston DJ, Brill JE, et al. Infectious complications in liver transplantation. Arch Surg. 123:360-364, 1988.

Cunha BA. Community-acquired pneumonia in HIV patients. Clinical Infectious Diseases. 28:410, 1999.

Cunha BA. Community-acquired pneumonia in patients with HIV. Drugs for Today. 31:739, 1998.

Cunha BA. Community-acquired pneumonias in SLE. Journal of Critical Illness 13:779-783, 1997.

Cunha BA. Infections in the nonleukopenic compromised host in critical care. Crit Care Clin. 14:263-282, 1998.

Cunha BA. Pneumonias in the compromised host. Infect Dis Clin North Am. 15:591-612, 2001.

Denning DW. Invasive aspergillosis. Clin Infect Dis. 26:781-803, 1998.

Dowell ST, Bresee JS. Severe varicella associated with steroid use. Pediatrics. 92:1223-1228, 1993.

Emery VC. Human herpes viruses 6 and 7 in solid organ transplant recipients. Clin Infect Dis. 32:1357-1360, 2001.

Englund JA, Whimbey E, Atmar RL. Diagnosis of respiratory viruses in cancer and transplant patients. Curr Clin Top Infect Dis. 19:30-59, 2003.

Feldman S. Varicella zoster virus pneumonitis. Chest 106:

(Suppl):22S-27S, 1994.

Fishman JA, Rubin RH. Infection in organ-transplant recipients. N Engl J Med. 338:1741-1751, 1998.

Flynn JD, Akers WS, Jones M, et al. Treatment of respiratory syncytial virus pneumonia in a lung transplant recipient: case review of the literature. Pharmacotherapy. 24:932-938, 2004.

Fraser TG, Zembower TR, Lynch P, et al. Cavitary Legionella pneumonia in a liver transplant recipient. Transpl Infect Dis. 6:77-80, 2004.

Gallant JE, Chaisson RE, Moore RD. The effect of adjunctive corticosteroids for the treatment of Pneumocystis carinii pneumonia on mortality and subsequent complications. Chest 114:1258, 1998.

Gregg A, Chapman R, Szer J. Fatal CMV pneumonia associated with steroid therapy after autologous transplantation in patients previously treated with fludarabine. Bone Marrow Transplant. 21:619-621, 1998.

Gustafson TL, Schaffner W, Lavely GB, et al. Invasive aspergillosis in renal transplant recipients: Correlation with corticosteroid therapy. J Infect Dis. 148:230-238, 1983.

Hammer SM, Saag MS, Schechter M, et al. Treatment for Adult HIV Infection. JAMA 296:827-843, 2006.

Hardy WD, Feinberg J, Finkelstein DM, et al. For the AIDS Clinical Trials Group. A controlled trial of trimethoprim-sulfamethoxazole or aerosolized pentamidine for secondary prophylaxis of Pneumocystis carinii pneumonia in patients with the acquired immunodeficiency syndrome: AIDS Clinical Trials Group protocol 021. N Engl J Med. 327:1842-1848, 1992.

Igra-Siegman Y, Kapila R, Sen P, et al. Syndrome of hyperinfection with Strongyloides stercoralis. Respir Infect Dis. 3:397-407, 1981.

Kasper WJ, Howe PM. Fatal varicella after a single course of corticosteroids. Pediatr Infect Dis J. 9:729-732, 1999.

Keenan GF. Management of complications of glucocorticoid therapy. Clin Chest Med. 18:507-520, 1997.

Kim HA, Yoo CD, Balk HJ, et al. Mycobacterium tuberculosis infection in a corticosteroid treated rheumatic disease patient population. Clin Exp Rheumatol. 16:9-13, 1998.

Klein NC, Go CH, Cunha BA. Infections associated with steroid use. Infect Dis Clin North Am. 15:423-432, 2001.

Leather HL, Wingard JR. Infectious following hematopoietic stem cell transplantation. Infect Dis Clin North Am. 15:483-520, 2001.

Lederman ER, Crum NF. A case series and focused review of nocardiosis: clinical and microbiologic aspects. Medicine (Baltimore). 83:300-313, 2004.

Lester RS, Knowles SR, Shear NH. The risk of systemic corticosteroid use. Dermatol Clin. 16:277-288, 1998.

Luft BJ, Naot Y, Araujo FG, et al. Primary and reactivated Toxoplasma infection in patients with cardiac transplants. Ann Intern Med. 99:27-31, 1983.

McEvoy CE, Niewoehner DE. Adverse effects of corticosteroid therapy for COPD: A critical review. Chest. 111:732-743, 1997.

Montoya JG, Giraldo LF, Efron B, et al. Infectious complications among 620 consecutive heart transplant patients at Stanford University Medical Center. Clin Infect Dis. 33:629-640, 2001.

Nenoff P, Horn LC, Mierzwa M, et al. Peracute disseminated fatal Aspergillus fumigatus sepsis as a complication of corticoid treated systemic lupus erythematosus. Mycoses. 38:467-471, 1995.

Ng TT, Robson GD, Denning DW. Hydrocortisone enhanced growth of Aspergillus spp: Implications for pathogenesis. Microbiology. 140:2475-2479, 1994.

Nicholson KG, Wood JM, Zambon M. Influenza. Lancet 362:1733-45, 2003.

Patterson JE. Epidemiology of fungal infectious in solid organ transplant patients. Transpl Infect Dis. 1:229-236, 1999.

Patterson TF. Approaches to fungal diagnosis in transplantation. Transpl Infect Dis. 1:262-272, 1999.

Paya CV, Hermans PE, Washington JA II, et al. Incidence, distribution, and outcome of episodes of infection in 100 orthotopic liver transplantations. Mayo Clin Proc. 64:555-564, 1989.

Paya CV. Prevention of cytomegalovirus disease in recipients of solid-organ transplants. Clin Infect Dis. 15:596-603, 2001.

Petri WA Jr. Infections in heart transplant recipients. Clin Infect Dis. 18:141-148, 1994.

Ramsey PG, Rubin RH, Tolkoff-Rubin NE, et al. The renal transplant patient with fever and pulmonary infiltrates: Etiology, clinical manifestations, and management. Medicine (Baltimore). 59:206-222, 1980.

Rubin RH. Impact of cytomegalovirus infections on organ transplant recipients. Rev Infect Dis. 12:754-766, 1990.

Rubin RH. Preemptive therapy in immunocompromised hosts. N Engl J Med. 324:1057-1059, 1991.

Sax PE. Opportunistic infections in HIV disease: down but not out. Infectious Disease Clinics of North America. 15:433-455, 2001.

Schaeffer MW, Buell JF, Gupta M, et al. Strongyloides hyperinfection syndrome after heart transplantation: case report and review of the literature. J Heart Lung Transpl. 23:905-911, 2004.

Scowden EB, Schaffner W, Stone WJ. Overwhelming strongyloidiasis: An unappreciated opportunistic infection. Medicine (Baltimore). 57:527-544, 1978.

Sia IG, Wilson KA, Groettum CM, et al. Cytomegalovirus (CMV) DNA load predicts relapsing CMV infection after solid organ transplantation. J Infect Dis. 181:717-720, 2000.

Simon DM, Levin S. Infectious complications of solid organ transplantations. Infect Dis Clin North Am. 15:521-549, 2001.

Stanbury RM, Graham EM. Systemic corticosteroid therapy: Side effects and their management. Br J Ophthalmol. 82:704-708, 1988.

Star SE. Varicella in children receiving steroids for asthma: Risks and management. Pediatr Infect Dis J. 11:419-420, 1992.

Stein DK, Sugar AM. Fungal infections in the immuno-compromised host. Diagn Microbiol Infect Dis. 12:221S-228S, 1989.

Stuck AE, Minder CE, Frey FJ. Risk of infectious complications in patients taking glucocorticosteroid. Rev Infect Dis. 11:954-963, 1989.

Sterneck M, Ferrell L, Ascher N, et al. Mycobacterial infection after liver transplantation: A report of three cases and review of the literature. Clin Transplant. 6:55-61, 1992.

Tarver RD, Teague SD, Heitkamp DE, et al. Radiology of community-acquired pneumonia. Radiol Clin North Am. 43:497-512, 2005.

Thomas, CF Jr., Limper AH. Pneumocystis pneumonia. N Engl J Med. 350:2487-98, 2004.

Tolkoff-Rubin NE, Rubin RH. Recent advances in the diagnosis and management of infection in the organ transplant recipient. Semin Nephrol. 20:148-163, 2000.

Wallace JR, Luchi M. Fatal cytomegalovirus pneumonia in a patient receiving corticosteroids and methotrexate for mixed connective tissue diseases. South Med J. 89:726-728, 1996.

Wang BY, Krishnan S, Isenberg HD. Mortality associated with concurrent strongyloidosis and cytomegalovirus infection in a patient on steroid therapy. Mt Sinai J Med. 66:128-132, 1999.

Wiggins RE Jr. Invasive aspergillosis: A complication of treatment of temporal arteritis. J Neuroophthalmol. 15:36-38, 1995.

Winston DJ, Gale RP, Meyer DV, et al. Infectious complications of human bone marrow transplantation. Medicine (Baltimore). 58:1-31, 1979.

Zaas AK, Alexander BD. New developments in the diagnosis and treatment of infections in lung transplant recipients. Respir Care Cline N Am. 10:531-547, 2004.

Zamora M. Cytomegalovirus and lung transplantation. Am J Transplant. 4:1219-1226, 2004.

GUIDELINES

Benson CA, Kaplan JE, Masur H, et al. Treating Opportunistic Infections Among HIV-Infected Adults and Adolescents: Recommendations from CDC, the National Institutes of Health, and the HIV Medicine Association/ Infectious Diseases Society of America. Clin Infect Dis 40:S131-235, 2005.

Panel on Clinical Practices for Treatment of HIV Infection. Guidelines for the Use of Antiretroviral Agents in HIV-Infected Adults and Adolescents. Department of Health and Human Services. www.aidsinfo.nih.gov/guidelines/. December 1, 2007.

TEXTBOOKS

Bartlet JG (ed). The Johns Hopkins hospital guide to medical care of patients with HIV infection, 10th Edition, Lippincott Williams & Wilkins, Philadelphia, 2002.

Bartlet JG, et al. A pocket guide to adult HIV/AIDS treatment, Health Resources and Services Administration, Fairfax, 2004.

Bowden RA, Ljungman P, Paya CV (eds). Transplant Infections, 2nd Edition. Philadelphia, Lippincott Williams & Wilkins, 2003.

Dolin R, Masur H, Saag MS (eds). AIDS Therapy, 2nd Edition. Churchill Livingstone, New York, 2003.

Gorbach SL, Bartlett JG, Blacklow NR, et al. Infectious Diseases, 3rd Edition. Philadelphia, Lippincott, Williams & Wilkins, 2004.

Grieco MH. Infections in the abnormal host. New York, Yorke Medical Books, 1980.

Ho M. Cytomegalovirus: Biology and Infection, 2nd Edition. Plenum Medical Book Co, New York, 1991.

Mandell GL, Bennett JE, Dolin R, et al. Mandell, Douglas, and Bennett's principles and practice of infectious diseases, 6th Edition. Philadelphia, Elsevier, 2005.

Parrillo JE, Masur H. The critically ill immunosuppressed patient: diagnosis and management. Rockville, MD, Aspen Publishers, Inc., 1987.

Rubin RH, Young LS, et al. Clinical approach to infection in the compromised host, 3rd Edition. Plenum Medical Book Co, New York, 1994.

Sax P, Cohen C, Kuritzkes D (eds). HIV Essentials, Physicians' Press, Royal Oak, MI, 2007.

Singh N, Aguado JM, et al. Infectious complications in transplant patients. Kluwer Academic Publishers, 2000.

St. Georgiev V. Infectious diseases in the immuno-compromised host. Boca Raton, CRC Press, 1998.

Tenholder MF (ed). Approach to pulmonary disease in the immunocompromised host. Mount Kisco, NY, Futura Publishing Company, Inc., 1991.

Wingard RJ, Bowden RA. Management of infection in oncology patients. London, Martin Dunitz Taylor & Francis Group, 2003.

Wormser GP (ed). AIDS, 4th Edition, Elsevier, Philadelphia, 2004.

Chapter 10

Pneumonias in Children

Leonard R. Krilov, MD
George H. McCracken, Jr, MD

Community-Acquired Pneumonia (CAP) in Children

Subset (age)	Usual Pathogens	IV Therapy[†]	PO Therapy or IV-to-PO Switch[†]
Birth to 20 days	Group B streptococci Gram-negative enteric bacteria CMV	Ampicillin **plus either** gentamicin **or** cefotaxime x 10-21 days	Not applicable
3 weeks to 3 months	RSV Parainfluenza 3	None (supportive care)	None
	C. trachomatis S. pneumoniae B. pertussis S. aureus	Cefotaxime **or** ceftriaxone **or** cefuroxime x 10-14 days*. Alternative: ampicillin or clindamycin*	<u>Afebrile:</u> Erythromycin x 14 days **or** azithromycin x 5-7 days. <u>Lobar, febrile:</u> Amoxicillin **or** amoxicillin/ clavulanic acid **or** cefdinir **or** cefuroxime **or** cefpodoxime x 10-14 days
> 3 months to < 5 years	Viruses (RSV, parainfluenza, influenza, adenovirus, rhinoviruses)	<u>RSV:</u> consider ribavirin. For infants at highest risk for severe RSV infection, consider palivizumab 15 mg/kg/month x 1-2 seasons for prevention <u>Influenza:</u> amantadine (influenza A) or oseltamivir (influenza A, B). Routine immunization for infants 6-23 months of age	
	S. pneumoniae H. influenzae M. pneumoniae M. tuberculosis	Cefuroxime **or** ceftriaxone **or** cefotaxime x 10-14 days*	Amoxicillin **or** amoxicillin-clavulanate **or** clarithromycin **or** azithromycin x 10-14 days
5-15 years	M. pneumoniae C. pneumoniae S. pneumoniae M. tuberculosis	Cefuroxime **or** ceftriaxone **or** cefotaxime x 10-14 days*	Erythromycin **or** clarithromycin **or** azithromycin **or** doxycycline (age > 8 years) x 10-14 days
Pertussis	Bordetella spp.[‡] Adenovirus M. pneumoniae C. trachomatis C. pneumoniae	Erythromycin x 14 days **or** azithromycin x 5 days	Erythromycin x 14 days **or** clarithromycin x 7 days **or** azithromycin x 5 days. If macrolide-intolerant: TMP-SMX x 14 days

Duration of therapy represents total time IV or IV, PO, or IV + PO.
† **See pp. 141-143 for drug dosages**
* If chronic cough of more insidious onset, consider adding IV or PO macrolide (azithromycin, clarithromycin, erythromycin) to cover Pertussis/C. trachomatis (3 weeks-3 months of age), Mycoplasma (3 months - 5 years of age), or Mycoplasma/C. pneumoniae (5-15 years of age)
‡ B. pertussis, B. parapertussis, B. bronchiseptica

Community-Acquired Pneumonia

Clinical Presentation: Fever ± dyspnea, cough, tachypnea with infiltrates on chest x-ray
Diagnostic Considerations: Usual pathogens differ by age. In neonates, pneumonia is typically diffuse and part of early-onset sepsis. In young infants, there is significant overlap between signs and symptoms of bronchiolitis (due to RSV) and pneumonia. Severe pneumonia is usually due to bacterial infection, although the organism is frequently not isolated (e.g., blood cultures are positive in only 10-20% of children < 2 years of age with bacterial pneumonia). In young infants, Chlamydia trachomatis can be detected by antigen assay or culture of nasopharyngeal (NP) secretions. Mycoplasma pneumonia, diagnosed by cold agglutinins and IgG/IgM serologies, peaks at 5-15 years of age, although cases in children < 5 years have been reported. Respiratory viruses (RSV, influenza, adenoviruses, parainfluenza viruses) can also be detected in NP secretions. If child lives in area with high prevalence of tuberculosis, consider tuberculosis in the differential diagnosis of primary pneumonia
Pitfalls: Reliance on upper airway specimen for gram stain/culture leads to misdiagnosis and mistreatment, as true deep sputum specimen is rarely obtainable in children
Therapeutic Considerations: Therapy is primarily empiric based on child's age, clinical/epidemiologic features and chest x-ray findings. Mycoplasma requires 2-3 weeks of treatment; C. pneumoniae may require up to 6 weeks of treatment. Routine use of conjugated pneumococcal vaccine (Prevnar) has decreased the incidence of pneumococcal pneumonia
Prognosis: Varies with pathogen, clinical condition at presentation, and underlying health status. Prognosis is worse in children with chronic lung disease, congenital heart disease, immunodeficiency, neuromuscular disease, hemoglobinopathy

Lower Respiratory Tract Viral Infections

Clinical Presentation: Viruses cause the majority of lower respiratory tract infections (LRTIs) in children. Respiratory syncytial virus (RSV) is the leading cause of LRTI in young infants, manifesting as bronchiolitis/viral pneumonia and causing annual mid-winter epidemics. The risk of secondary bacterial infection (other than possibly otitis media) is very low. Fever is typically low grade and usually improves over 3-5 days, even if hospitalized. Influenza viruses are another major cause of winter epidemic LRTIs in children of all ages. Hospitalization rates in infants under one year of age rival those in the > 65 year old population. Characteristic findings include high fever and diffuse inflammation of the airways. Young infants may have prominent GI symptoms as well. Secondary bacterial infection (otitis media, pneumonia, sepsis) are frequent complications of influenza. Primary influenza pneumonia, encephalopathy, and myocarditis are rare, severe complications. Other respiratory viruses associated with LRTIs in children include parainfluenza type 3 (viral pneumonia), parainfluenza types 1 and 2 (croup), adenoviruses, and the newly identified human metapneumovirus (hmpv)
Diagnostic Considerations: Viral syndromes are often diagnosed based on clinical assessment alone. For confirmation or in more severe cases, rapid diagnosis by antigen detection (direct fluorescent antibody staining, ELISA, PCR) and/or viral culture are readily available
Pitfalls: Routine use of corticosteroids or bronchodilators in RSV bronchiolitis are not supported by clinical evidence. Overuse of the diagnosis of "flu" (e.g., stomach flu, summer flu) has led to diluted appreciation for true influenza and its severity. Influenza vaccine has been traditionally underutilized in high-risk children

Therapeutic Considerations: For most viral LRTIs treatment is primarily supportive (e.g., adequate hydration, fever control, supplemental oxygen for severe illness). Ribavirin is approved for RSV infection but is rarely used due to uncertain clinical benefit, high cost, and cumbersome method of administration (prolonged aerosol). For infants at greatest risk of severe RSV disease (e.g., premature infants, infants with underlying chronic lung disease or congenital heart disease), monthly prophylaxis with palivizumab (Synagis) 15 mg/kg/month (IM) decreases RSV hospitalization rates. Per American Academy of Pediatrics guidelines, palivizumab is indicated for infants with chronic lung disease or congenital heart disease who are ≤ 24 months of age at start of RSV season. For premature infants, palivizumab is considered based on a combination of gestational age (GA) and chronological age (CA): GA ≤ 28 weeks plus CA ≤ 12 months; GA 29-32 weeks plus CA ≤ 6 months; GA 33-35 weeks plus CA ≤ 6 months plus 2 or more additional risk factors, including day care attendance, school-age siblings, cigarette smoke exposure, neuromuscular disease, or congenital airway anomalies. Annual influenza vaccination is indicated for high-risk children, including those > 6 months of age with asthma, metabolic disease, hemoglobinopathies, immunocompromised state, renal disease, or heart disease. Children who live with high-risk individuals (e.g., adult > 65 years of age, infant < 6 months of age, immunocompromised host) should also receive influenza vaccine. Additionally the ACIP, AAP, and AAFP recommend routine immunization for all children 6-23 months of age. The antiviral drugs amantadine (influenza A only) and oseltamivir (influenza A and B strains) have pediatric indications and can be used for treatment or prophylaxis as in adults

Prognosis: Most children with viral LRTIs do well and recover without sequelae. Infants hospitalized with RSV infection have higher rates of wheezing episodes over the next 10 years. The highest rates of hospitalization from influenza occur in children < 2 years of age and in the elderly

Pertussis

Clinical Presentation: Upper respiratory tract symptoms (congestion, rhinorrhea) over 1-2 weeks (catarrhal stage) progressing to paroxysms of cough (paroxysmal stage) lasting 2-4 weeks, often with a characteristic inspiratory whoop, followed by a convalescent stage lasting 1-2 weeks during which cough paroxysms decrease in frequency and severity. Fever is low grade or absent. In children < 6 months, whoop is frequently absent and apnea may occur. Duration of classic pertussis is 6-10 weeks. Older children and adults may present with persistent cough (without whoop) lasting 2-6 weeks. Complications include seizures, secondary bacterial pneumonia, encephalopathy, death; risk of complications is greatest in children < 1 year

Diagnostic Considerations: Diagnosis is usually based on nature of cough and duration of symptoms. Laboratory diagnosis may be difficult. A positive culture for Bordetella pertussis from a nasopharyngeal swab inoculated on fresh selective media is diagnostic, but the organism is difficult to recover after 3-4 weeks of illness. Direct fluorescent antibody (DFA) staining of nasopharyngeal secretions is available, but sensitivities/specificities are variable to poor. Leukocytosis with lymphocytosis may be present in pertussis but can occur in response to other respiratory pathogens

Pitfalls: Be sure to consider pertussis in older children and adults with prolonged coughing illness. Family contacts of index case should receive post-exposure antimicrobial prophylaxis. Virtually all children should be vaccinated against pertussis. Rare contraindications to pertussis vaccination include anaphylaxis to a prior dose or encephalopathy within 7 days of a dose. Relative precautions to further pertussis immunization include: seizure within 3 days of a dose; persistent, severe, inconsolable crying for ≥ 3 hours within 48 hours of a dose; collapse or shock-like state within 48 hours of a dose; or temperature of ≥ 40.5 C without other cause within 48 hours of a dose

Therapeutic Considerations: Infants < 6 months frequently require hospitalization. By the paroxysmal stage, antibiotics have minimal effect on the course of the illness but are still indicated to decrease transmission. An association has been made between oral erythromycin and infantile hypertrophic pyloric stenosis in infants < 6 weeks of age; consider an alternative macrolide (azithromycin or clarithromycin) in these cases

Prognosis: Good. Despite the prolonged course, long-term pulmonary sequelae have not been described after pertussis. Children < 1 year are at greatest risk of morbidity and mortality, although mortality rates remain very low

Tuberculosis

Subset	Pathogen	PO or IM Therapy (see next page for drug dosages)
Latent infection (positive PPD, clinically well, negative chest x-ray)	M. tuberculosis	INH x 9 months **or** rifampin x 6 months (if INH-resistant)
Pulmonary and extrapulmonary TB (except meningitis)	M. tuberculosis	INH **plus** rifampin **plus** PZA x 2 months followed by INH **plus** rifampin x 4 months[†]
Meningitis	M. tuberculosis	INH **plus** rifampin **plus** PZA **plus either** streptomycin (IM) **or** ethionamide x 2 months, followed by INH **plus** rifampin x 7-10 months (i.e., 9-12 months total therapy)
Congenital	M. tuberculosis	INH **plus** rifampin **plus** PZA **plus** streptomycin (IM)

Duration of therapy represents total time IV or IV, PO, or IV + PO. Most patients on IV therapy able to take PO meds should be switched to PO therapy after clinical improvement

† *If drug resistance is a concern, EMB or streptomycin (IM) is added to the initial regimen until drug susceptibilities are determined*

Pneumonia Essentials

TB Drug	Daily dosage (mg/kg)	Twice weekly dosage (mg/kg)
Isoniazid (INH)	10-15	20-30
Rifampin	10-20	10-20
Ethambutol (EMB)	15-25	50
Pyrazinamide (PZA)	20-40	50
Streptomycin	20-40 (IM)	—
Ethionamide	15-20 (in 2-3 divided doses/day)	—

Alternative drugs (capreomycin, ciprofloxacin, levofloxacin, cycloserine, kanamycin, para-aminosalicylic acid) are used less commonly and should be administered in consultation with an expert in the treatment of tuberculosis

Clinical Presentation: Most children diagnosed with tuberculosis have asymptomatic infection detected by tuberculin skin testing. Symptomatic disease typically presents 1-6 months after infection with fever, growth delay, weight loss, night sweats, and cough. Extrapulmonary involvement may present with meningitis, chronic mastoiditis, lymphadenopathy, bone, joint, or skin involvement. Renal tuberculosis and reactivation cavitary disease are rare in children but may be seen in adolescents

Diagnostic Considerations: A positive tuberculin skin test indicates likely infection with M. tuberculosis. Tuberculin reactivity develops 2-12 weeks after infection. The definition of a positive skin test reaction is based on age, immune status, risk of exposure, and degree of suspicion of tuberculosis disease. Children < 8 years old cannot produce sputum for AFB smear and culture; specimens for analysis can be obtained by collecting 3 consecutive morning gastric aspirates

Pitfalls: Tuberculosis may be missed if not considering the diagnosis in children at increased epidemiological risk for exposure. Tuberculous meningitis often presents insidiously with nonspecific irritability and lethargy weeks prior to the development of frank neurological defects

Therapeutic Considerations: Choice of initial therapy depends on stage of disease and likelihood of resistant organisms (based on index case, geographical region of acquisition). For HIV-infected patients, duration of therapy is prolonged to ≥ 12 months. For tuberculosis meningitis and miliary disease, the addition of corticosteroids to anti-TB therapy is beneficial

Prognosis: Varies with extent of disease, drug resistance and underlying immune status, but is generally good for pulmonary disease in children. Bone infection may result in orthopedic sequelae (e.g., Pott's disease of the spine with vertebral collapse). The prognosis for meningitis is guarded once focal neurological deficits and persistent depression of mental status occur

Common Pediatric Antimicrobial Drugs

Drug	Dosage in Neonates	Dosage in Infants/Children*
Amoxicillin	Not indicated	22.5-45 mg/kg (PO) q12h
Amoxicillin-clavulanate	Not indicated	22.5-45 mg/kg (of amoxicillin component) (PO) q12h
Ampicillin	25-50 mg/kg/dose (IV or IM). <u>Severe Group B streptococcal sepsis</u>: 100 mg/kg/dose. Dosing interval is based on gestational age (GA) and chronological age (CA):	25-50 mg/kg (IV or IM) q6h

GA + CA (weeks)	CA (days)	Interval (hours)
≤ 29	0-28 > 28	12 8
30-36	0-14 >14	12 8
≥ 37	0-7 > 7	12 8

Drug	Dosage in Neonates	Dosage in Infants/Children*
Azithromycin	Not indicated	<u>Otitis media/sinusitis</u>: 30 mg/kg (PO) x 1 dose **or** 10 mg/kg (PO) q24h x 3 days **or** 10 mg/kg (PO) on day 1 followed by 5 mg/kg (PO) q24h on days 2-5 <u>Pharyngitis/tonsillitis</u>: 12 mg/kg (PO) q24h x 5 days <u>Community-acquired pneumonia</u> (not indicated for moderate or severe disease): 10 mg/kg (IV or PO) on day 1 followed by 5 mg/kg (IV or PO) q24h on days 2-5
Cefdinir	Not indicated	7 mg/kg (PO) q12h **or** 14 mg/kg (PO) q24h
Cefotaxime	50 mg/kg (IV or IM). (25 mg/kg/dose is adequate for gonococcal infection). See *ampicillin* for dosing interval	25-50 mg/kg (IV or IM) q6-8h
Cefpodoxime	Not indicated	5 mg/kg (PO) q12h

Common Pediatric Antimicrobial Drugs

Drug	Dosage in Neonates	Dosage in Infants/Children*
Ceftriaxone[‡]	<u>Sepsis and disseminated gonococcal infection</u>: 50 mg/kg (IV or IM) q24h. <u>Meningitis</u>: 100 mg/kg loading dose followed by 80 mg/kg (IV or IM) q24h	50 mg/kg (IV or IM) q24h. <u>Meningitis</u>: 50 mg/kg (IV or IM) q12h. <u>Acute otitis media</u>: 50 mg/kg (IM) x 1 dose (or 3 doses IM q24h in high-risk patients)
Cefuroxime axetil	Not indicated	10-15 mg/kg (PO) q12h 25-50 mg/kg (IV or IM) q8h
Clarithromycin	Not indicated	7.5 mg/kg (PO) q12h
Clindamycin	5.0-7.5 mg (IV or PO). Dosing interval is based on gestational age (GA) and chronological age (CA):	5-10 mg/kg (IV or IM) q6-8h or 10-30 mg/kg/day (PO) divided q6-8h

GA + CA (weeks)	CA (days)	Interval (hours)
< 29	0-28 > 28	12 8
30-36	0-14 > 14	12 8
37-44	0-7 > 7	8 6

Drug	Dosage in Neonates	Dosage in Infants/Children*
Doxycycline	Contraindicated	> 45 kg: 100 mg (PO) q12h ≤ 45 kg: 1.1-2.5 mg/kg (PO) q12h Use only in children > 8 years 1-2 mg/kg (IV) q12-24h
Erythromycin	<u>Chlamydia pneumonitis/conjunctivitis or pertussis</u>: 12.5 mg/kg (PO) q6h (E. estolate preferred). <u>Other infections</u>: E. estolate 10 mg/kg (PO) q8h **or** E. ethylsuccinate 10 mg/kg (PO) q6h <u>Severe infections and PO not possible</u>: 5-10 mg/kg (IV over ≥ 60 min) q6h	10-12.5 mg/kg (PO) q6-8h 5-12.5 mg/kg (IV) q6h

Common Pediatric Antimicrobial Drugs

Drug	Dosage in Neonates	Dosage in Infants/Children*
Gentamicin**	*During first week of life* dosing is based on gestational age (administer IV dose over 30 min): • ≤ 29 weeks (or asphyxia, PDA, or indomethacin): 5 mg/kg (IV) q48h • 30-33 weeks: 4.5 mg/kg (IV) q48h • 34-37 weeks: 4 mg/kg (IV) q36h • ≥ 38 weeks: 4 mg/kg (IV) q24h *After first week of life*: Initial dose of 4 mg/kg, then draw serum concentrations 30 min after end of infusion (peak) and 12-24 hours later (trough) to determine dosing interval. Aim for peak of 5-12 mcg/mL and trough of 0.5-1 mcg/mL.	2-2.5 mg/kg (IV or IM) q8h
Trimethoprim-sulfameth-oxazole	Contraindicated	Pneumocystis carinii pneumonia (PCP) 5 mg/kg (PO) q6h (typically after initial IV therapy). *IV dosing*: PCP or severe infection: 5 mg/kg (of trimethoprim component) (IV) q6h; minor infections: 4-6 mg/kg (of trimethoprim component) (IV) q12h

* Dosages are generally based on weight (mg/kg), up to adult dose as maximum
** Drug can be given IM but absorption may be variable

REFERENCES AND SUGGESTED READINGS

Cunha BA. Therapeutic implications of antibacterial resistance in community-acquired respiratory tract infections in children. Infection 32:98-108, 2004.

Donnelly LF. Imaging in immunocompetent children who have pneumonia. Radiol Clin North Am 43:253-65, 2005.

Haas H. Antibiotic therapy in children with atypical bacterial infections. Arch Pediatr 12(Suppl1)S45-8, 2005.

Hammerschlag MR. Pneumonia due to chlamydia pneumoniae in children: epidemiology, diagnosis, and treatment. Pediatr Pulmonol 36:384-90, 2003.

Korppi M. Community-acquired pneumonia in children: issues in optimizing antibacterial treatment. Paediatr Drugs 5:821-32. 2003.

McCracken GH Jr. Diagnosis and management of pneumonia in children. Pediatr Infect Dis J 19:924-8, 2000.

McCracken GH Jr. Etiology and treatment of pneumonia. Pediatr Infect Dis J. 19:373-7, 2000.

McIntosh K. Community-acquired pneumonia in children. N Engl J Med 7;346:429-37, 2002.

Ostapchuk M, Roberts DM, Haddy R. Community-acquired pneumonia in infants and children. Am Fam Physician. 1;70:899-908, 2004.

Panitch HB. Evaluation of recurrent pneumonia. Pediatr Infect Dis J 24:265-6, 2005.

Pelton SI, Hammerschlag MR. Overcoming current obstacles in the management of bacterial community-acquired pneumonia in ambulatory children. Clin Pediatr (Phila) 44:1-17, 2005.

Schuchat A, Dowell SF. Pneumonia in children in the developing world: new challenges, new solutions. Semin Pediatr Infect Dis 15:181-9, 2004.

Scola BL, Maltezou H. Legionella and Q fever community acquired pneumonia in children. Paediatr Respir Rev 5(Suppl A):S171-7, 2004.

Sinaniotis CA, Sinaniotis AC. Community-acquired pneumonia in children. Curr Opin Pulm Med 11:218-225, 2005.

Steinhoff M, Black R. Childhood pneumonia: we must move forward. Lancet 369:1409-10, 2007.

TEXTBOOKS

Christian CG (ed). Infections in immunocompromised infants and children. New York, Churchill Livingstone, 1992.

Feigin RD, Cherry JD (eds). Textbook of pediatric infectious diseases. 2nd Edition, Philadelphia, WB Saunders Company, 1987.

Krugman S, Katz SL, Gershon AA (eds), et al. Infectious diseases of children. 9th Edition, St. Louis, Mosby Year Book, 1992.

Long SS, Pickering LK, Prober CG. Principles and practice of pediatric infectious diseases. 2nd Edition, New York, Churchill Livingstone, 2003.

Remington JS, Klein JO (eds). Infectious Diseases of the fetus and newborn infant. 6th Edition, Philadelphia, WB Saunders Company, 2006.

Chapter 11
Chest X-Ray Atlas

Burke A. Cunha, MD
Douglas S. Katz, MD

This atlas has been developed to assist in the management of patients who present with respiratory symptoms and chest x-ray abnormalities. Sixteen common chest x-ray patterns are provided. Common infectious and noninfectious etiologies are followed by usual clinical features, which can be used to identify the disorder and help guide empiric/specific therapy.

Chest X-Ray Patterns

REFERENCES AND SUGGESTED READINGS

Burgener FA, Kormano M. Differential Diagnosis in Conventional Radiology, 2nd ed. Stuttgart, Georg Thieme Verlag, 1991.

Chapman S, Nakielny R. Aids to Radiological Differential Diagnosis, 2nd ed. London, Bailliere Tindall, 1990.

Conn RB, Borer WZ, Snyder JW. Current Diagnosis 9. Philadelphia, W. B. Saunders Company, 1997.

Crapo JD, Glassroth J, Karlinsky JB, King TE. Baum's Textbook of Pulmonary Diseases, 7th ed. Philadelphia, Lippincott Williams & Wilkins, 2004.

Eisenberg RL. Clinical Imaging. An Atlas of Differential Diagnosis, 2nd ed. Gaithersburg, Aspen Publishers, Inc., 1992.

Gorbach SL, Bartlett JG, Blacklow NR. Infectious Diseases, 3rd ed. Philadelphia, Lippincott Williams & Wilkins, 2004.

Karetzky M, Cunha BA, Brandstetter. The Pneumonias. New York, Springer-Verlag, 1993.

Kasper L, Braunwald E, Fauci AS, Hauser SL, Longo DL, Jameson JL. Harrison's Principles of Internal Medicine, 16th ed. New York, The McGraw Hill Companies, 2004.

Levison ME. The Pneumonias: Clinical Approaches to Infectious Diseases of the Lower Respiratory Tract. Boston, John Wright, PSG Inc., 1984.

Lillington GA, Jamplis RW. A Diagnostic Approach to Chest Diseases, 2nd ed. Baltimore, The Williams & Wilkins Company, 1977.

Mandell GL, Bennet JE, Dolin R. Mandell, Douglas, and Bennett's Principles and Practice of Infectious Diseases, 6th ed., Elsevier, 2005.

Murray JF, Nadel JA. Textbook of Respiratory Medicine, 3rd ed. Philadelphia, W.B. Saunders Company, 2000.

Teplick JE, Haskin ME. Roentgenologic Diagnosis, 3rd ed. Philadelphia, W. B. Saunders Company, 1976.

Wright FW. Radiology of the Chest and Related Conditions. London, Taylor & Francis, 2002.

UNILATERAL FOCAL SEGMENTAL/LOBAR INFILTRATE WITHOUT EFFUSION

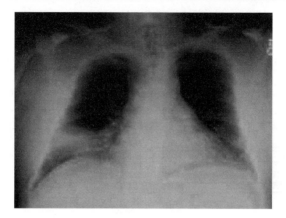

Infectious Causes

Causes	Features (may have some, none, or all)			
	History	**Physical**	**Laboratory**	**Chest X-Ray**
S. pneumoniae	Elderly, smokers, COPD, ↓ humoral immunity (multiple myeloma, SLE, CLL, hyposplenism).	Fever, chills, no relative bradycardia. Chest signs related to extent of consolidation.	↑ WBC, ↓ platelets (overwhelming infection/ hyposplenism), normal LFTs. Sputum with abundant PMNs and gram-positive diplococci. Blood cultures usually positive.	Consolidation usually limited to one lobe (RLL most common) ± air bronchogram. Pleural effusion very common. Empyema uncommon. No cavitation.
H. influenzae	Recent contact with H. influenzae URI.	Fever, chills.	↑ WBC. Sputum/ pleural effusion with gram-negative pleomorphic bacilli. Blood cultures often positive.	Usually RLL with small/moderate effusion. No empyema. No cavitation.
M. catarrhalis	Chronic/heavy smoker, COPD.	Nonspecific.	Sputum with gram-negative/variable diplococci. Blood cultures negative.	Usually lower lobe ± consolidation. No pleural effusion or cavitation.

Infectious Causes

Causes	Features (may have some, none, or all)			
	History	Physical	Laboratory	Chest X-Ray
K. pneumoniae	Nosocomial pneumonia or history of alcoholism in patient with community-acquired pneumonia.	Fever, chills, signs of alcoholic cirrhosis, signs of consolidation over involved lobe.	↑ WBC, ↓ platelets, ↑ SGOT/SGPT (2° to alcoholism). "Red currant jelly" sputum with PMNs and plump gram-negative encapsulated bacilli.	"Bulging fissure" sign secondary to expanded lobar volume. Empyema rather than pleural effusion. Cavitation in 5-7 days (thick walled).
Legionella	Recent contact with Legionella containing water. Usually elderly. May have watery diarrhea, abdominal pain, mental confusion.	Fever/chills, relative bradycardia. Hepatic/splenic enlargement goes against the diagnosis. ↓ breath sounds if consolidation or pleural effusion.	↑ WBC, ↑SGOT/SGPT, ↓PO_4^-, ↓Na^+, ↑CPK, ↑ESR, ↑CPR, proteinuria, microscopic hematuria, L. pneumophila antigenuria (serotype I only) may not be positive early. Mucoid/purulent sputum with few PMNs. Positive sputum DFA (before therapy) is diagnostic. ↑ Legionella titer ≥ 1:256 or ≥ 4-fold rise between acute and convalescent titers.	Rapidly progressive asymmetrical infiltrates clue to Legionella. Consolidation and pleural effusion not uncommon. Cavitation rare.
Psittacosis	Recent bird contact with psittacine birds. Severe headache.	Fever/chills, ± relative bradycardia, Horder's spots on face, epistaxis, ± splenomegaly. Signs of consolidation common.	↑/normal WBC, ↑LFTs. Sputum with few PMNs. Positive C. psittaci serology.	Dense infiltrate. Consolidation common. Pleural effusion/cavitation rare.
Q fever	Recent contact with sheep or parturient cats.	Fever/chills, ± relative bradycardia, splenomegaly, ± hepatomegaly.	↑/normal WBC, ↑LFTs. Sputum with no bacteria/few PMNs (caution–biohazard). Acute Q fever with ↑ in phase II ELISA antigens.	Dense consolidation. Cavitation/pleural effusion rare.

Non-Infectious Causes

Causes	Features (may have some, none, or all)			
	History	Physical	Laboratory	Chest X-Ray
Atelectasis	Ineffectual moist recurrent cough characteristic of post-operative atelectasis.	Fevers ≤ 102°F. If large, signs of volume loss (↓ respiratory excursion, ↑ diaphragm, mediastinum shift toward affected side). If small, ↓ breath sounds over affected segment/lobe.	↑ WBC (left shift), normal platelets. Other lab results related to underlying cause of atelectasis.	Segmental infiltrate. RUL/RML atelectasis obscures right heart border. In LUL atelectasis, may be triangular infiltrate extending to upper anterior mediastinum mimicking malignancy. LLL atelectasis causes ↑ density of heart shadow. No cavitation or pleural effusion.
Pulmonary embolus/ infarct	Acute onset dyspnea/pleuritic chest pain. History of lower extremity trauma, stasis or hypercoagulable disorder.	↑ pulse/ respiratory rate.	↑ fibrin split products and D-dimers ± ↑ total bilirubin. Bloody pleural effusion. ECG with RV strain/P-pulmonale (large embolus). Positive V/Q scan and CT pulmonary angiogram.	Normal or show non-specific pleural-based infiltrates resembling atelectasis. Focal segmental/lobar hyperlucency (Westermark's sign) in some. "Hampton's hump" with infarct. Resolving infarcts ↓ in size but maintain shape/density ("melting ice cube").
Lymphoma	Fever, ↓ appetite with weight loss, night sweats, fatigue.	Adenopathy ± splenomegaly.	Normal WBC, ↑ basophils, ↑ eosinophilia, ↓ lymphocytes, ↑ platelets, ↑ESR, ↑ alkaline phosphatase, ↑ $\propto_{1,2}$ globulins on SPEP.	Unilateral or asymmetrical bilateral hilar adenopathy. Lung infiltrate may appear contiguous with hilar adenopathy. No clear channel between mediastinum and hilar nodes. Small pleural effusions rare.

Non-Infectious Causes

Causes	Features (may have some, none, or all)			
	History	Physical	Laboratory	Chest X-Ray
Alveolar cell carcinoma	Fever, ↑ appetite with weight loss, night sweats.	± dullness over lobe with large lower lobe lesions.	Positive cytology by BAL/lung biopsy.	Well/ill-defined circumscribed peripheral infiltrates ± air bronchograms. May be multifocal/multilobar. Hilar adenopathy present. Stranding to the hilum ("pleural tail" sign). ± pleural effusion if lower lobe infiltrate. No cavitation.
Aspiration pneumonia	Swallowing disorder 2° to CNS/GI disorder; impaired consciousness; recent aspiration 2° to dental, upper GI, or pulmonary procedure.	Unremarkable.	↑ WBC, ↑ESR.	Infiltrate usually involves superior segments of lower lobes (or posterior segments of upper lobes if aspiration occurred supine). Focal infiltrate initially, which may be followed in 7 days by cavitation/lung abscess.

UNILATERAL FOCAL SEGMENTAL/LOBAR INFILTRATE WITH EFFUSION

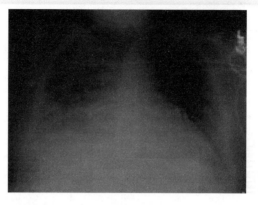

Infectious Causes

Causes	Features (may have some, none, or all)			
	History	**Physical**	**Laboratory**	**Chest X-Ray**
Klebsiella pneumoniae	Nosocomial pneumonia or history of alcoholism in patient with community-acquired pneumonia.	Fever, chills, signs of alcoholic cirrhosis, signs of consolidation over involved lobe.	↑ WBC, ↓ platelets, ↑SGOT/SGPT (2° to alcoholism). "Red currant jelly" sputum with PMNs and plump gram-negative encapsulated bacilli.	"Bulging fissure" sign secondary to expanded lobar volume. Empyema rather than pleural effusion. Usually cavitation in 5-7 days (thick walled).
H. influenzae	Recent contact with H. influenzae URI.	Fever, chills.	↑ WBC. Sputum/ pleural effusion with gram-negative pleomorphic bacilli. Blood cultures often positive.	Usually RLL with small/moderate effusion. No empyema. No cavitation.
TB (primary)	Recent TB contact.	Unilateral lower lobe dullness related to size of pleural effusion.	PPD (−)/anergic. Exudative pleural effusion (pleural fluid with ↑ lymphocytes, ↑ glucose, ± RBCs).	Lower lobe infiltrate with small/moderate pleural effusion. No cavitation or apical infiltrates. Hilar adenopathy asymmetrical when present.

Infectious Causes

Causes	Features (may have some, none, or all)			
	History	Physical	Laboratory	Chest X-Ray
Coccidio-mycosis (chronic)	Previous exposure in endemic coccidiomycosis areas. Asymptomatic.	± E. nodosum.	Normal WBC, no eosinophilia in chronic phase. Complement fixation IgG titer ≥ 1:32 indicates active disease.	Thick/thin-walled cavities < 3 cm ± calcifications. Air fluid level rare unless secondarily infected. Cavities usually in anterior segments of upper lobes (vs. posterior segments with TB). No surrounding tissue reaction. Pleural effusion common.
Tularemia	History of recent deer fly, rabbit, or tick exposure. Tularemia pneumonia may complicate any of the clinical presentations of tularemia.	Fever, chills, no relative bradycardia. Chest findings related to extent of infiltrate/ consolidation and pleural effusion.	Normal/↑ WBC, normal LFTs. Sputum/pleural effusion with gram-negative coccobacilli (caution – biohazard). Bloody pleural effusion. Tularemia serology with ↑ microagglutination titer ≥ 1:160 acutely and ≥ 4-fold rise between acute and convalescent titers.	Pleural effusion ± hilar adenopathy.
Adenovirus	Recent URI.	Fever, chills, myalgias. Sore throat and conjunctivitis not associated with adenoviral pneumonia. Chest exam with signs of consolidation.	↑ adenoviral titers and positive adenoviral cultures of respiratory secretions.	Ill-defined infiltrate(s) without cavitation ± pleural effusion.

Infectious Causes

Causes	Features (may have some, none, or all)			
	History	Physical	Laboratory	Chest X-Ray
Legionella	Recent contact with Legionella containing water. Usually elderly. May have watery diarrhea, abdominal pain, mental confusion.	Fever/chills, relative bradycardia. Hepatic/ splenic enlargement goes against the diagnosis. ↓ breath sounds if consolidation or pleural effusion.	↑ WBC, ↑SGOT/SGPT, ↓PO_4^-, ↓Na^+, ↑CPK, ↑ESR, ↑CPR, proteinuria, microscopic hematuria, L. pneumophila antigenuria (serotype I only) may not be positive early. Mucoid/purulent sputum with few PMNs. Positive sputum DFA (before therapy) is diagnostic. ↑ Legionella titer ≥ 1:256 or ≥ 4-fold rise between acute/convalescent titers.	Rapidly progressive asymmetrical infiltrates clue to Legionella. Consolidation and pleural effusion not uncommon. Cavitation rare.
Group A streptococci	Recent exposure or recent blunt chest trauma ± chest pain.	Fever/chills. Physical signs related to size of pleural effusion.	↑ WBC. Pleural fluid is serosanguineous. Sputum/pleural fluid with gram-positive cocci in pairs/chains. Positive pleural fluid/blood cultures.	Unilateral infiltrate may be obscured by large pleural effusion. No empyema. No cavitation.
Rhodococcus equi	Insidious onset of fever, dyspnea, chest pain, ± hemoptysis. Immuno-suppressed patients with ↓ cell-mediated immunity or exposure to cattle, horses, pigs.	Unremarkable.	Normal/↑ WBC. Sputum/pleural fluid with gram-positive pleomorphic weakly acid-fast bacilli. Sputum, pleural fluid, blood cultures positive for R. equi.	Segmental infiltrate with upper lobe predominance ± cavitation. Air-fluid levels and pleural effusion common.

Non-Infectious Causes

Causes	Features (may have some, none, or all)			
	History	Physical	Laboratory	Chest X-Ray
Pulmonary embolus/ infarct	Acute onset dyspnea/pleuritic chest pain. History of lower extremity trauma, stasis or hypercoagulable disorder.	↑ pulse/ respiratory rate.	↑ fibrin split products and D-dimers ± ↑ total bilirubin. Bloody pleural effusion. ECG with RV strain/P-pulmonale (large embolus). Positive V/Q scan and CT pulmonary angiogram.	Normal or show non-specific pleural-based infiltrates resembling atelectasis. Focal segmental/lobar hyperlucency (Westermark's sign) in some. "Hampton's hump" with infarct. Resolving infarcts ↓ in size but maintain shape/density ("melting ice cube").
Lymphoma	Fever, ↓ appetite with weight loss, night sweats, fatigue.	Adenopathy ± splenomegaly.	Normal WBC, ↑ basophils, ↑ eosinophilia, ↓ lymphocytes, ↑ platelets, ↑ESR, ↑ alkaline phosphatase, ↑ $\propto_{1,2}$ globulins on SPEP.	Unilateral or asymmetrical bilateral hilar adenopathy. Lung infiltrate may appear contiguous with hilar adenopathy. No clear channel between mediastinum and hilar nodes. Small pleural effusions rare.
Alveolar cell carcinoma	Fever, ↑ appetite with weight loss, night sweats.	± dullness over lobe with large lower lobe lesions.	Positive cytology by BAL/lung biopsy.	Well/ill-defined circumscribed peripheral infiltrates ± air bronchograms. May be multifocal/multilobar. Hilar adenopathy present. Stranding to the hilum ("pleural tail" sign). ± pleural effusion if lower lobe infiltrate. No cavitation.
Radiation pneumonitis	History of mantle radiation for lymphoma, lung cancer, or breast cancer.	Nonspecific.	Nonspecific.	Symmetrical infiltrates in the distribution of radiation therapy after 1 month. Infiltrates have "straight edges" ± air bronchograms. Fibrosis common over radiation field after 9-12 months. Usually no pleural effusions (small, if present).

UNILATERAL ILL-DEFINED INFILTRATES WITHOUT EFFUSION

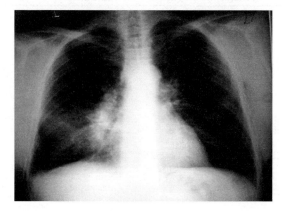

Infectious Causes

Causes	Features (may have some, none, or all)			
	History	**Physical**	**Laboratory**	**Chest X-Ray**
Mycoplasma pneumoniae	Prolonged dry/nonproductive cough. No laryngitis. Mild sore throat/ear. Watery diarrhea.	Usually fevers ≤ 102° F without relative bradycardia. Myalgias, bullous myringitis or otitis, non-exudative pharyngitis, E. multiforme. Chest exam with rales and no signs of consolidation or effusion.	Normal/↑ WBC; normal platelets, LFTs, PO_4^-, CPK. ↑ cold agglutinins (early). ↑ IgM (not IgG) Mycoplasma pneumoniae titers. Respiratory secretions culture positive for Mycoplasma pneumoniae.	Ill-defined usually lower lobe indistinct infiltrates. No consolidation or air bronchograms. Small/no pleural effusion.

Infectious Causes

| Causes | Features (may have some, none, or all) | | | |
	History	Physical	Laboratory	Chest X-Ray
Chlamydophilia (Chlamydia) pneumoniae	Prolonged "mycoplasma-like" illness with laryngitis.	Low-grade fevers, myalgias, non-exudate pharyngitis, laryngitis. No relative bradycardia, ear findings, or rash. Chest exam without signs of consolidation or pleural effusion.	↑ WBC, normal platelets, normal LFTs. No cold agglutinins. ↑ IgM (not IgG) C. pneumoniae titers. Respiratory secretions culture positive for C. pneumoniae.	Ill-defined, usually lower lobe indistinct infiltrate(s). May be "funnel shaped." No consolidation, cavitation, or pleural effusion.
Adenovirus	Recent URI.	Fever, chills, myalgias. Sore throat and conjunctivitis not associated with adenoviral pneumonia. Chest exam with signs of consolidation.	↑ adenoviral titers and positive adenoviral cultures of respiratory secretions.	Ill-defined infiltrate(s) without cavitation ± pleural effusion.
Legionella	Recent contact with Legionella containing water. Usually elderly. May have watery diarrhea, abdominal pain, mental confusion.	Fever/chills, relative bradycardia. Hepatic/ splenic enlargement goes against the diagnosis. ↓ breath sounds if consolidation or pleural effusion.	↑ WBC, ↑SGOT/SGPT, ↓PO$_4^-$, ↓Na$^+$, ↑CPK, ↑ESR, ↑CPR, proteinuria, microscopic hematuria, L. pneumophila antigenuria (serotype I only) may not be positive early. Mucoid/purulent sputum with few PMNs. Positive sputum DFA (before therapy) is diagnostic. ↑ Legionella titer ≥ 1:256 or ≥ 4-fold rise between acute/convalescent titers.	Rapidly progressive asymmetrical infiltrates clue to Legionella. Consolidation and pleural effusion not uncommon. Cavitation rare.

Infectious Causes

Causes	Features (may have some, none, or all)			
	History	Physical	Laboratory	Chest X-Ray
Psittacosis	Recent bird contact with psittacine birds. Severe headache.	Fever/chills, ± relative bradycardia, ± Horder's spots on face, epistaxis, ± splenomegaly. Signs of consolidation common.	↑/normal WBC, ↑LFTs. Sputum with few PMNs. Positive C. psittaci serology.	Dense infiltrate. Consolidation common. Pleural effusion/ cavitation rare.
Q fever	Recent contact with sheep or parturient cats.	Fever/chills, ± relative bradycardia, splenomegaly, ± hepatomegaly.	↑/normal WBC, ↑LFTs. Sputum with no bacteria/few PMNs (caution– biohazard). Acute Q fever with ↑ in phase II ELISA antigens.	Dense consolidation. Cavitation/pleural effusion rare.
Nocardia	Fevers, night sweats, fatigue, ↓ cell-mediated immunity (e.g., HIV, organ transplant, immunosuppressive therapy).	Unremarkable.	Normal/↑ WBC, ↑ESR. Sputum with gram-positive AFB.	Dense large infiltrates. May cavitate and mimic TB, lymphoma, or squamous cell carcinoma. No calcification ± pleural effusion.
Actinomycosis	Recent dental work.	± chest wall sinus tracts.	Normal/↑ WBC, ↑ESR. Sputum with gram-positive filamentous anaerobic bacilli.	Dense infiltrates extending to chest wall. No hilar adenopathy. Cavitation rare. ± pleural effusion rare.
Cryptococcus neoformans	Exposure to air conditioner or pigeons.	Unremarkable.	Normal WBC. Cryptococcal serology with ↑ C. neoformans antigen levels.	Dense lower nodular mass lesions. No calcification or cavitation. ± pleural effusion.

Infectious Causes

Causes	Features (may have some, none, or all)			
	History	Physical	Laboratory	Chest X-Ray
Aspiration pneumonia	Swallowing disorder 2° to CNS/GI disorder; impaired consciousness; recent aspiration 2° to dental, upper GI, or pulmonary procedure.	Unremarkable.	↑ WBC, ↑ESR.	Infiltrate usually involves superior segments of lower lobes (or posterior segments of upper lobes if aspiration occurred supine). Focal infiltrate initially, which may be followed in 7 days by cavitation/ lung abscess.

Non-Infectious Causes

Causes	Features (may have some, none, or all)			
	History	Physical	Laboratory	Chest X-Ray
Bronchogenic carcinoma	Fever, ↓ appetite with weight loss, cough ± hemoptysis. Cough with copious clear/ mucoid sputum in large cell anaplastic carcinoma. Increased risk in smokers, aluminum/ uranium miners, cavitary lung disease (adeno-carcinoma), previous radiation therapy from lymphoma/breast cancer.	Paraneoplastic syndromes especially with small (oat) cell/squamous cell carcinoma ± hypertrophic pulmonary osteoarthropathy.	Normal/↑ WBC, ↑ platelets, ↑ESR, findings related to underlying malignancy, ± clubbing.	Small/squamous cell carcinomas present as central lesions/ hilar masses. Adenocarcinoma/ large cell anaplastic carcinomas are usually peripheral initially. "Tumor tendrils" extending into surrounding lung tissue is characteristic. No calcifications (may be present on chest CT). Cavitation with squamous cell carcinoma. ± pleural effusions.

Non-Infectious Causes

Causes	Features (may have some, none, or all)			
	History	Physical	Laboratory	Chest X-Ray
Lymphangitic metastases	History of breast, thyroid, pancreas, cervical, prostate, or lung carcinoma.	Findings related to underlying malignancy.	Normal/↑ WBC, ↑ESR.	Interstitial indistinct pulmonary infiltrates (may be reticulonodular) with lower lobe predominance Usually unilateral but may be bilateral. No consolidation or cavitation ± pleural effusions.
Lung contusion	Recent closed chest trauma, chest pain.	Chest wall contusion over infiltrate.	↑ WBC (left shift).	Patchy ill-defined infiltrate(s) ± rib fractures/ pneumothorax in area of infiltrate. Infiltrate clears within 1 week.
Congestive heart failure	Coronary heart disease, valvular heart disease, cardiomyopathy.	No/low-grade fevers ↑ pulse and respiratory rate, positive jugular venous distension and hepatojugular reflex, cardio-megaly, S_3, ascites, hepatomegaly, pedal edema.	↑ WBC (left shift), normal platelets, mildly ↑ SGOT/ SGPT.	Cardiomegaly, pleural effusion (R > [R + L] > L). Kerley B lines with vascular redistribution to upper lobes. Typically bilateral rather than unilateral.
Alveolar cell carcinoma	Fever, ↑ appetite with weight loss, night sweats.	± dullness over lobe with large lower lobe lesions.	Positive cytology by BAL/lung biopsy.	Well/ill-defined circumscribed peripheral infiltrates ± air bronchograms. May be multifocal/ multilobar. Hilar adenopathy present. Stranding to the hilum ("pleural tail" sign). ± pleural effusion if lower lobe infiltrate. No cavitation.

Non-Infectious Causes

Causes	Features (may have some, none, or all)			
	History	Physical	Laboratory	Chest X-Ray
Lymphoma	Fever, ↓ appetite with weight loss, night sweats, fatigue.	Adenopathy ± splenomegaly.	Normal WBC, ↑ basophils, ↑ eosinophilia, ↓ lymphocytes, ↑ platelets, ↑ESR, ↑ alkaline phosphatase, ↑ $\propto_{1,2}$ globulins on SPEP.	Unilateral or asymmetrical bilateral hilar adenopathy. Lung infiltrate may appear contiguous with hilar adenopathy. No clear channel between mediastinum and hilar nodes. Small pleural effusions rare.
Pulmonary hemorrhage	History of closed chest trauma or hemorrhagic disorder.	↑ WBC (left shift), ↑ pulse rate, ↑ respiratory rate. Signs of closed chest trauma.	Anemia plus findings secondary to underlying hemorrhagic disorder.	Localized or diffuse fluffy alveolar infiltrate(s). No cavitation, consolidation, or effusion.
Systemic lupus erythematosus (SLE)	Fatigue, chest pain. History of SLE.	Fever/myalgias, alopecia, malar rash, "cytoid bodies" in retina, painless oral ulcers, synovitis, splenomegaly, generalized adenopathy, Raynaud's phenomenon.	↑ ANA, ↑ DS-DNA, ↓ C_3, polyclonal gammopathy on SPEP, ↑ ferritin. Pleural fluids with ↑ ANA, ↓ C_3	Migratory ill-defined non-segmental infiltrates ± small pleural effusions. No consolidation or cavitation.
Aspiration pneumonia	Swallowing disorder 2° to CNS/GI disorder; impaired consciousness; recent aspiration 2° to dental, upper GI, or pulmonary procedure.	Unremarkable.	↑ WBC, ↑ESR.	Infiltrate usually involves superior segments of lower lobes (or posterior segments of upper lobes if aspiration occurred supine). Focal infiltrate initially, which may be followed in 7 days by cavitation/ lung abscess.

UNILATERAL ILL-DEFINED INFILTRATES WITH EFFUSION

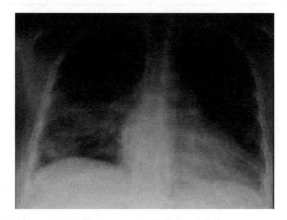

Infectious Causes

Causes	Features (may have some, none, or all)			
	History	Physical	Laboratory	Chest X-Ray
TB (primary)	Recent TB contact.	Unilateral lower lobe dullness related to size of pleural effusion.	PPD anergic. Exudative pleural effusion (pleural fluid with ↑ lymphocytes, ↑ glucose, ± RBCs).	Lower lobe infiltrate with small/moderate pleural effusion. No cavitation or apical infiltrates. Hilar adenopathy asymmetrical when present.
Nocardia	Fevers, night sweats, fatigue, ↓ cell-mediated immunity (e.g., HIV, organ transplant, immuno-suppressive therapy).	Unremarkable.	Normal/↑ WBC, ↑ESR. Sputum with gram-positive AFB.	Dense large infiltrates. May cavitate and mimic TB, lymphoma, or squamous cell carcinoma. No calcification ± pleural effusion.

Infectious Causes

Causes	Features (may have some, none, or all)			
	History	Physical	Laboratory	Chest X-Ray
Legionella	Recent contact with Legionella containing water. Usually elderly. May have watery diarrhea, abdominal pain, mental confusion.	Fever/chills, relative bradycardia. Hepatic/ splenic enlargement goes against the diagnosis. ↓ breath sounds if consolidation or pleural effusion.	↑ WBC, ↑SGOT/SGPT, ↓PO$_4^-$, ↓Na$^+$, ↑CPK, ↑ESR, ↑CPR, proteinuria, microscopic hematuria, L. pneumophila antigenuria (serotype I only) may not be positive early. Mucoid/purulent sputum with few PMNs. Positive sputum DFA (before therapy) is diagnostic. ↑ Legionella titer ≥ 1:256 or ≥ 4-fold rise between acute/convalescent titers.	Rapidly progressive asymmetrical infiltrates clue to Legionella. Consolidation and pleural effusion not uncommon. Cavitation rare.

Non-Infectious Causes

Causes	Features (may have some, none, or all)			
	History	Physical	Laboratory	Chest X-Ray
Lymphangitic metastases	History of breast, thyroid, pancreas, cervical, prostate, or lung carcinoma.	Findings related to underlying malignancy.	Normal/ ↑ WBC, ↑ESR.	Interstitial indistinct pulmonary infiltrates (may be reticulonodular) with lower lobe predominance Usually unilateral but may be bilateral. No consoli- dation or cavitation ± pleural effusions.

Non-Infectious Causes

Causes	Features (may have some, none, or all)			
	History	Physical	Laboratory	Chest X-Ray
Pulmonary embolus/ infarct	Acute onset dyspnea/pleuritic chest pain. History of lower extremity trauma, stasis or hypercoagulable disorder.	↑ pulse/ respiratory rate.	↑ fibrin split products and D-dimers ± ↑ total bilirubin. Bloody pleural effusion. ECG with RV strain/ P-pulmonale (large embolus). Positive V/Q scan and CT pulmonary angiogram.	Normal or show non-specific pleural-based infiltrates resembling atelectasis. Focal segmental/lobar hyperlucency (Westermark's sign) in some. "Hampton's hump" with infarct. Resolving infarcts ↓ in size but maintain shape/density ("melting ice cube").
Lymphoma	Fever, ↓ appetite with weight loss, night sweats, fatigue.	Adenopathy ± splenomegaly.	Normal WBC, ↑ basophils, ↑ eosinophilia, ↓ lymphocytes, ↑ platelets, ↑ESR, ↑ alkaline phosphatase, ↑ $\alpha_{1,2}$ globulins on SPEP.	Unilateral or asymmetrical bilateral hilar adenopathy. Lung infiltrate may appear contiguous with hilar adenopathy. No clear channel between mediastinum and hilar nodes. Small pleural effusions rare.
Bronchogenic carcinoma	Fever, ↓ appetite with weight loss, cough ± hemoptysis. Cough with copious clear/ mucoid sputum in large cell anaplastic carcinoma. Increased risk in smokers, aluminum/ uranium miners, cavitary lung disease (adeno-carcinoma), previous radiation therapy from lymphoma/breast cancer.	Paraneoplastic syndromes especially with small (oat) cell/squamous cell carcinoma ± hypertrophic pulmonary osteoarthropathy.	Normal/ ↑ WBC, ↑ platelets, ↑ESR, findings related to underlying malignancy, ± clubbing.	Small/squamous cell carcinomas present as central lesions/hilar masses. Adenocarcinoma/ large cell anaplastic carcinomas are usually peripheral initially. "Tumor tendrils" extending into surrounding lung tissue is characteristic. No calcifications (may be present on chest CT). Cavitation with squamous cell carcinoma. ± pleural effusions.

Non-Infectious Causes

Causes	Features (may have some, none, or all)			
	History	Physical	Laboratory	Chest X-Ray
Alveolar cell carcinoma	Fever, ↑ appetite with weight loss, night sweats.	± dullness over lobe with large lower lobe lesions.	Positive cytology by BAL/lung biopsy.	Well/ill-defined circumscribed peripheral infiltrates ± air bronchograms. May be multifocal/ multilobar. Hilar adenopathy present. Stranding to the hilum ("pleural tail" sign). ± pleural effusion if lower lobe infiltrate. No cavitation.
Metastatic carcinoma	History of breast, thyroid, renal cell, colon, pancreatic cancer or osteogenic sarcoma.	Findings related to underlying malignancy and, when present, to bone, hepatic, CNS metastases.	Secondary to effects of primary neoplasm, metastases, paraneoplastic syndrome.	Nodular lesions that vary in size. Metastatic lesions are usually well circumscribed with lower lobe predominance. Usually no bronchial obstruction (obstruction suggests colon, renal, or melanoma metastases). Usually no cavitation (except for squamous cell metastases). Calcification usually suggests osteosarcoma (rarely adenocarcinoma). Pleural effusion rare (except for breast cancer).

BILATERAL INFILTRATES
WITHOUT EFFUSION

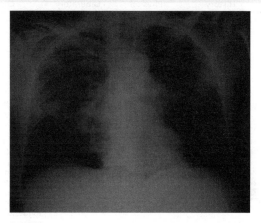

Infectious Causes

Causes	Features (may have some, none, or all)			
	History	Physical	Laboratory	Chest X-Ray
Viral influenza	Acute onset of fever, myalgias, headache, fatigue, sore throat, rhinorrhea, dry cough, ± pleuritic chest pain.	↑ respiratory rate, cyanosis in severe cases.	↓WBC, ↓ platelets, few/no atypical lymphocytes, ↑A-a gradient. Influenza in respiratory secretions by culture/DFA. ↑ influenza titers.	Very early with normal/near normal appearance. Later with diffuse bilateral interstitial infiltrates. No focal/segmental infiltrates unless secondary bacterial pneumonia present. No pleural effusions.
SARS	Acute onset of fever, myalgia, dry cough ± diarrhea.	↑ respiratory rate, cyanosis in severe cases.	N/↓ WBC, N/↓ platelets, ↓ pO$_2$, ↑ A-a gradient.	Culture of SARS - CoV from respiratory secretions.

Infectious Causes

| Causes | Features (may have some, none, or all) | | | |
	History	Physical	Laboratory	Chest X-Ray
HSV-1	Fever. Often presents in normal hosts as "failure to wean" from ventilator.	Unremarkable.	↑ WBC, ↓ pO₂, ↑A-a gradient. HSV-1 in respiratory secretions by culture/DFA. Cytology with cytopathic changes of HSV.	Minimal bilateral diffuse infiltrates without cavitation or effusion.
RSV	Recent URI contact, dry cough, wheezing.	Mild lower respiratory tract infection in normal host. Moderate/severe pneumonia in organ transplants.	Normal WBC; ↓pO₂/↑A-a gradient in severe RSV. RSV in respiratory secretions by culture/DFA.	Near normal chest x-ray or bilateral symmetrical patchy infiltrates. Consolidation uncommon. No cavitation or effusion.
VZV	VZV pneumonia occurs 2-3 days after rash. ↑ risk with pregnancy, smoking.	Healing vesicles, dry cough. Mild pneumonia in normal hosts. Moderate/severe pneumonia in organ transplants.	↑ WBC, ↑ platelets, ↑ basophils; ↓pO₂/↑A-a gradient in severe chickenpox pneumonia. ↑ VZV titers.	Minimal diffuse fluffy interstitial infiltrates. Diffuse small calcifications may develop years later. No calcification of hilar nodes (in contrast to TB/histoplasmosis).
CMV	↓ cell-mediated immunity (HIV, organ transplants, immunosuppressive therapy). Increasing dyspnea over 1 week	Fever ≤ 102°F.	↓pO₂, ↑A-a gradient, ↑LDH (PCP). PCP cysts or CMV "Cowdry Owl eye" inclusion bodies in respiratory secretions or transbronchial open lung biopsy.	Most HIV patients with PCP also have underlying CMV. Organ transplants with CMV usually do not have underlying PCP.
P. carinii (PCP)	↓ cell-mediated immunity (e.g., HIV, immuno-suppressive therapy). Increasing dyspnea over 1 week. Chest pain with shortness of breath suggests pneumothorax.	↓ breath sounds bilaterally. Other findings depend on size/location of pneumothorax (if present).	Normal/↑ WBC (left shift), ↓ lymphocytes, ↑LDH. ↓pO₂, ↓DL_CO, ↑A-a gradient. PCP cysts in sputum/respiratory secretions.	Bilateral perihilar symmetrical fluffy infiltrates ± pneumothorax. No calcification, cavitation, or pleural effusion.

Infectious Causes

Causes	Features (may have some, none, or all)			
	History	Physical	Laboratory	Chest X-Ray
TB (reactivation)	Fevers, night sweats, normal appetite with weight loss, cough ± hemoptysis.	± bilateral apical dullness.	Normal WBC, ↑ platelets, ↑ESR (≤ 70 mm/h). Positive PPD. AFB in sputum smear/culture.	Slowly progressive bilateral infiltrates. No pleural effusion. Usually in apical segment of lower lobes or apical/posterior segments of upper lobes. Calcifications common.
Legionella	Recent contact with Legionella containing water. Usually elderly. May have watery diarrhea, abdominal pain, mental confusion.	Fever/chills, relative bradycardia. Hepatic/splenic enlargement goes against the diagnosis. ↓ breath sounds if consolidation or pleural effusion.	↑ WBC, ↑SGOT/SGPT, ↓PO_4^-, ↓Na^+, ↑CPK, ↑ESR, ↑CPR, proteinuria, microscopic hematuria, L. pneumophila antigenuria (serotype I only) may not be positive early. Mucoid/purulent sputum with few PMNs. Positive sputum DFA (before therapy) is diagnostic. ↑ Legionella titer ≥ 1:256 or ≥ 4-fold rise between acute/convalescent titers.	Rapidly progressive asymmetrical infiltrates clue to Legionella. Consolidation and pleural effusion not uncommon. Cavitation rare.
Psittacosis	Recent bird contact with psittacine birds. Severe headache.	Fever/chills, ± relative bradycardia, ± Horder's spots on face, epistaxis, ± splenomegaly. Signs of consolidation common.	↑/normal WBC, ↑LFTs. Sputum with few PMNs. Positive C. psittaci serology.	Dense infiltrate. Consolidation common. Pleural effusion/cavitation rare.

Infectious Causes

Causes	Features (may have some, none, or all)			
	History	Physical	Laboratory	Chest X-Ray
Q fever	Recent contact with sheep or parturient cats.	Fever/chills, ± relative bradycardia, splenomegaly, ± hepato-megaly.	↑/normal WBC, ↑LFTs. Sputum with no bacteria/few PMNs (caution–biohazard). Acute Q fever with ↑ in phase II ELISA antigens.	Dense consolidation. Cavitation/pleural effusion rare.
Nosocomial pneumonia (hema-togenous)	Fever/pulmonary symptoms ≥ 7 days in hospital. Increased risk with antecedent heart failure in previous 1-2 weeks.	Bilateral rales ± purulent respiratory secretions (tracheo-bronchitis).	↑ WBC (left shift). Normal pO_2/A-a gradient. Blood cultures positive for pulmonary pathogens. Respiratory secretions with WBCs ± positive culture of S. aureus, Enterobacter, P. aeruginosa, B. cepacia, Acinetobacter, Citrobacter, Klebsiella, or Serratia. Definitive diagnosis by lung biopsy/culture.	Bilateral symmetrical diffuse infiltrates. May be focal/segmental in aspiration nosocomial pneumonia. ↑ lung volumes (vs. ARDS). Klebsiella cavitation in 3-5 days; S. aureus and P. aeruginosa cavitation in 72 hours. No pleural effusion.

Non-Infectious Causes

Causes	Features (may have some, none, or all)			
	History	Physical	Laboratory	Chest X-Ray
Adult respiratory distress syndrome (ARDS)	Intubated on ventilator, multi-organ system failure.	± rales.	↑ WBC (left shift), normal ESR, ↓pO_2, ↓D_LCO, ↑A-a gradient.	Bilateral fluffy infiltrates appearing ≥ 12 hours after profound hypoxemia. No cardiomegaly or pleural effusion. Reduced lung volumes (vs. nosocomial pneumonia or CHF). Bilateral consolidation ≥ 48 hours after appearance of infiltrates.

Non-Infectious Causes

Causes	Features (may have some, none, or all)			
	History	Physical	Laboratory	Chest X-Ray
Goodpasture's Syndrome	Often preceded by a URI. Most common in 20-30 year old adults. Fever, weight loss, fatigue, cough, hemoptysis, hematuria.	Findings secondary to iron deficiency anemia.	↑WBC, anemia, ↑ creatinine, urine with RBCs/RBC casts. Positive pANCA. Linear IgG pattern on alveolar/ glomerular basement membrane.	Bilateral fine reticulonodular infiltrates predominantly in lower lobes. No cavitation.
Wegener's granulo-matosis	Most common in middle-aged adults. Cough, fever, fatigue.	Findings of chronic sinusitis, bloody nasal discharge.	↑WBC, anemia, ↑ platelets, ↑ESR, ↑RF, negative ANA, proteinuria, hematuria. Positive cANCA.	Bilateral asymmetrical nodular infiltrates of varying size with irregular margins. Cavitation common. Inner lining of cavities irregular. Air-fluid levels rare. ± pleural effusions. No calcifications.
Pulmonary hemorrhage	History of closed chest trauma or hemorrhagic disorder.	↑WBC (left shift), ↑ pulse rate, ↑ respiratory rate. Signs of closed chest trauma.	Anemia plus findings secondary to underlying hemorrhagic disorder.	Localized or diffuse fluffy alveolar infiltrates. No cavitation, consolidation, or effusion.
Chronic renal failure	Chronic renal failure on dialysis.	Findings related to uremia.	Normal/↑ WBC (left shift) plus findings related to renal failure.	Bilateral symmetrical fluffy perihilar infiltrates (butterfly pattern) ± pleural effusions. No cardiomegaly (unlike CHF), but large pericardial effusion can mimic cardiomegaly.
Lung contusion	Recent closed chest trauma, chest pain.	Chest wall contusion over infiltrate.	↑WBC (left shift).	Patchy ill-defined infiltrate(s) ± rib fractures/ pneumothorax in area of infiltrate. Infiltrate clears within 1 week.
Fat emboli	1-2 days post long bone fracture/ trauma.	↑ respiratory rate.	Urinalysis with "Maltese crosses."	Bilateral predominantly peripheral lower lobe infiltrates. Usually clears within 1 week.

Non-Infectious Causes

Causes	Features (may have some, none, or all)			
	History	Physical	Laboratory	Chest X-Ray
Loeffler's Syndrome	Drug or parasitic exposure.	Unremarkable	Normal WBC, ↑ eosinophilia, ↑ESR.	Characteristic "reversed bat-wing" pattern (i.e., peripheral infiltrates). Upper lobe predominance.
Sarcoidosis (Stage III)	Dyspena, fatigue, nasal stuffiness	Waxy/yellowish papules on face/upper trunk. Funduscopic exam with "candle wax drippings."	↑ESR, normal LFTs, ↑ creatinine (if renal involvement), ↑ ACE levels, hypercalciuria, hypercalcemia, polyclonal gammopathy on SPEP. Anergic.	Bilateral nodular infiltrates of variable size without hilar adenopathy. Cavitation/ pleural effusion rare.
Alveolar cell carcinoma	Fever, ↑ appetite with weight loss, night sweats.	± dullness over lobe with large lower lobe lesions.	Positive cytology by BAL/lung biopsy.	Well/ill-defined circumscribed peripheral infiltrates ± air bronchograms. May be multifocal/ multilobar. Hilar adenopathy present. Stranding to the hilum ("pleural tail" sign). ± pleural effusion if lower lobe infiltrate. No cavitation.
Metastatic carcinoma	History of breast, thyroid, renal cell, colon, pancreatic cancer or osteogenic sarcoma.	Findings related to underlying malignancy and, when present, to bone, hepatic, CNS metastases.	Secondary to effects of primary neoplasm, metastases, paraneoplastic syndrome.	Nodular lesions that vary in size. Metastatic lesions are usually well circum-scribed with lower lobe predominance. Usually no bronchial obstruction (obstruction suggests colon, renal, or melanoma metastases). Usually no cavitation (except for squamous cell metastases). Calcification usually suggests osteo-sarcoma (rarely adeno-carcinoma). Pleural effusion rare (except for breast cancer).

Non-Infectious Causes

Causes	Features (may have some, none, or all)			
	History	Physical	Laboratory	Chest X-Ray
Lymphoma	Fever, ↓ appetite with weight loss, night sweats, fatigue.	Adenopathy ± splenomegaly.	Normal WBC, ↑ basophils, ↑ eosinophilia, ↓ lymphocytes, ↑ platelets, ↑ESR, ↑ alkaline phosphatase, ↑ $\propto_{1,2}$ globulins on SPEP.	Unilateral or asymmetrical bilateral hilar adenopathy. Lung infiltrate may appear contiguous with hilar adenopathy. No clear channel between mediastinum and hilar nodes. Small pleural effusions rare.
Leukostasis (AML)	Untreated acute myelogenous leukemia (AML).	Fever, sternal tenderness, petechiae, ecchymosis.	↑WBC (≥ 100 K/ mm^3) with blasts in peripheral smear/bone marrow, ↓ platelets.	Diffuse symmetrical fluffy infiltrates without pleural effusion.
Drug-induced	Exposure to chemo-therapeutic agents (e.g., BCNU, busulfan, methotrexate, cyclophospham-ide, bleomycin) or other drugs (e.g., nitro-furantoin, sulfasalazine, amiodarone, opiates, cocaine).	Unremarkable.	Normal WBC ± ↑ eosinophilia, normal/↑ ESR/LFTs. Eosinophils in pleural effusion.	Bilateral coarse symmetrical patchy infiltrates/fibrosis ± pleural effusions. Hilar adenopathy only with drug-induced pseudolymphoma (secondary to dilantin). No cavitation.
Idiopathic pulmonary hemosiderosis (IPH)	Hemoptysis ± cough.	Findings of iron deficiency anemia.	Iron deficiency anemia. Hemosiderin in alveolar macrophages and urine.	Diffuse, bilateral ill-defined opacities or multiple "stellate" shaped infiltrates that clear between attacks. Recent hemorrhage may be superimposed on a fine reticular pattern that occurs after repeated bleeds.

Non-Infectious Causes

Causes	Features (may have some, none, or all)			
	History	Physical	Laboratory	Chest X-Ray
Bronchiolitis obliterans with organizing pneumonia (BOOP)	Fever, dyspnea, cough.	Unremarkable.	↑WBC (left shift), ↑LDH, ↓pO$_2$, ↑A-a gradient	Classically bilateral patchy peripheral infiltrates. Often lower lobe predominance. No cavitation or pleural effusion.
Pulmonary alveolar proteinosis (PAP)	Asymptomatic if not infected with Nocardia.	Unremarkable.	Normal/↑ WBC, ↑LDH	Bilateral granular or peripheral infiltrates in butterfly pattern. No hilar adenopathy, cardiomegaly, or pleural effusion.

BILATERAL INFILTRATES
WITH EFFUSION

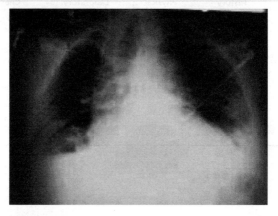

Infectious Causes

Causes	Features (may have some, none, or all)			
	History	Physical	Laboratory	Chest X-Ray
Legionella	Recent contact with Legionella containing water. Usually elderly. May have watery diarrhea, abdominal pain, mental confusion.	Fever/chills, relative bradycardia. Hepatic/ splenic enlargement goes against the diagnosis. ↓ breath sounds if consolidation or pleural effusion.	↑WBC, ↑SGOT/SGPT, ↓PO_4^-, ↓Na^+, ↑CPK, ↑ESR, ↑CPR, proteinuria, microscopic hematuria, L. pneumophila antigenuria (serotype I only) may not be positive early. Mucoid/purulent sputum with few PMNs. Positive sputum DFA (before therapy) is diagnostic. ↑ Legionella titer ≥ 1:256 or ≥ 4-fold rise between acute/convalescent titers.	Rapidly progressive asymmetrical infiltrates clue to Legionella. Consolidation and pleural effusion not uncommon. Cavitation rare.

Infectious Causes

Causes	Features (may have some, none, or all)			
	History	Physical	Laboratory	Chest X-Ray
Hantavirus	Subacute onset, shortness of breath, substernal chest discomfort. Interim improvement followed by rapid deterioration.	↑ respiratory rate, cyanosis in severe cases.	↓WBC, ↓ platelets ↓ pO₂, ↑ A-a gradient. ↑ hantavirus titers.	Large pleural effusions.
Measles	Recent airborne exposure.	Measles rash, Koplik's spots.	Normal/↑ WBC (left shift), normal/↓ platelets, ↑LFTs, ↑CPK, normal/↓pO₂. If ↓pO₂, then ↑A-a gradient. ↑IgM measles titer. Warthin-Finkeldey cells in respiratory secretions.	Bilateral diffuse fine reticulonodular infiltrates ± hilar adenopathy. Lower lobe predominance. Consolidation/ pleural effusion uncommon. No cavitation. Focal infiltrate indicates superimposed bacterial pneumonia.
Strongyloides	Strongyloides exposure. 1/3 asymptomatic; 2/3 with fever, dyspnea, cough. Hyperinfection syndrome with abdominal pain, diarrhea ± GI bleed.	With hyperinfection syndrome, fever, ↓ BP, abdominal tenderness ± rebound, ± meningitis.	↑WBC (left shift), ↑ eosinophilia, ± anemia. Blood/CSF cultures positive for enteric gram-negative bacilli. Rhabditiform larvae in sputum/stool.	Diffuse hilar patchy infiltrates without consolidation or cavitation. Eosinophilic pleural effusion common.

Non-Infectious Causes

Causes	Features (may have some, none, or all)			
	History	Physical	Laboratory	Chest X-Ray
Congestive heart failure	Coronary heart disease, valvular heart disease, cardiomyopathy.	No/low grade fevers, ↑ pulse/ respiratory rate, positive jugular venous distension and hepatojugular reflex, cardio-megaly, S₃, ascites, hepatomegaly, pedal edema.	↑WBC (left shift), normal platelets, mildly ↑SGOT/SGPT.	Cardiomegaly, pleural effusion (R > [R + L] > L). Kerley B lines with vascular redistribution to upper lobes. Typically bilateral rather than unilateral.

Non-Infectious Causes

Causes	Features (may have some, none, or all)			
	History	Physical	Laboratory	Chest X-Ray
Chronic renal failure	Chronic renal failure on dialysis.	Findings related to uremia.	Normal/↑ WBC (left shift) plus findings related to renal failure.	Bilateral symmetrical fluffy perihilar infiltrates (butterfly pattern) ± pleural effusions. No cardiomegaly (unlike CHF), but large pericardial effusion can mimic cardiomegaly.
SLE	Fatigue, chest pain. History of SLE.	Fever/myalgias, alopecia, malar rash, "cytoid bodies" in retina, painless oral ulcers, synovitis, splenomegaly, generalized adenopathy, Raynaud's phenomenon.	↑ ANA, ↑ DS-DNA, ↓ C_3, polyclonal gammopathy on SPEP, ↑ ferritin. Pleural fluids with ↑ ANA, ↓ C_3	Migratory ill-defined non-segmental infiltrates. No signs of consolidation or cavitation. ± small pleural effusions.
Goodpasture's Syndrome	Often preceded by a URI. Most common in 20-30 year old adults. Fever, weight loss, fatigue, cough, hemoptysis, hematuria.	Findings secondary to iron deficiency anemia.	↑WBC, anemia, ↑ creatinine, urine with RBCs/RBC casts. Positive pANCA. Linear IgG pattern on alveolar/glomerular basement membrane.	Bilateral fine reticulonodular infiltrates predominantly in lower lobes. No cavitation.
Wegener's granulomatosis	Most common in middle-aged adults. Cough, fever, fatigue.	Findings of chronic sinusitis, bloody nasal discharge.	↑WBC, anemia, ↑ platelets, ↑ESR, ↑RF, negative ANA, proteinuria, hematuria. Positive cANCA.	Bilateral asymmetrical nodular infiltrates of varying size with irregular margins. Cavitation common. Inner lining of cavities irregular. Air-fluid levels rare. ± pleural effusions. No calcifications.

Non-Infectious Causes

Causes	Features (may have some, none, or all)			
	History	Physical	Laboratory	Chest X-Ray
Sarcoidosis (Stage III)	Dyspnea, fatigue, nasal stuffiness	Waxy/yellowish papules on face/upper trunk. Funduscopic exam with "candle wax drippings."	↑ESR, normal LFTs, ↑ creatinine (if renal involvement), ↑ ACE levels, hypercalciuria, hypercalcemia, polyclonal gammopathy on SPEP. Anergic.	Bilateral nodular infiltrates of variable size without hilar adenopathy. Cavitation/pleural effusion rare.
Lymphoma	Fever, ↓ appetite with weight loss, night sweats, fatigue.	Adenopathy ± splenomegaly.	Normal WBC, ↑ basophils, ↑ eosinophilia, ↓ lymphocytes, ↑ platelets, ↑ESR, ↑ alkaline phosphatase, ↑ $\propto_{1,2}$ globulins on SPEP.	Unilateral or asymmetrical bilateral hilar adenopathy. Lung infiltrate may appear contiguous with hilar adenopathy. No clear channel between mediastinum and hilar nodes. Small pleural effusions rare.
Lymphangitic metastases	History of breast, thyroid, pancreas, cervical, prostate, or lung carcinoma.	Findings related to underlying malignancy.	Normal/↑ WBC, ↑ESR.	Interstitial indistinct pulmonary infiltrates (may be reticulonodular) with lower lobe predominance Usually unilateral but may be bilateral. No consolidation or cavitation ± pleural effusions.

Non-Infectious Causes

Causes	Features (may have some, none, or all)			
	History	Physical	Laboratory	Chest X-Ray
Drug-induced	Exposure to chemotherapeutic agents (e.g., BCNU, busulfan, methotrexate, cyclophosphamide, bleomycin) or other drugs (e.g., nitrofurantoin, sulfasalazine, amiodarone, opiates, cocaine).	Unremarkable.	Normal WBC ± ↑ eosinophilia, normal/↑ ESR/LFTs. Eosinophils in pleural effusion.	Bilateral coarse symmetrical patchy infiltrates/fibrosis ± pleural effusions. Hilar adenopathy only with drug-induced pseudolymphoma (secondary to dilantin). No cavitation.

CAVITARY INFILTRATES
(THICK WALLED)

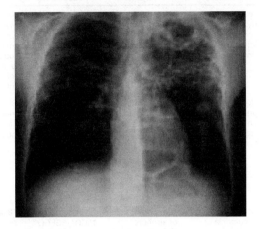

Infectious Causes Based on Speed of Cavitation

Speed of Cavitation	Causes
Very rapid cavitation (3 days)	S. aureus, P. aeruginosa
Rapid cavitation (5-7 days)	K. pneumoniae
Slow cavitation (> 7 days)	Pyogenic lung abscess, septic pulmonary emboli
Chronic cavitation	TB (reactivation), histoplasmosis (reactivation), melioidosis, nocardia, actinomycosis, Rhodococcus equi, amebic abscess, alveolar echinococcosis (hydatid cysts)

Infectious Causes

Causes	Features (may have some, none, or all)			
	History	Physical	Laboratory	Chest X-Ray
S. aureus	Fever, cough, dyspnea. Recent/concurrent influenza pneumonia.	↓ breath sounds ± cyanosis.	↑WBC (left shift), ↓PO₂, ↑A-a gradient. Sputum positive for S. aureus. ↑IgM influenza titers.	Multiple thick-walled cavitary lesions super-imposed on normal looking lung fields or early minimal infiltrates of influenza.
P. aeruginosa	Nosocomial pneumonia usually on ventilator. Nearly always rapidly fatal.	Unremarkable.	↑WBC (left shift). Respiratory secretions culture ± for P. aeruginosa. Blood cultures positive for P. aeruginosa (hematogenous nosocomial pneumonia).	Bilateral diffuse infiltrates with rapid cavitation (≤ 72 hours).
Klebsiella pneumoniae	Nosocomial pneumonia or history of alcoholism in patient with community-acquired pneumonia.	Fever, chills, signs of alcoholic cirrhosis, signs of consolidation over involved lobe.	↑WBC, ↓ platelets, ↑SGOT/SGPT (2° to alcoholism). "Red currant jelly" sputum with PMNs and plump gram-negative encapsulated bacilli.	"Bulging fissure" sign secondary to expanded lobar volume. Empyema rather than pleural effusion. Usually cavitation in 5-7 days (thick walled).
Pyogenic lung abscess	Recent aspiration. Fevers, chills, weight loss. Swallowing disorder secondary to CNS/GI disorder.	Foul (putrid lung abscess) breath.	↑WBC, ↑ESR. Sputum with normal oropharyngeal anaerobic flora in putrid lung abscess.	Thick-walled cavity in portion of lung dependent during aspiration (usually basilar segment of lower lobes if aspiration occurred supine). Cavitation occurs > 7 days.
Septic pulmonary emboli	Usually IV drug abuser with fever/chills. Tricuspid regurgitation murmur or recent OB/GYN surgical procedure.	Fever > 102°F. Tricuspid valve regurgitant murmur with cannon A waves in neck.	Blood cultures positive for acute bacterial endocarditis pathogens.	Multiple peripheral nodules of varying size. Lower lobe predominance. Cavitation > 7 days characteristic of septic pulmonary emboli.

Infectious Causes

Causes	Features (may have some, none, or all)			
	History	Physical	Laboratory	Chest X-Ray
TB (reactivation)	Fevers, night sweats, normal appetite with weight loss, cough ± hemoptysis.	± bilateral apical dullness.	Normal WBC, ↑ platelets, ↑ESR (≤ 70 mm/h). Positive PPD. AFB in sputum smear/culture.	Slowly progressive bilateral infiltrates. No pleural effusion. Usually in apical segment of lower lobes or apical/posterior segments of upper lobes. Calcifications common.
Histoplasmosis (reactivation)	Fever, night sweats, cough, weight loss, histoplasmosis exposure (River valleys of Central/ Eastern United States).	± E. nodosum; otherwise unremarkable.	Normal WBC, normal/↑ eosinophilia, anemia, ↑ platelets, PPD negative. Immunodiffusion test with positive H precipitin band (diagnostic of active/chronic histoplasmosis).	Unilateral/bilateral multiple patchy infiltrates with upper lobe predilection. Bilateral hilar adenopathy uncommon. Calcifications common. No pleural effusion. Chest x-ray resembles reactivation TB.
Melioidosis	Past travel to Asia (usually > 10 years). Fever, cough, hemoptysis.	Unremarkable.	↑WBC (left shift), ↑ESR, PPD negative. Sputum/ blood cultures positive for B. (pseudomonas) pseudomallei.	Resembles reactivation TB, but lesions not apical and predominantly in middle/lower lung fields. No pleural effusion.
Nocardia	Fevers, night sweats, fatigue, ↓ cell-mediated immunity (e.g., HIV, organ transplant, immuno-suppressive therapy).	Unremarkable.	Normal/↑ WBC, ↑ESR. Sputum with gram-positive AFB.	Dense large infiltrates. May cavitate and mimic TB, lymphoma, or squamous cell carcinoma. No calcification ± pleural effusion.
Actinomycosis	Recent dental work.	± chest wall sinus tracts.	Normal/↑WBC, ↑ESR. Sputum with Gram-positive filamentous anaerobic bacilli.	Dense infiltrates extending to chest wall. No hilar adenopathy. Cavitation ± pleural effusion rare.

Infectious Causes

Causes	Features (may have some, none, or all)			
	History	Physical	Laboratory	Chest X-Ray
Rhodococcus equi	Insidious onset of fever, dyspnea, chest pain, ± hemoptysis. Immuno-suppressed patients with ↓ cell-mediated immunity or exposure to cattle, horses, pigs.	Unremarkable.	Normal/↑WBC. Sputum/pleural fluid with gram-positive pleomorphic weakly acid-fast bacilli. Sputum, pleural fluid, blood cultures positive for R. equi.	Segmental infiltrate with upper lobe predominance ± cavitation. Air-fluid levels and pleural effusion common.
Amebic cysts	Hepatic amebic abscess. Remote history of usually mild amebic dysentery.	± hepatomegaly.	Normal WBC and ESR. ↑ E. histolytica HI titers.	Well-circumscribed cavitary lesions adjacent to right diaphragm. ± calcifications. Sympathetic pleural effusion above hepatic amebic abscess.
Alveolar echinococcosis (hydatid cysts)	Symptoms related to cyst size/ location: 1/3 asymptomatic; 2/3 with fever, malaise, chest pain ± hemoptysis. RUQ abdominal pain may occur.	Hepatomegaly common.	Normal/↑ WBC, no eosinophilia, ↑ alkaline phosphate/SGPT with hepatic cysts. Abdominal ultrasound/CT with calcified hepatic irregularly shaped cysts ("Swiss cheese" calcification characteristic). ↑ E. multilocularis IHA titers.	RLL usual location (hepatic cysts penetrate diaphragm into RLL). Nodules are 70% solitary, 30% multiple. Pleural effusion rare. Endocyst membrane on surface of cyst fluid ("water lilly" sign) is characteristic.

Non-Infectious Causes

Causes	Features (may have some, none, or all)			
	History	Physical	Laboratory	Chest X-Ray
Wegener's granulomatosis	Most common in middle-aged adults. Cough, fever, fatigue.	Findings of chronic sinusitis, bloody nasal discharge.	↑WBC, anemia, ↑ platelets, ↑ESR, ↑RF, negative ANA, proteinuria, hematuria. Positive cANCA.	Bilateral asymmetrical nodular infiltrates of varying size with irregular margins. Cavitation common. Inner lining of cavities irregular. Air-fluid levels rare. ± pleural effusions. No calcifications.
Squamous cell carcinoma	Long term smoking history.	Clubbing, hypertrophic pulmonary osteoarthropathy ± findings 2° to superior vena caval syndrome and CNS/bone metastases.	↑ Ca^{++} (without bone metastases).	Unilateral perihilar mass lesion. Cavitation common. No pleural effusion.
Lymphoma	Fever, ↓ appetite with weight loss, night sweats, fatigue.	Adenopathy ± splenomegaly.	Normal WBC, ↑ basophils, ↑ eosinophilia, ↓ lymphocytes, ↑ platelets, ↑ESR ↑ alkaline phosphatase, ↑ $\propto_{1,2}$ globulins on SPEP.	Unilateral or asymmetrical bilateral hilar adenopathy. Lung infiltrate may appear contiguous with hilar adenopathy. No clear channel between mediastinum and hilar nodes. Small pleural effusions rare.
Metastatic carcinoma	History of breast, thyroid, renal cell, colon, pancreatic cancer or osteogenic sarcoma.	Findings related to underlying malignancy and, when present, to bone, hepatic, CNS metastases.	Secondary to effects of primary neoplasm, metastases, paraneoplastic syndrome.	Nodular lesions that vary in size. Metastatic lesions are usually well circumscribed with lower lobe predominance. Usually no bronchial obstruction (obstruction suggests colon, renal, or melanoma metastases). Usually no cavitation (except for squamous cell metastases). Calcification usually suggests osteosarcoma (rarely adenocarcinoma). Pleural effusion rare (except for breast cancer).

Non-Infectious Causes

Causes	Features (may have some, none, or all)			
	History	Physical	Laboratory	Chest X-Ray
Rheumatoid nodules	Usually in severe rheumatoid arthritis (RA); ± history of silicosis.	Findings secondary to RA. Rheumatoid nodules on exterior surfaces of arms.	Normal WBC, ↑ESR, ↑ANA, ↑RF (high titer). Pleural fluid with ↓ glucose	Lung nodules are round and well circumscribed, predominantly in lower lobes and typically superimposed on interstitial lung disease ("rheumatoid lung"). Cavitation is common. ± pulmonary fibrosis, pleural effusion. Silicosis + RA nodules = Caplan's syndrome.

CAVITARY INFILTRATES
(THIN WALLED)

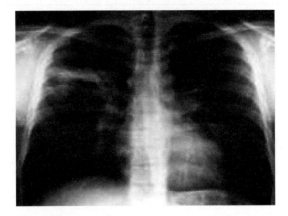

Infectious Causes

Causes	Features (may have some, none, or all)			
	History	**Physical**	**Laboratory**	**Chest X-Ray**
Atypical TB	Often occurs in setting of previous lung disease.	Unremarkable.	Normal WBC, ↑ESR. Weakly positive PPD. Positive sputum AFB/culture.	Multiple cavitary lesions ± calcifications usually involving both lungs. Resembles reactivation TB except that cavities are thin walled. No pleural effusion.
Coccidiomycosis (reactivation)	Previous exposure in endemic coccidiomycosis areas (e.g., Southwest USA). Asymptomatic.	± E. nodosum.	Normal WBC. Eosinophilia acutely but not in chronic phase, and eosinophils in pleural fluid. CF IgG titer ≥ 1:32 indicates active disease.	Thick/thin walled cavities (< 3 cm) usually in anterior segments of lower lobes ± calcifications/ bilateral hilar adenopathy. Air-fluid levels rare unless secondarily infected. Pleural effusion rare.

Infectious Causes

| Causes | Features (may have some, none, or all) | | | |
	History	Physical	Laboratory	Chest X-Ray
Paragonimiasis	Ingestion of fresh-water crabs/crayfish. Acute symptoms (< 6 months): fevers, abdominal pain, diarrhea followed by episodes of pleuritic chest pain. Chronic symptoms (> 6 months): fevers, night sweats, cough ± hemoptysis. Asymptomatic in some.	Wheezing, ± urticaria (acutely).	↑WBC, eosinophilia. Eosinophils in pleural fluid. Sputum with Charot-Leyden crystals. Sputum/feces with operculated P. Westermani eggs.	Cavitary patchy or well-defined infiltrates predominantly in mid-lung fields. Hydropneumothorax common. Calcifications and pleural effusion common.
Sporotrichosis	Fever, cough, weight loss. No hemoptysis. Antecedent lymphocutaneous or skeletal sporotrichosis.	Secondary to residual of lympho-cutaneous sporotrichosis, ± E. nodosum.	Normal WBC, no eosinophilia.	Bilateral lower lobe nodular densities/thin walled cavities ± hilar adenopathy. No pleural effusion.
Pneumatoceles	Common in S. aureus pneumonia in children. Fever, cough, dyspnea. ± antecedent influenza.	Unremarkable unless pneumatocele ruptures, then signs of pneumothorax.	↑WBC (left shift), ↓pO$_2$ (secondary to influenza).	Multiple thin-walled cavities in areas of S. aureus pneumonia. Common in children; rare in adults.

Non-Infectious Causes

Causes	Features (may have some, none, or all)			
	History	Physical	Laboratory	Chest X-Ray
Emphysema (blebs/cyst)	Long history of smoking. Rupture of apical bleb common in males > 30 years. Pneumonia rare in severe emphysema (vs. chronic bronchitis) but may occur early in unaffected areas of lung.	Asthenic "pink puffers." Barrel chest. Diaphragmatic excursions < 2 cm.	Normal WBC, ↓pO$_2$.	↓ lung markings ("vanishing lung") ± blebs. Hyperlucent lungs with upper lobe predominance. Flattened diaphragms, vertically elongated cardiac silhouette, ↑ retrocardiac and retrosternal airspaces. No infiltrates or pleural effusions. (In upper lobe emphysema, no vascular redistribution to upper lobes with CHF).
Bronchogenic cyst	Congenital anomaly. Usually asymptomatic. Cough if symptomatic.	Unremarkable unless secondarily infected, then signs 2° to mediastinal abscess.	Normal WBC/ESR.	Circumscribed cystic lesion originates in lung but appears high in mediastinum. If filled with fluid, appears as solitary tumor. If near the trachea, may rupture into bronchus/trachea and cyst may contain air. If communicates openly with bronchus, appears as thin walled cavitary nodule. If infected, presents as mediastinal abscess.

Non-Infectious Causes

Causes	Features (may have some, none, or all)			
	History	Physical	Laboratory	Chest X-Ray
Cystic bronchiectasis	Recurrent pulmonary infections with purulent sputum ± hemoptysis.	Unremarkable unless dextrocardia with sinusitis (Kartagener's syndrome).	↑WBC, normal ESR.	Bilateral large cystic lucencies at lung bases. Upper lobes relatively spared (unless secondary chronic aspiration). Thickened bronchial markings at bases. Bronchiectasis of cystic fibrosis predominantly involves upper lobes.
Sequestered lung	Usually asymptomatic. Productive cough ± hemoptysis if communicates with bronchus or if infected.	Unremarkable.	Normal WBC, ↑ESR	Solid nodule unless communicates with bronchus, then thin-walled cavity ± air fluid levels. Usually posterior based segment of lower lobes (LLL > RLL). If > 3 cm, presents as mass lesion.
Histiocytosis X (eosinophilic granuloma, Langerhan's cell histio-cytosis)	Patients usually 20-40 years. Usually asymptomatic. Fever, cough, dyspnea in some. Diabetes insipidus rare.	Hepato-splenomegaly, skin lesions, hemoptysis (rare).	Normal WBC, eosinophilia.	Pneumothorax superimposed on diffuse pulmonary fibrosis. Cystic bone lesions. Usually mid/upper lung fields with nodules/ thin-walled cysts or infiltrates. No hilar adenopathy or pleural effusion.

SOLITARY PULMONARY NODULE

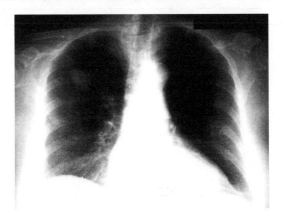

Infectious Causes

Causes	Features (may have some, none, or all)			
	History	Physical	Laboratory	Chest x-ray
TB (tuberculoma)	Asymptomatic. ± history of TB contact.	Unremarkable.	Normal WBC and ESR. No eosinophilia. Positive PPD.	Smooth well-circumscribed nodule (0.5-4 cm). Calcification common. No cavitation or pleural effusion.
Histoplasmosis (histoplasmoma)	Asymptomatic. ± history of histoplasmosis exposure.	Unremarkable.	Normal WBC and ESR. No eosinophilia. Histoplasmosis serology positive or negative.	Smooth well-circumscribed nodule (0.5-4 cm). Calcification common. No cavitation or pleural effusion.
Dirofilaria immitis	Contact with soil/dogs. Presents as asymptomatic pulmonary nodules in humans and heartworm in dogs.	Unremarkable.	Normal WBC and ESR. No eosinophilia. D. immitis serology positive or negative.	Single nodule usually 1-3 cm. No lobar predilection. No cavitation. Calcification common.

Infectious Causes

Causes	Features (may have some, none, or all)			
	History	Physical	Laboratory	Chest x-ray
Coccidiomycosis (coccidioma)	Asymptomatic. Exposure to C. immitis.	Unremarkable.	Normal WBC, no eosinophilia, normal ESR. Coccidiomycosis serology positive or negative.	Smooth well-circumscribed nodule (0.5-4 cm). No calcification of nodules. No cavitation or pleural effusion.
Aspergillus (aspergilloma)	Asymptomatic. If symptomatic, then cough ± hemoptysis. Occurs in pre-existing lung cavities.	± signs secondary to anemia.	Normal WBC, no eosinophilia, normal ESR. ↑ Aspergillus precipitins.	Round lesion within pre-existing lung cavity. Dense fungus ball silhouetted against black crescent shaped air space in cavity is characteristic ("crescent" sign).
Aspergillus (invasive)	Fever, cough, ± hemoptysis only in compromised hosts (organ transplants, patients on steroids, prolonged/ profound leukopenia, or immunosuppressive drugs).	Unremarkable unless skin lesions of disseminated aspergillosis.	↓WBC in leukopenia in patients receiving chemotherapy. ↑WBC/lymphopenia with steroids.	Usually irregular nodular infiltrates. Aspergillus nodules often have fuzzy borders ("halo sign") surrounding nodule. Cavitation common. A "crescent sign" develops later as nodules cavitate.
Alveolar echinococcosis (hydatid cysts)	Symptoms related to cyst size/location. 1/3 asymptomatic; 2/3 with fever, malaise, chest pain, ± hemoptysis. RUQ abdominal pain may occur.	Hepatomegaly common.	Normal/↑WBC, no eosinophilia, ↑ alkaline phosphate/SGPT with hepatic cysts. Abdominal ultrasound/CT with calcified hepatic irregularly shaped cysts ("Swiss cheese" calcification characteristic).↑ Echinococcus multilocularis IHA titers.	RLL usual location (hepatic cysts penetrate diaphragm into RLL). Nodules are 70% solitary, 30% multiple. Pleural effusion rare. Endocyst membrane on surface of cyst fluid ("water lilly" sign) is characteristic.

Non-Infectious Causes

Causes	Features (may have some, none, or all)			
	History	Physical	Laboratory	Chest x-ray
Bronchogenic carcinoma	Fever, ↓ appetite with weight loss, cough ± hemoptysis. Cough with copious clear/ mucoid sputum in large cell anaplastic carcinoma. Increased risk in smokers, aluminum/ uranium miners, cavitary lung disease (adeno-carcinoma), previous radiation therapy from lymphoma/breast cancer.	Paraneoplastic syndromes especially with small (oat) cell/squamous cell carcinoma ± hypertrophic pulmonary osteoarthro-pathy.	Normal/↑ WBC, ↑ platelets, ↑ESR, findings related to underlying malignancy, ± clubbing.	Small/squamous cell carcinomas present as central lesions/ hilar masses. Adenocarcinoma/ large cell anaplastic carcinomas are usually peripheral initially. "Tumor tendrils" extending into surrounding lung tissue is characteristic. No calcifications (may be present on chest CT). Cavitation with squamous cell carcinoma. ± pleural effusions; if present, usually with RBCs/bloody.
Alveolar cell carcinoma	Fever, ↑ appetite with weight loss, night sweats.	± dullness over lobe with large lower lobe lesions.	Positive cytology by BAL/lung biopsy.	Well/ill-defined circumscribed peripheral infiltrates ± air bronchograms. May be multifocal/ multilobar. Hilar adenopathy present. Stranding to the hilum ("pleural tail" sign). ± pleural effusion if lower lobe infiltrate; if present, usually with RBCs/bloody. No cavitation.
Bronchial adenoma	Cough, hemoptysis.	Findings secondary to anemia.	Normal WBC, ↑ESR.	Well-circumscribed peripheral nodules. Smooth margins. Usually in lower lobes. Nodules are 25% single, 75% multiple. Slow growing. No cavitation or calcification.

Non-Infectious Causes

Causes	Features (may have some, none, or all)			
	History	Physical	Laboratory	Chest x-ray
Bronchogenic cyst	Congenital anomaly. Usually asymptomatic. Cough if symptomatic.	Unremarkable unless secondary infected, then signs secondary to mediastinal abscess.	Normal WBC and ESR.	Circumscribed cystic lesion originates in lung but appears high in mediastinum. If filled with fluid, appears as solitary tumor. If near the trachea, may rupture into bronchus/trachea and cyst may contain air. If communicates openly with bronchus, appears as thin walled cavitary nodule. If infected, presents as mediastinal abscess.
Hamartoma	Asymptomatic. Most common cause of granulomatous coin lesions.	Unremarkable.	Normal WBC and ESR.	Sharply defined smooth or lobulated borders. Calcification common and may be single or multiple ("popcorn calcification" characteristic).
Sequestered lung	Asymptomatic.	Productive cough ± hemoptysis if communicates with bronchus or if infected.	Normal WBC and ESR.	Usually posterior based segment of lower lobes (LLL > RLL). Solid nodule unless communicates with bronchus, then thin walled cavities ± air fluid levels. If > 3 cm, presents as dense infiltrate/mass lesion.
Arteriovenous malformation (AVM)	Asymptomatic.	Chest auscultation with venous hum over AVM.	Normal WBC and ESR.	RLL > LLL. Venous feeder vessel connects to hilum ("scimitar" sign).

Non-Infectious Causes

Causes	Features (may have some, none, or all)			
	History	Physical	Laboratory	Chest x-ray
Metastatic carcinoma	History of breast, thyroid, renal cell, colon, or pancreatic cancer or osteogenic sarcoma.	Findings related to underlying malignancy and, when present, to bone, hepatic, CNS metastases.	Secondary to effects of primary neoplasm metastases, paraneoplastic syndrome.	Nodular lesions that vary in size. Metastatic lesions tend to be well circumscribed with a lower lobe predominance. Usually no bronchial obstruction (bronchial obstruction suggests colon, renal, or melanoma metastases). Usually no cavitation (except with squamous cell metastases). Calcification usually suggests osteosarcoma (rarely adenocarcinoma). Pleural effusion rare (except for breast cancer).

MULTIPLE PULMONARY NODULES

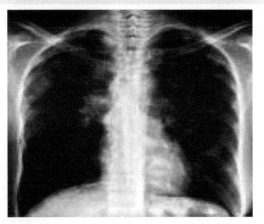

Infectious Causes

Causes	Features (may have some, none, or all)			
	History	Physical	Laboratory	Chest x-ray
Lung abscess	Recent aspiration or swallowing disorder secondary to CNS/GI disorder. Fevers, chills, weight loss.	Foul breath (putrid lung abscess).	↑ WBC, ↑ ESR. Sputum with normal oropharyngeal anaerobic flora in putrid lung abscess.	Thick-walled cavity in portion of lung dependent during aspiration; usually basilar segment of lower lobes if aspiration occurred supine. Cavitation occurs > 7 days.
TB (reactivation)	Fevers, night sweats, Normal appetite with weight loss, cough, ± hemoptysis.	± bilateral apical dullness.	Normal WBC, no eosinophilia, ↑ platelets, ↑ ESR (≤ 70 mm/h). Positive PPD. AFB in sputum smear/culture.	Slowly progressive bilateral apical/lung infiltrates. No pleural effusion. Usually in apical segment of lower lobes or segments of upper lobes. Calcifications common.

Infectious Causes

Causes	Features (may have some, none, or all)			
	History	Physical	Laboratory	Chest x-ray
Coccidio-mycosis (reactivation)	Previous exposure in endemic coccidiomycosis areas. Asymptomatic.	± E. nodosum.	Normal WBC. Eosinophilia acutely but not in chronic phase, and eosinophils in pleural fluid. CF IgG titer ≥ 1:32 indicates active disease.	Thick/thin walled cavities < 3 cm ± calcifications. Air fluid level rare. Lower lobe predilection ± bilateral hilar adenopathy. Cavities characteristically in anterior segments (vs. posterior segments). Pleural effusion rare.
Histoplasmosis (reactivation)	Fever, night sweats, cough, weight loss, histoplasmosis exposure (River valleys of Central/ Eastern United States).	± E. nodosum; otherwise unremarkable.	Normal WBC, ± eosinophilia, anemia, ↑ platelets, PPD negative. Immunodiffusion test with positive H precipitin band (diagnostic of active/chronic histoplasmosis).	Unilateral/bilateral multiple patchy infiltrates with upper lobe predilection. Bilateral hilar adenopathy uncommon. Calcifications common. No pleural effusion. Chest x-ray resembles reactivation TB.
Alveolar echinococcosis (hydatid cysts)	Symptoms related to cyst size/ location: 1/3 asymptomatic; 2/3 with fever, malaise, chest pain ± hemoptysis. RUQ abdominal pain may occur.	Hepatomegaly common.	Normal/↑ WBC, no eosinophilia, ↑ alkaline phosphate/SGPT with hepatic cysts. Abdominal ultrasound/CT with calcified hepatic irregularly shaped cysts ("Swiss cheese" calcification characteristic). ↑ E. multilocularis IHA titers.	RLL usual location (hepatic cysts penetrate diaphragm into RLL). Nodules are 70% solitary, 30% multiple. Pleural effusion rare. Endocyst membrane on surface of cyst fluid ("water lilly" sign) is characteristic.

Infectious Causes

| Causes | Features (may have some, none, or all) | | | |
	History	Physical	Laboratory	Chest x-ray
Aspergillus (invasive)	Fever, cough, ± hemoptysis only in compromised hosts (organ transplants, patients on steroids, prolonged/ profound leukopenia, or immunosuppressive drugs).	Unremarkable unless skin lesions of disseminated aspergillosis.	↓WBC in leukopenia in patients receiving chemotherapy. ↑WBC/lymphopenia with steroids.	Usually irregular nodular infiltrates. Aspergillus nodules often have fuzzy borders ("halo sign") surrounding nodule. Cavitation common. A "crescent sign" develops later as nodules cavitate.

Non-Infectious Causes

| Causes | Features (may have some, none, or all) | | | |
	History	Physical	Laboratory	Chest x-ray
Metastatic carcinoma	History of breast, thyroid, renal cell, colon, pancreatic cancer or osteogenic sarcoma.	Findings related to underlying malignancy and, when present, to bone, hepatic, CNS metastases.	Secondary to effects of primary neoplasm, metastases, paraneoplastic syndrome.	Nodular lesions that vary in size. Metastatic lesions are usually well circumscribed with lower lobe predominance. Usually no bronchial obstruction (obstruction suggests colon, renal, or melanoma metastases). Usually no cavitation (except for squamous cell metastases). Calcification usually suggests osteosarcoma (rarely adenocarcinoma). Pleural effusion rare (except for breast cancer).

Non-Infectious Causes

Causes	Features (may have some, none, or all)			
	History	Physical	Laboratory	Chest x-ray
Lymphoma	Fever, ↓ appetite with weight loss, night sweats, fatigue.	Adenopathy ± splenomegaly.	Normal WBC, ↑ basophils, ↑ eosinophilia, ↓ lymphocytes, ↑ platelets, ↑ESR, ↑ alkaline phosphatase, ↑ $\alpha_{1,2}$ globulins on SPEP.	Unilateral or asymmetrical bilateral hilar adenopathy. Lung infiltrate may appear contiguous with hilar adenopathy. No clear channel between mediastinum and hilar nodes. Small pleural effusions rare.
Goodpasture's Syndrome	Often preceded by a URI. Most common in 20-30 year old adults. Fever, weight loss, fatigue, cough, hemoptysis, hematuria.	Findings secondary to iron deficiency anemia.	↑WBC, anemia, ↑ creatinine, urine with RBCs/RBC casts. Positive pANCA. Linear IgG pattern on alveolar/glomerular basement membrane.	Bilateral fine reticulonodular infiltrates predominantly in lower lobes. No cavitation.
Wegener's granulomatosis	Most common in middle-aged adults. Cough, fever, fatigue.	Findings of chronic sinusitis, bloody nasal discharge.	↑WBC, anemia, ↑ platelets, ↑ESR, ↑RF, negative ANA, proteinuria, hematuria. Positive cANCA.	Bilateral asymmetrical nodular infiltrates of varying size with irregular margins. Cavitation common. Inner lining of cavities irregular. Air-fluid levels rare. ± pleural effusions. No calcifications.
Rheumatoid nodules	Usually in severe rheumatoid arthritis (RA). ± history of silicosis.	Findings secondary to RA. Rheumatoid nodules on exterior surfaces of arms.	Normal WBC, ↑ESR, ↑ANA, ↑RF (high titer). Pleural fluid with ↓ glucose	Nodules are round and well circumscribed, predominantly in lower lobes. Cavitation is common. Superimposed on interstitial lung disease ("rheumatoid lung"). ± pulmonary fibrosis, pleural effusion. Silicosis + RA nodules = Caplan's syndrome.

Non-Infectious Causes

| Causes | Features (may have some, none, or all) | | | |
	History	Physical	Laboratory	Chest x-ray
Arteriovenous malformation (AVM)	Asymptomatic	Chest auscultation with venous hum over AVM.	Normal WBC and ESR.	RLL > LLL. Venous feeder vessel connects to hilum ("scimitar" sign).
Sarcoidosis (Stage III)	Dyspena, fatigue, nasal stuffiness	Waxy/yellowish papules on face/upper trunk. Funduscopic exam with "candle wax drippings."	↑ESR, normal LFTs, ↑ creatinine (if renal involvement), ↑ ACE levels, hypercalciuria, hypercalcemia, polyclonal gammopathy on SPEP. Anergic.	Bilateral nodular infiltrates of variable size without hilar adenopathy. Cavitation/ pleural effusion rare.
Churg-Strauss granulomatosis	In most, history of fever, weight loss, malaise, myalgias, arthralgias.	Bilateral wheezing.	↑ WBC (left shift), eosinophilia, ↑ESR, ↑IgE, (+) p-ANCA.	Bilateral peripheral multiple nodular densities. No calcification or pleural effusion.

UNILATERAL HILAR ADENOPATHY
WITH OR WITHOUT INFILTRATES

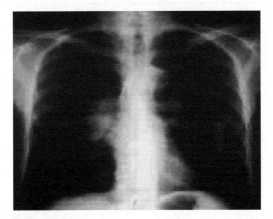

Infectious Causes

Causes	Features (may have some, none, or all)			
	History	Physical	Laboratory	Chest x-ray
TB (primary)	Recent TB contact.	Unilateral lower lobe dullness related to size of pleural effusion.	PPD anergic. Exudative pleural effusion (pleural fluid with ↑ lymphocytes, ↑ glucose, ± RBCs).	Lower lobe infiltrate with small/moderate pleural effusion. No cavitation or apical infiltrates. Hilar adenopathy asymmetrical when present.

Infectious Causes

Causes	Features (may have some, none, or all)			
	History	Physical	Laboratory	Chest x-ray
Tularemia	History of recent deer fly, rabbit, or tick exposure. Tularemia pneumonia may complicate any of the clinical presentations of tularemia.	Fever, chills, no relative bradycardia. Chest findings related to extent of infiltrate/ consolidation and pleural effusion.	Normal/↑WBC, normal LFTs. Sputum/pleural effusion with gram-negative coccobacilli (caution – biohazard). Bloody pleural effusion. Tularemia serology with ↑ microagglutination titer ≥ 1:160 acutely and ≥ 4-fold rise between acute and convalescent titers.	Pleural effusion ± hilar adenopathy.
Sporotrichosis	Fever, cough, weight loss usual. No hemoptysis. Antecedent history of skeletal or lymphocutaneous sporotrichosis.	Secondary to residual of lymphocutaneous sporotrichosis. ± E. nodosum.	Normal WBC, no eosinophilia.	Bilateral lower lobe nodular densities/thin-walled cavities. ± hilar adenopathy. No pleural effusion.

Non-Infectious Causes

Causes	Features (may have some, none, or all)			
	History	Physical	Laboratory	Chest x-ray
Lymphoma	Fever, ↓ appetite with weight loss, night sweats, fatigue.	Adenopathy ± splenomegaly.	Normal WBC, ↑ basophils, ↑ eosinophilia, ↓ lymphocytes, ↑ platelets, ↑ESR, ↑ alkaline phosphatase, ↑ ∝$_{1, 2}$ globulins on SPEP.	Unilateral or asymmetrical bilateral hilar adenopathy. Lung infiltrate may appear contiguous with hilar adenopathy. No clear channel between mediastinum and hilar nodes. Small pleural effusions rare.

Non-Infectious Causes

Causes	Features (may have some, none, or all)			
	History	Physical	Laboratory	Chest x-ray
Squamous cell carcinoma	Long term smoking history.	Clubbing, hypertrophic pulmonary osteoarthropathy ± findings 2° to superior vena caval syndrome and CNS/bone metastases.	↑ Ca^{++} (without bone metastases).	Unilateral perihilar mass lesion. Cavitation common. No pleural effusion.
Small cell carcinoma	Non-smokers. Early metastases to bone marrow/CNS.	Hypertrophic pulmonary osteoarthropathy ± findings secondary to SVC syndrome and/or CNS/bone marrow invasion.	Secondary to bone marrow invasion.	Unilateral perihilar mass lesion. No cavitation, calcification, or pleural effusion.

BILATERAL HILAR ADENOPATHY
WITH OR WITHOUT INFILTRATES

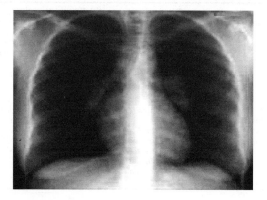

Infectious Causes

Causes	Features (may have some, none, or all)			
	History	Physical	Laboratory	Chest x-ray
TB (primary)	Recent TB contact.	Unilateral lower lobe dullness related to size of pleural effusion.	Normal WBC, no eosinophilia. PPD anergic. Exudative pleural effusion (pleural fluid with ↑ lymphocytes, ↑ glucose, ± RBCs).	Lower lobe infiltrate with small/moderate pleural effusion. No cavitation or apical infiltrates. Hilar adenopathy asymmetrical when present.
Histoplasmosis (primary)	Fever, dry cough, flu-like illness, myalgias, arthralgias. Recent exposure to River valleys of Central/Eastern United States.	± E. nodosum.	↑WBC, eosinophilia, anemia, ↓ platelets. Immunodiffusion test positive for M (mycelial) precipitin band (diagnostic of acute histoplasmosis).	Unilateral/bilateral multiple patchy infiltrates with bilateral hilar adenopathy No pleural effusion.

Infectious Causes

Causes	Features (may have some, none, or all)			
	History	Physical	Laboratory	Chest x-ray
Coccidiomycosis (chronic)	Previous exposure in endemic coccidiomycosis areas. Asymptomatic.	± E. nodosum.	Normal WBC. No eosinophilia in chronic phase. CF IgG titer ≥ 1:32 indicates active disease.	Thick/thin-walled cavities < 3 cm ± calcifications. Air fluid level rare unless secondarily infected. Cavities usually in anterior segments of upper lobes (vs. posterior segments with TB). No surrounding tissue reaction. Pleural effusion common.
Pertussis	Paroxysmal bouts of dry cough. Non/partial immunization against pertussis.	Conjunctival hemorrhages. secondary to severe coughing.	↑WBC and lymphocytosis (> 60%). Culture of nasopharynx/cough positive for B. pertussis. Blood cultures negative.	Bilateral perihilar fuzzy infiltrates. "Shaggy heart sign." No pleural effusion or cavitation. ± unilateral hilar adenopathy.
Plague (pneumonic)	Acute onset of fever, headache, myalgias, chest pain, dyspnea, and cough. Patients rapidly become critically ill. Sputum thin at onset but rapidly becomes purulent/bloody.	Fever/diaphoresis, tachypnea, hypotension ± cyanosis.	↑WBC (left shift). Sputum with pleomorphic plump gram-negative bacilli.	Begins with as focal infiltrate with rapid progression to multilobar involvement. Bilateral hilar adenopathy. No cavitation. Consolidation and pleural effusions common.

Non-Infectious Causes

Causes	Features (may have some, none, or all)			
	History	Physical	Laboratory	Chest x-ray
Metastatic carcinoma	History of breast, thyroid, renal cell, colon, pancreatic cancer or osteogenic sarcoma.	Findings related to underlying malignancy and, when present, to bone, hepatic, CNS metastases.	Secondary to effects of primary neoplasm, metastases, paraneoplastic syndrome.	Nodular lesions that vary in size. Metastatic lesions are usually well circumscribed with lower lobe predominance. Usually no bronchial obstruction (obstruction suggests colon, renal, or melanoma metastases). Usually no cavitation (except for squamous cell metastases). Calcification usually suggests osteosarcoma (rarely adenocarcinoma). Pleural effusion rare (except for breast cancer).
Sarcoidosis (Stage I–II)	Shortness of breath, fatigue, nasal stuffiness	Waxy/yellowish papules on face/upper trunk. Uveitis, parotid swelling, E. nodosum	↑ESR, normal LFTs, ↑ creatinine (if renal involvement), ↑ACE levels, hypercalciuria/ hypercalcemia, polyclonal gammopathy on SPEP. Anergic.	Bilateral nodular infiltrates of variable size. Cavitation rare. Symmetrical/smooth bilateral hilar adenopathy ± right paratracheal adenopathy. Clear channel between nodes and mediastinum. Pleural effusion rare.

Non-Infectious Causes

Causes	Features (may have some, none, or all)			
	History	Physical	Laboratory	Chest x-ray
Silicosis	Foundry workers, quarry workers, sandblasters, stone cutters, coal miners with ≥ 10 years exposure. PPD positive if superimposed TB (reactivation).	Healthy appearing.	Normal WBC, ESR, pO_2. If complicated by superimposed TB, then findings related to TB.	Bilateral hilar adenopathy with "eggshell" calcification. Upper lobe predominance. Bilateral diffuse nodules (2-10 mm) sparing lung bases. Nodules may calcify, coalesce, or cavitate. ± peripheral emphysema. If superimposed TB, findings of reactivation TB will also be present.
Lymphoma	Fever, ↓ appetite with weight loss, night sweats, fatigue.	Adenopathy ± splenomegaly.	Normal WBC, ↑ basophils, ↑ eosinophilia, ↓ lymphocytes, ↑ platelets, ↑ESR, ↑ alkaline phosphatase, ↑ $\propto_{1,2}$ globulins on SPEP.	Unilateral or asymmetrical bilateral hilar adenopathy. Lung infiltrate may appear contiguous with hilar adenopathy. No clear channel between mediastinum and hilar nodes. Small pleural effusions rare.
ALL/CLL	Fever, malaise, ↓ appetite with weight loss, fatigue, weakness.	Generalized adenopathy. ± sternal tenderness, hepatomegaly/ splenomegaly.	Peripheral smear/bone marrow with abnormal lymphocytes. If CNS findings with ALL, ± CSF cytology. With CLL, anemia, ↓ platelets (late). Hypogamma-globulinemia globulins on SPEP.	Symmetrical enlargement of hilum/mediastinum ± diffuse infiltrates/pleural effusion.

Non-Infectious Causes

Causes	Features (may have some, none, or all)			
	History	Physical	Laboratory	Chest x-ray
Atypical measles	Previous immunization with killed measles vaccine.	Petechial rash peripheral on trunk/extremities. No conjunctival injection or Koplik's spots.	Normal/↑WBC (left shift), eosinophilia. Negative IgM and positive IgG measles titers.	Bilateral symmetrical infiltrates with hilar adenopathy.

DIFFUSE RETICULAR INFILTRATES

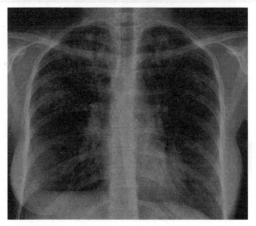

Infectious Causes

Causes	Features (may have some, none, or all)			
	History	Physical	Laboratory	Chest x-ray
TB (miliary)	FUO, intact appetite with weight loss, night sweats, fatigue. More common in elderly and those on chronic/high-dose steroids.	Asthenic habitus. ± signs of TB basilar meningitis. TB endophthal-mitis is diagnostic of miliary TB.	↑/↓WBC, anemia, ↑ platelets, ↑ ESR. Granulomas in liver/bone marrow biopsy.	Widespread multiple opacities of uniform (1-4 mm) size that slowly increase on serial films. Bilateral/diffuse small opacities larger in upper lung fields. Opacities have "snow storm" appearance.
Coccidiomycosis (miliary)	Previous exposure in endemic coccidiomycosis areas. Asymptomatic.	Unremarkable unless E. nodosum present (disappears with disseminated infection).	Normal WBC. No eosinophilia in chronic phase. CF IgG titer ≥ 1:32 indicates active disease.	Bilateral diffuse small opacities with lower lobe predilection. Resembles TB (miliary). Thick/thin-walled cavities < 3 cm ± calcifications. Air fluid level rare.

Non-Infectious Causes

Causes	Features (may have some, none, or all)			
	History	Physical	Laboratory	Chest x-ray
Idiopathic pulmonary fibrosis/ fibrosing alveolitis	Slowly progressive dyspnea (months-to-years). Usually 50-70 years of age. Chronic non-productive cough.	Clubbing, dry/crackling rales bilaterally.	Normal WBC and ESR. PFTs with restrictive pattern.	Early lower lobe predominance later spreads upward. Vascular lung marking obliterated by fibrosis ("honeycombed lungs"). Bilateral subpleural reticular/nodular infiltrates. ± traction bronchiectasis. Upper lung fibrosis suggests TB, sarcoidosis, histoplasmosis, allergic alveolitis, or ankylosing spondylitis.
Silicosis	Foundry workers, quarry workers, sandblasters, stone cutters, coal miners with ≥ 10 years exposure. PPD positive if superimposed TB (reactivation).	Healthy appearing.	Normal WBC, ESR, pO_2. If complicated by superimposed TB, then findings related to TB.	Bilateral hilar adenopathy with "eggshell" calcification. Upper lobe predominance. Bilateral diffuse nodules (2-10 mm) sparing lung bases. Nodules may calcify, coalesce, or cavitate. ± peripheral emphysema. If superimposed TB, findings of reactivation TB will also be present.
Sarcoidosis (Stage III)	Shortness of breath, fatigue.	Waxy/yellowish papules on the face/upper trunk. No fever. Funduscopic "candle wax drippings".	↑ ESR, normal LFT's, ↑ creatinine if renal involvement, ↑ACE levels, hypercalciuria, hypercalcemia, polyclonal gammopathy on SPEP. Anergic.	Bilateral nodular/ reticulonodular infiltrates/fibrosis. No hilar adenopathy.

Non-Infectious Causes

Causes	Features (may have some, none, or all)			
	History	Physical	Laboratory	Chest x-ray
Rheumatoid nodules	Usually in severe rheumatoid arthritis (RA). ± history of silicosis.	Findings secondary to RA. Rheumatoid nodules on exterior surfaces of arms.	Normal WBC, ↑ESR, ↑ANA, ↑RF (high titer). Pleural effusion ↓ glucose	Nodules are round and well circumscribed, predominantly in lower lobes. Cavitation is common. Superimposed on interstitial lung disease ("rheumatoid lung"). ± pulmonary fibrosis, pleural effusion. Silicosis + RA nodules = Caplan's syndrome.
Systemic lupus erythematosus (SLE)	Fatigue, chest pain. History of SLE.	Fever/myalgias, alopecia, malar rash, "cytoid bodies" in retina, painless oral ulcers, synovitis, splenomegaly, generalized adenopathy, Raynaud's phenomenon.	↑ ANA, ↑ DS-DNA, ↓ C_3, polyclonal gammopathy on SPEP, ↑ ferritin. Pleural fluid with ↑ ANA, ↓ C_3	Migratory ill-defined non-segmental infiltrates ± small pleural effusions. No consolidation or cavitation.
Allergic alveolitis	Inhalation of organic dusts (pigeon breeder's disease), cotton/line dust disease (byssinosis), farmer's lung secondary to moldy hay/grain, sugar cane dust disease (bagassosis), maple bark (strippers disease).	Unremarkable.	Normal WBC and ESR.	Typically in mid lung fields. Chronic dust exposure predisposes to fibrosis.

Non-Infectious Causes

Causes	Features (may have some, none, or all)			
	History	Physical	Laboratory	Chest x-ray
Histiocytosis X (eosinophilic granuloma/ Langerhan's cell histiocytosis)	Patients usually 20-40 years. Most are asymptomatic. Fever, cough, dyspnea in some. Diabetes insipidus rare.	Hepato-splenomegaly, skin lesions, hemoptysis (rare).	Normal WBC, eosinophilia.	Pneumothorax superimposed on diffuse pulmonary fibrosis. Cystic bone lesions. Usually mid/upper lung fields with nodules or infiltrates. Thin-walled cysts. No hilar adenopathy or pleural effusion.
Leukostasis (AML)	Untreated acute myelogenous leukemia (AML).	Fever, sternal tenderness, petechiae, ecchymosis.	↑WBC (≥ 100 K/mm^3) with blasts in peripheral smear/bone marrow, ↓ platelets.	Diffuse symmetrical fluffy infiltrates without pleural effusion.
Lymphangitic metastases	History of breast, thyroid, pancreas, cervical, prostate, or lung carcinoma.	Findings related to underlying malignancy.	Normal/↑ WBC, ↑ESR.	Interstitial indistinct pulmonary infiltrates (may be reticulonodular) with lower lobe predominance Usually unilateral but may be bilateral. No consolidation or cavitation ± pleural effusions.
Drug-induced	Exposure to chemotherapeutic agents (e.g., BCNU, busulfan, methotrexate, cyclophospham-ide, bleomycin) or other drugs (e.g., nitro-furantoin, sulfasalazine, amiodarone, opiates, cocaine).	Unremarkable.	Normal WBC ± eosinophilia. Normal/↑ ESR/LFTs. Eosinophils in pleural effusion.	Bilateral coarse symmetrical patchy infiltrates/fibrosis ± pleural effusions. Hilar adenopathy only with drug-induced pseudolymphoma (secondary to dilantin). No cavitation.

Non-Infectious Causes

Causes	Features (may have some, none, or all)			
	History	Physical	Laboratory	Chest x-ray
Bronchiolitis obliterans with organizing pneumonia (BOOP)	Fever, dyspnea, cough.	Unremarkable.	↑WBC (left shift), ↑LDH, ↓pO$_2$, ↑A-a gradient	Classically bilateral patchy peripheral infiltrates. Often lower lobe predominance. No cavitation or pleural effusion.

MILIARY INFILTRATES

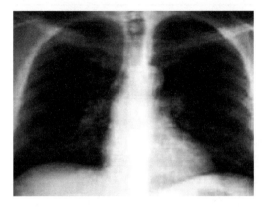

Infectious Causes

Causes	Features (may have some, none, or all)			
	History	Physical	Laboratory	Chest x-ray
TB (miliary)	FUO, intact appetite with weight loss, night sweats, fatigue. More common in elderly and those on chronic/high-dose steroids.	Asthenic habitus. ± signs of TB basilar meningitis. TB endophthalmitis is diagnostic of miliary TB.	↑/↓WBC, no eosinophilia, anemia, ↑ platelets, ↑ESR. Granulomas in liver/bone marrow biopsy.	Widespread multiple opacities of uniform (1-4 mm) size that slowly increase on serial films. Bilateral/diffuse small opacities larger in upper lung fields. Opacities have "snow storm" appearance.

Infectious Causes

Causes	Features (may have some, none, or all)			
	History	Physical	Laboratory	Chest x-ray
Histoplasmosis (miliary)	Fever, night sweats, cough, weight loss, histoplasmosis exposure (River valleys of Central/Eastern United States).	± E. nodosum; unremarkable.	Normal WBC, ± eosinophilia, anemia, ↑ platelets, PPD negative. Immunodiffusion test positive for H precipitin band (diagnostic of acute/chronic histoplasmosis).	Unilateral/bilateral multiple patchy infiltrates (consolidation in some areas, clear in others). Upper lobe predilection. Bilateral hilar adenopathy uncommon. Calcifications common. ± ipsilateral pleural effusion. Resembles reactivation TB.
Coccidiomycosis (miliary)	Previous exposure in endemic coccidiomycosis areas. Asymptomatic.	± E. nodosum.	Normal WBC. No eosinophilia in chronic phase. CF IgG titer ≥ 1:32 indicates active disease.	Bilateral diffuse small opacities with lower lobe predilection. No cavitation or pleural effusion. Thick/thin walled cavities < (3 cm) ± calcifications. Air fluid level rare.

Non-Infectious Causes

Causes	Features (may have some, none, or all)			
	History	Physical	Laboratory	Chest x-ray
Sarcoidosis (Stage III)	Shortness of breath, fatigue, nasal stuffiness	Waxy/yellowish papules on face/upper trunk. Funduscopic exam with "candle wax drippings."	↑ ESR, normal LFTs, ↑ creatinine (if renal involvement), ↑ACE levels, hypercalciuria/ hypercalcemia, polyclonal gammopathy on SPEP. Anergic.	Bilateral nodular infiltrates of variable size. Cavitation rare. No hilar adenopathy. Pleural effusion rare.

Non-Infectious Causes

Causes	Features (may have some, none, or all)			
	History	Physical	Laboratory	Chest x-ray
Silicosis	Foundry workers, quarry workers, sandblasters, stone cutters, coal miners with ≥ 10 years exposure. PPD positive if superimposed TB (reactivation).	Healthy appearing.	Normal WBC, ESR, pO$_2$. If complicated by superimposed TB, then findings related to TB.	Bilateral hilar adenopathy with "eggshell" calcification. Upper lobe predominance. Bilateral diffuse nodules (2-10 mm) sparing lung bases. Nodules may calcify, coalesce, or cavitate. ± peripheral emphysema. If superimposed TB, findings of reactivation TB will also be present.
Allergic alveolitis	Inhalation of organic dusts. (pigeon breeder's disease), cotton/line dust disease (byssinosis) farmer's lung secondary to moldy hay/grain, sugar cane dust disease (bagassosis), maple bark (strippers disease).	Unremarkable.	Normal WBC and ESR	Typically in mid lung fields. Chronic dust exposure predisposes to fibrosis.
Alveolar cell carcinoma	Fever, ↑ appetite with weight loss, night sweats.	± dullness over lobe with large lower lobe lesions.	Positive cytology by BAL/lung biopsy.	Well/ill-defined circumscribed peripheral infiltrates ± air bronchograms. May be multifocal/ multilobar. Hilar adenopathy present. Stranding to the hilum ("pleural tail" sign). ± pleural effusion if lower lobe infiltrate. No cavitation.

Non-Infectious Causes

Causes	Features (may have some, none, or all)			
	History	Physical	Laboratory	Chest x-ray
Metastatic carcinoma	History of breast, thyroid, renal cell, colon, pancreatic cancer or osteogenic sarcoma.	Findings related to underlying malignancy and, when present, to bone, hepatic, CNS metastases.	Secondary to effects of primary neoplasm, metastases, paraneoplastic syndrome.	Nodular lesions that vary in size. Metastatic lesions are usually well circumscribed with lower lobe predominance. Usually no bronchial obstruction (obstruction suggests colon, renal, or melanoma metastases). Usually no cavitation (except for squamous cell metastases). Calcification usually suggests osteosarcoma (rarely adenocarcinoma). Pleural effusion rare (except for breast cancer).
Lymphoma	Fever, ↓ appetite with weight loss, night sweats, fatigue.	Adenopathy ± splenomegaly.	Normal WBC, ↑ basophils, ↑ eosinophilia, ↓ lymphocytes, ↑ platelets, ↑ESR, ↑ alkaline phosphatase, ↑ $\propto_{1,2}$ globulins on SPEP.	Unilateral or asymmetrical bilateral hilar adenopathy. Lung infiltrate may appear contiguous with hilar adenopathy. No clear channel between mediastinum and hilar nodes. Small pleural effusions rare.
Histiocytosis X (eosinophilic granuloma/ Langerhan's cell histiocytosis)	Patients usually 20-40 years. Most are asymptomatic. Fever, cough, dyspnea in some. Diabetes insipidus rare.	Hepato-splenomegaly, skin lesions, hemoptysis (rare).	Normal WBC, eosinophilia.	Pneumothorax superimposed on diffuse pulmonary fibrosis. Cystic bone lesions. Usually mid/upper lung fields with nodules or infiltrates. Thin-walled cysts. No hilar adenopathy or pleural effusion.
Pulmonary alveolar microlithiasis	Asymptomatic. Positive family history.	Unremarkable unless signs of cor pulmonale.	Normal WBC and ESR.	Bilateral miliary calcified nodular densities most pronounced at lung bases. No hilar adenopathy or pleural effusion. More densely calcified than miliary TB nodules. Lung detail obscured by density of calcifications ("black diaphragm" sign).

UNILATERAL HYPERLUCENT LUNG

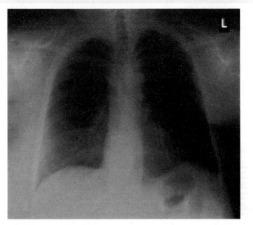

Infectious Causes

Causes	Features (may have some, none, or all)			
	History	Physical	Laboratory	Chest x-ray
TB (reactivation)	Fevers, night sweats, normal appetite with weight loss, cough ± hemoptysis.	± bilateral apical dullness.	Normal WBC, no eosinophilia, ↑ platelets, ↑ESR (≤ 70 mm/h). Positive PPD. AFB in sputum smear/culture.	Slowly progressive bilateral infiltrates. No pleural effusion. Usually in apical segment of lower lobes or apical/posterior segments of upper lobes. Calcifications common.

Non-Infectious Causes

Causes	Features (may have some, none, or all)			
	History	Physical	Laboratory	Chest x-ray
Pneumothorax	Recent history of central line insertion, tracheostomy, thoracentesis, thoracotomy. May be spontaneous or secondary to Legionella, PCP, TB, coccidiomycosis, emphysema, histiocytosis X, metastatic osteogenic carcinoma, esophageal perforation.	Findings related to location/size of pneumothorax. ↓ breath sounds, tracheal shift away from midline.	↓pO$_2$ if pneumothorax is large.	No lung markings above lobar/lung collapse.
Mastectomy/ absent pectoralis muscle	Mastectomy of breast cancer on affected side/surgically removed pectoralis muscle.	Mastectomy scar. Resected pectoralis muscle/scar.	Normal WBC and ESR.	Absent breast/pectoralis muscle shadow appears as unilateral hyperlucent lung.
Compensatory emphysema	History of lobectomy for lung malignancy.	↓ breath sounds/↑ resonance on affected side. Thoracotomy scar.	Normal WBC and ESR.	No lung markings unilaterally.
Scoliosis	Congential or acquired severe scoliosis.	Findings secondary to scoliosis.	Normal WBC and ESR.	Chest deformity of scoliosis. Affected lung has ↓ but present lung markings.

Non-Infectious Causes

Causes	Features (may have some, none, or all)			
	History	Physical	Laboratory	Chest x-ray
Pulmonary embolus/ infarct	Acute onset dyspnea/pleuritic chest pain. History of lower extremity trauma, stasis or hypercoagulable disorder.	↑ pulse/ respiratory rate.	↑ fibrin split products and D-dimers ± ↑ total bilirubin. Bloody pleural effusion. ECG with RV strain/P-pulmonale (large embolus). Positive V/Q scan and CT pulmonary angiogram.	Normal or show non-specific pleural-based infiltrates resembling atelectasis. Focal segmental/lobar hyperlucency (Westermark's sign) in some. "Hampton's hump" with infarct. Resolving infarcts ↓ in size but maintain shape/density ("melting ice cube").
Pulmonary artery agenesis	If left-sided, usually associated tetralogy of Fallot. Recurrent respiratory infection, cough, ± hemoptysis.	Mediastinum shifted to affected side.	Normal/↑WBC, normal ESR.	Affected lung with small volume, not translucent. Usual hilar shadow absent.
Swyer-James/ Macleod's Syndrome	Asymptomatic or chronic purulent cough, dyspnea.	↑ resonance on affected side. Mediastinal shift to affected side during inspiration and away in expiration.	Normal WBC and ESR.	Resembles obstructive emphysema, but normal lung volume.

SPONTANEOUS PNEUMOTHORAX

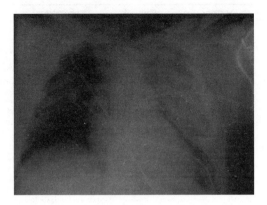

Infectious Causes

Causes	Features (may have some, none, or all)			
	History	Physical	Laboratory	Chest x-ray
Legionella	Recent contact with Legionella containing water. Usually elderly. May have watery diarrhea, abdominal pain, mental confusion.	Fever/chills, relative bradycardia. Hepatic/ splenic enlargement goes against the diagnosis. ↓ breath sounds if consolidation or pleural effusion.	↑WBC, ↑SGOT/SGPT, ↓$PO_4^{=}$, ↓Na^+, ↑CPK, ↑ESR, ↑CPR, proteinuria, microscopic hematuria, L. pneumophila antigenuria (serotype I only) may not be positive early. Mucoid/ purulent sputum with few PMNs. Positive sputum DFA (before therapy) is diagnostic. ↑ Legionella titer ≥ 1:256 or ≥ 4-fold rise between acute/convalescent titers.	Rapidly progressive asymmetrical infiltrates clue to Legionella. Consolidation and pleural effusion not uncommon. Cavitation rare.

Infectious Causes

Causes	Features (may have some, none, or all)			
	History	Physical	Laboratory	Chest x-ray
TB (reactivation)	Fevers, night sweats, normal appetite with weight loss, cough ± hemoptysis.	± bilateral apical dullness.	Normal WBC, no eosinophilia, ↑ platelets, ↑ESR (≤ 70 mm/h). Positive PPD. AFB in sputum smear/culture.	Slowly progressive bilateral infiltrates. NO pleural effusion. Usually in apical segment of lower lobes or apical/ posterior segments of upper lobes. Calcifications common.
Coccidiomycosis (reactivation)	Previous exposure in endemic coccidiomycosis areas. Asymptomatic.	± E. nodosum.	Normal WBC. Eosinophilia acutely but not in chronic phase, and no eosinophilia in pleural fluid. CF IgG titer = 1:32 indicates active disease.	Thick/thin walled cavities < 3 cm ± calcifications. Air fluid level rare. Lower lobe predilection ± bilateral hilar adenopathy. Cavities characteristically in anterior segments (vs. posterior segments). Pleural effusion rare.
P. (carinii) jiroveci (PCP)	↓ cell-mediated immunity (e.g., HIV, immuno-suppressive therapy). Increasing dyspnea over 1 week. Chest pain with shortness of breath suggests pneumothorax.	↓ breath sounds bilaterally. Other findings depend on size/location of pneumothorax (if present).	Normal/↑ WBC (left shift), ↓ lymphocytes, ↑LDH. ↓pO$_2$, ↓DL$_{CO}$, ↑A-a gradient. PCP cysts in sputum/ respiratory secretions.	Bilateral perihilar symmetrical fluffy infiltrates ± pneumothorax. No calcification, cavitation, or pleural effusion.

Non-Infectious Causes

Causes	Features (may have some, none, or all)			
	History	Physical	Laboratory	Chest x-ray
Iatrogenic	Recent history of central line insertion, tracheostomy, thoracentesis, thoracotomy. May also be ventilator related (barotrauma) or post chest surgery.	Findings related to location/size of pneumothorax. ↓ breath sounds, tracheal shift away from midline.	↓pO₂ if pneumothorax large.	No lung markings above/lateral to lobar lung collapse on upright PA chest x-ray.
Emphysema (ruptured bleb/cyst)	Long history of smoking. Rupture of apical bleb common in males > 30 years. CAP may occur in unaffected areas of lung.	Asthenic "pink puffers." Barrel chest. Diaphragmatic excursions < 2 cm.	Normal WBC. ↓pO₂.	↓ lung markings ("vanishing lung") ± blebs. Hyperlucent lungs with upper lobe predominance. Flattened diaphragms, vertically elongated cardiac silhouette, ↑ retrocardiac and retrosternal airspaces. No infiltrates or pleural effusions. No vascular redistribution to upper lobes with CHF in upper lobe emphysema.
Histiocytosis X (eosinophilic granuloma/ Langerhan's cell histiocytosis)	Patients usually 20-40 years. Most are asymptomatic. Fever, cough, dyspnea in some. Diabetes insipidus rare.	Hepato-splenomegaly, skin lesions, hemoptysis (rare).	Normal WBC, eosinophilia.	Pneumothorax superimposed on diffuse pulmonary fibrosis. Cystic bone lesions. Usually mid/upper lung fields with nodules or infiltrates. Thin-walled cysts. No hilar adenopathy or pleural effusion.
Osteogenic sarcoma	Low-grade fevers. Long bone pain/mass. Primary malignant bone tumor of young adults. ↑ incidence in the elderly with Paget's disease.	Bone swelling/ tenderness.	Normal WBC, ↑ESR, positive bone scan.	Metastases nearly always nodular. Large/well-rounded "cannon ball" nodules characteristic.

Non-Infectious Causes

| Causes | Features (may have some, none, or all) | | | |
	History	Physical	Laboratory	Chest x-ray
Esophageal perforation	Acute onset of upper abdominal/chest pain following recent upper GI endoscopy or violent vomiting/retching.	± anterior chest wall crepitus.	↑WBC (left shift), ↑↑↑ amylase in pleural fluid.	Pneumomediastinum. Unilateral pleural effusion typically left sided.

Chapter 12

Other Respiratory Tract Infections and Complications of Pneumonia

Burke A. Cunha, MD

Acute Bacterial Exacerbation of Chronic Bronchitis (AECB)

Subset	Pathogens	PO Therapy
AECB	S. pneumoniae H. influenzae M. catarrhalis	Levofloxacin 500 mg (PO) q24h x 5 days **or** Moxifloxacin 400 mg q24h x 5 days **or** Gemifloxacin 320 mg(PO) q24h x 5 days **or** Telithromycin 800 mg (PO) q24h x 5 days **or** Doxycycline 100 mg (PO) q12h x 5 days **or** Amoxicillin/clavulanic acid 500/125 mg (PO) q12h x 5 days **or** Clarithromycin XL 1 gm (PO) q24h x 5 days **or** Azithromycin 500 mg (PO) x 3 days, or 500 mg (PO) on day 1 followed by 250 mg (PO) q24h on days 2-5

Clinical Presentation: Productive cough and negative chest x-ray in a patient with chronic bronchitis

Diagnostic Considerations: Diagnosis by productive cough, purulent sputum, and chest x-ray negative for pneumonia. H. influenzae is relatively more common than other pathogens

Pitfalls: Do not obtain sputum cultures in chronic bronchitis; cultures usually reported as normal/mixed flora and should not be used to guide therapy

Therapeutic Considerations: Treated with same antibiotics as for community-acquired pneumonia, since pathogens are the same (even though H. influenzae is relatively more frequent). Respiratory viruses/C. pneumoniae may initiate AECB, but AECB is usually followed by bacterial infection, which is responsible for symptoms and is the aim of therapy. Bronchodilators are helpful to treat bronchospasm. Macrolide-resistant S. pneumoniae is an important clinical problem (prevalence ≥ 30%)

Prognosis: Related to underlying cardiopulmonary status

Bacterial Sinusitis

Subset	Usual Pathogens	IV Therapy (Hospitalized)	PO Therapy or IV-to-PO Switch (Ambulatory)
Acute	S. pneumoniae H. influenzae M. catarrhalis	Levofloxacin 750 mg (IV) q24h x 5 days **or** Moxifloxacin 400 mg (IV) q24h x 7 days **or** Ceftriaxone 1 gm (IV) q24h x 1- 2 weeks **or** Doxycycline 200 mg (IV) q12h x 3 days, then 100 mg (IV) q12h x 11 days	Levofloxacin 750 mg (PO) q24h x 5 days **or** Moxifloxacin 400 mg (PO) q24h x 7 days **or** Doxycycline 200 mg (PO) q12h x 3 days, then 100 mg (PO) q12h x 11 days* **or** Telithromycin 800 mg (PO) q24h x 5 days **or** Amoxicillin/clavulanic acid XR 2 tablets (PO) q12h x 10 days **or** Cephalosporin[‡] (PO) q12h x 2 weeks **or** Clarithromycin XL 1 gm (PO) q24h x 2 weeks
Chronic	Same as acute plus oral anaerobes	Requires prolonged antimicrobial therapy (2-4 weeks)	

Duration of therapy represents total time IV, PO, or IV + PO in adults. Most patients on IV therapy able to take PO meds should be switched to PO therapy soon after clinical improvement (usually < 72 hours). See Chapter 7 for pediatric therapy
*   *Loading dose is not needed PO if given IV with the same drug*
‡   *Cefdinir 300 mg or cefditoren 400 mg or cefixime 400 mg or cefpodoxime 200 mg*

Acute Sinusitis

Clinical Presentation: Nasal discharge and cough frequently with headache, facial pain, and low-grade fever lasting > 10-14 days. Can also present acutely with high fever (≥ 104° F) and purulent nasal discharge ± intense headache lasting for ≥ 3 days. Other manifestations depend on the affected sinus: <u>maxillary sinus:</u> percussion tenderness of molars; maxillary toothache; local extension may cause osteomyelitis of facial bones with proptosis, retrobital cellulitis, ophthalmoplegia; direct intracranial extension is rare; <u>frontal sinus:</u> prominent headache; intracranial extension may cause epidural/brain abscess, meningitis, cavernous sinus/superior sagittal sinus thrombosis; orbital extension may cause periorbital cellulitis; <u>ethmoid sinus:</u> eyelid edema and prominent tearing; extension may cause retrobital pain/periorbital cellulitis and/or cavernous sinus/superior sagittal sinus thrombosis; <u>sphenoid sinus:</u> severe headache; extension into cavernous sinus may cause meningitis, cranial nerve paralysis [III, IV, VI], temporal lobe abscess, cavernous sinus thrombosis). Cough and nasal discharge are prominent in children

Diagnostic Considerations: Diagnosis by sinus x-rays or CT/MRI showing complete sinus opacification, air-fluid levels, mucosal thickening. Consider sinus aspiration in immunocompromised hosts or treatment failures. In children, acute sinusitis is a clinical diagnosis; imaging studies are not routine

Pitfalls: May present as periorbital cellulitis (obtain head CT/MRI to rule out underlying sinusitis). If CT/MRI demonstrates "post-septal" involvement, treat as acute bacterial meningitis. In children, transillumination, sinus tenderness to percussion, and color of nasal mucus are not reliable indicators of sinusitis

Therapeutic Considerations: Treat for full course to prevent relapses/complications. Macrolides and TMP-SMX may predispose to drug-resistant S. pneumoniae (DRSP), and 25% of S. pneumoniae are naturally resistant to macrolides. Consider local resistance rates before making empiric antibiotic selections

Prognosis: Good if treated for full course. Relapses may occur with suboptimal treatment. For frequent recurrences, consider radiologic studies and ENT consultation

---

COMPLICATIONS OF PNEUMONIA

The majority of normal hosts with CAP treated early with appropriate antimicrobial therapy on an ambulatory basis have an uncomplicated course and excellent prognosis (mortality < 1%). However, complications may occur, particularly in elderly patients, immunocompromised hosts, and individuals with underlying medical conditions, which may threaten survival (Table 12.1). Complications include pulmonary complications (e.g., respiratory failure in emphysema patients, vascular invasion with infarction, bronchopulmonary fistula, pleural adhesions, purulent pericarditis, empyema), systemic complications (e.g., patients, bacteremia), exacerbation of comorbid conditions (e.g., acute myocardial infarction from underlying coronary heart disease, diabetes mellitus), other complications related to the acute illness (e.g., stress ulcer), and failure to respond to therapy.

Table 12.1. Complications of Pneumonia

- Pulmonary complications: empyema, lung abscess/cavitation, bronchopleural fistula, necrotizing pneumonia, vascular invasion with infarction, pleural adhesions, bronchiolitis obliterans (BOOP)
- Systemic complications: sepsis, bacteremia with metastatic infection (e.g., meningitis, endocarditis, septic arthritis)
- Exacerbation of comorbid medical conditions: heart failure, angina/MI, diabetes mellitus, others
- Complications related to mechanical ventilation: pneumothorax, interstitial emphysema, ARDS
- Drug reactions
- Other complications related to acute illness: stress ulcer/GI bleed, DVT/pulmonary embolism
- Failure to respond to therapy (see Tables 1.23, 15.9)

Lung Abscess/Empyema

Subset	Usual Pathogens	Preferred IV Therapy	Alternate IV Therapy	PO Therapy or IV-to-PO Switch
Lung abscess/ empyema	Oral anaerobes S. aureus K. pneumoniae S. pneumoniae	Clindamycin 600 mg (IV) q8h* **or** Piperacillin/ tazobactam 3.375 gm (IV) q6h*	Meropenem 1 gm (IV) q8h* **or** Ertapenem 1 gm (IV) q24h*	Clindamycin 300 mg (PO) q8h* **or** Levofloxacin 500 mg (PO) q24h* **or** Moxifloxacin 400 mg (PO) q24h*
Bronchiectasis, cystic fibrosis	P. aeruginosa	Meropenem 2 gm (IV) q8h*	Cefepime 2 mg (IV) q8h* ± Amikacin 1 gm (IV) q24h*	Levofloxacin 750 mg (PO) q24h* **or** Ciprofloxacin 1 gm (PO) q24h*

Duration of therapy represents total time IV, PO, or IV + PO. Most patients on IV therapy able to take PO meds should be switched to PO therapy soon after clinical improvement (usually < 72 hours)
* *Treat until resolved/cured*

Clinical Presentation: Lung abscess presents as single/multiple cavitary lung lesion(s) with fever. Empyema presents as persistent fever/pleural effusion without layering on lateral decubitus chest x-ray

Diagnostic Considerations: In lung abscess, plain film/CT scan demonstrates cavitary lung lesions appearing > 1 week after pneumonia. Most CAPs are not associated with pleural effusion, and few develop empyema. In empyema, pleural fluid pH is ≤ 7.2; culture purulent exudate for pathogen

Pitfalls: Pleural effusions secondary to CAP usually resolve rapidly with treatment. Suspect empyema in patients with persistent pleural effusions with fever

Therapeutic Considerations: Chest tube/surgical drainage needed for empyema. Treat lung abscess until it resolves (usually 3-12 months)

Prognosis: Good if adequately drained

Mediastinitis

Subset	Usual Pathogens	Preferred IV Therapy	Alternate IV Therapy	IV-to-PO Switch
Following esophageal perforation or thoracic surgery	Oral anaerobes	Piperacillin/ tazobactam 3.375 gm (IV) q6h x 2 weeks **or** Ampicillin/sulbactam 3 gm (IV) q6h x 2 weeks	Meropenem 1 gm (IV) q8h x 2 weeks **or** Imipenem 500 mg (IV) q6h x 2 weeks **or** Ertapenem 1 gm (IV) q24h x 2 wks	Amoxicillin/ clavulanic acid 500/125 mg (PO) q8hx 2 weeks **or** Levofloxacin 500 mg (PO) q24h x 2 weeks **or** Moxifloxacin 400 mg (PO) q24h x 2 weeks

Duration of therapy represents total time IV or IV + PO. Most patients on IV therapy able to take PO meds should be switched to PO therapy after clinical improvement

Diagnostic Considerations: Chest x-ray usually shows perihilar infiltrate in mediastinitis. Pleural effusions from esophageal tears have elevated amylase levels
Pitfalls: Do not overlook esophageal tear in mediastinitis with pleural effusions
Therapeutic Considerations: Obtain surgical consult if esophageal perforation is suspected
Prognosis: Related to extent, location, and duration of esophageal tear/mediastinal infection

Sepsis/Septic Shock from Pneumonia

Source	Usual Pathogens	Preferred IV Therapy	Alternate IV Therapy	IV-to-PO Switch
Community-acquired pneumonia	S. pneumoniae H. influenzae K. pneumoniae	Quinolone* (IV) q24h x 2 weeks **or** Ceftriaxone 1 gm (IV) q24h x 2 weeks	Cefepime 2 gm (IV) q12h x 2 weeks **or** Any 2nd generation cephalosporin (IV) x 2 weeks	Quinolone* (PO) q24h x 2 weeks **or** Doxycycline 200 mg (PO) q12h x 3 days, then 100 mg (PO) q12h x 11 days
Nosocomial pneumonia	P. aeruginosa K. pneumoniae E. coli S. marcescens	Treat the same as for ventilator-associated pneumonia (Chapter 7)		

Duration of therapy represents total time IV or IV + PO. Most patients on IV therapy able to take PO meds should be switched to PO therapy after clinical improvement
*   *Levofloxacin 500 mg (IV or PO) q24h or ciprofloxacin 400 mg (IV) or 500 mg (PO) q12h or moxifloxacin 400 mg (IV or PO) q24h*

Sepsis, Lung Source

Clinical Presentation: Normal hosts with community-acquired pneumonia (CAP) do not present with sepsis. CAP with sepsis suggests the presence of impaired immunity/hyposplenic function (see "sepsis in hyposplenia/asplenia," below), a pneumonia mimic, or another serious medical problem (Tables 12.2, 12.3)

Diagnostic Considerations: Impaired splenic function may be inferred by finding Howell-Jolly bodies (small, round, pinkish or bluish inclusion bodies in red blood cells) in the peripheral blood smear. The number of Howell-Jolly bodies is proportional to the degree of splenic dysfunction

Pitfalls: CAP with hypotension/sepsis should suggest hyposplenic function, impaired immunity, or an alternate diagnosis that can mimic CAP/shock. Be sure to exclude acute MI, acute heart failure/COPD, PE/infarction, overzealous diuretic therapy, concomitant GI bleed, and acute pancreatitis

Therapeutic Considerations: Patients with malignancies, myeloma, or SLE are predisposed to CAP, which is not usually severe or associated with shock. Be sure patients with CAP receiving steroids at less than "stress doses" do not have hypotension/shock from relative adrenal insufficiency. In patients with SLE, try to distinguish between lupus pneumonitis and CAP; lupus pneumonitis usually occurs as part of a lupus flare, CAP usually does not

Prognosis: Related to underlying cardiopulmonary/immune status. Early treatment is important

Table 12.2. Approach to Severe Community-Acquired Pneumonia With Shock

CAP does *not* present with shock in *normal* hosts. If shock is present with CAP, look for:

- Mimics of pneumonia (acute MI, acute PE)
- Exacerbation of pre-existing advanced cardiopulmonary disease (e.g., acute MI, pneumothorax, emphysema)
- Impaired or absent splenic function (see Table 12.3) (degree of splenic dysfunction correlates with number of Howell-Jolly bodies in the peripheral blood smear)
- GI bleed, acute pancreatitis, volume depletion (diuretics, poor oral intake)

Table 12.3. Conditions Associated With Impaired Splenic Function/Humoral (B-Lymphocyte) Immunity

• Amyloidosis	• IV gamma globulin therapy	• Splenectomy
• Celiac disease	• Myeloproliferative disorders	• Splenic infarcts
• Chronic active hepatitis	• Non-Hodgkin lymphoma	• Splenic malignancies
• Chronic alcoholism	• Regional enteritis	• Steroid therapy
• Congenital asplenia	• Waldenstrom macroglobulinemia	• SLE
• Fanconi syndrome	• Rheumatoid arthritis	• Systemic mastocytosis
• Hyposplenism of old age	• Sézary syndrome	• Systemic necrotizing vasculitis
• IgA deficiency	• Sickle cell trait/disease	• Thyroiditis
• Intestinal lymphangiectasia		• Ulcerative colitis

REFERENCES AND SUGGESTED READINGS

AAD-Sinusitis, Sinus and Allergy Health Partnership. Antimicrobial treatment guidelines for acute bacterial rhinosinusitis. Otolaryngol Head Neck Surg 130:1-45. 2004.

Adams SG, Anzueto A. Antibiotic therapy in acute exacerbations of chronic bronchitis. Semin Respir Infect. 15:234-47, 2000.

Annane D, Bellissant E, Cavaillon J-M. Septic shock. Lancet 365:63-78, 2005.

Anon JB. Treatment of acute bacterial rhinosinusitis caused by antimicrobial-resistant Streptococcus pneumoniae. Am J Med 2;117(Suppl 3A):23S-28S, 2004.

Benninger MS. Amoxicillin/clavulanate potassium extended release tablets: a new antimicrobial for the treatment of acute bacterial sinusitis and community-acquired pneumonia. Expert Opin Pharmacother. 4:1839-46, 2003.

Brook I. Management of anaerobic infection. Expert Rev Anti Infect Ther 2:153-8, 2004.

Cunha BA. Antibiotic selection for the treatment of sinusitis, otitis media, and pharyngitis infectious disease in clinical practice 7:S324-S326, 1998.

Cunha BA. The diagnostic significance of increased ACE levels. Infectious Disease Practice 22:7-8, 1998.

Cunha BA. The extrapulmonary manifestations of community-acquired pneumonias. Chest 112:945, 1998.

Cunha BA. Fever following post-open heart surgery. Infectious Disease Practice 21:47-48, 1997.

Cunha BA. Newer antibiotics for the treatment of acute exacerbations of chronic bronchitis. Advances in Therapy 13:313-323, 1996.

Cunha BA. Severe community acquired pneumonia. Critical Care Clinics 8:105-117, 1998.

Cunha BA. Therapy of fulminant pneumonia. Emergency Medicine 6:107-110, 1994.

Dever LL, Shashikumar K, Johanson WG. Antibiotics in the treatment of acute exacerbations of chronic bronchitis. Expert Opin Investig Drugs. 11:911-25, 2002.

File TM Jr. New insights in the treatment by levofloxacin. Chemotherapy 50(Suppl1):22-8, 2004.

Godfried MH. Clarithromycin (Biaxin) extended-release tablet: a therapeutic review. Expert Rev Anti Infect Ther 1:9-20, 2003.

Johnson P, Cihon C, Herrington J, et al. Efficacy and tolerability of moxifloxacin in the treatment of acute bacterial sinusitis caused by penicillin-resistant Streptococcus pneumoniae: a pooled analysis. Clin Ther. 26:224-231, 2004.

Kasbekar N, Acharya PS. Telithromycin: the first ketolide for the treatment of respiratory infections. Am J Health Pharm 62:905-15, 2005.

Klossek JM, Federspil P. Update on treatment guidelines for acute bacterial sinusitis. Int J Clin Pract 59:230-8, 2005.

Martinez FJ, Anzueto A. Appropriate outpatient treatment of acute bacterial exacerbations of chronic bronchitis. Am J Med 118(Suppl 7A):39S-44S, 2005.

McCormack PL, Keating GM. Amoxicillin/clavulanic acid 2000 mg/125 mg extended release (XR): a review of its use in the treatment of respiratory tract infections in adults. Drugs 65:121-36, 2005.

Merrill WH, Akhter SA, Wolf RK, et al. Simplified treatment of postoperative mediastinitis. Ann Thorac Surg. 78:608-12, 2004.

Norrby SR. Optimal treatment strategies for acute exacerbations of chronic bronchitis: high-risk patients. Suppl 4:47-52, 2001.

[No authors listed]. Moxifloxacin–a new fluoroquinolone antibacterial. Drug Ther Bull 42:61-2, 2004.

Piccirillo JF. Clinical practice. Acute bacterial sinusitis. N Engl J Med 26;35:902-10, 2004.

Poole MD. Acute bacterial rhinosinusitis: clinical impact of resistance and susceptibility. Am J Med 2;117(Suppl 3A):29S-38S, 2004.

Poole MD, Portugal LG. Treatment of rhinosinusitis in the outpatient setting. Am J Med 118(Suppl 7A):45S-50S, 2005.

Poole M, Anon J, Paglia M, et al. A trial of high-dose, short-course levofloxacin for the treatment of acute bacterial sinusitis. Otolaryngol Head Neck Surg, 134:10-17, 2006.

Sande Ma, Gwaltney JM. Acute community-acquired bacterial sinusitis: continuing challenges and current management. Clin Infect Dis 1;39(Suppl3):S151-8, 2004.

Sethi S, File TM. Managing patients with recurrent acute exacerbations of chronic bronchitis: a common clinical problem. Curr Med Res Opin 20:1511-21, 2004.

Shams WE, Evans ME. Guide to selection of fluoroquinolones in patients with lower respiratory tract infections. Drugs 65:949-91, 2005.

Shea KW, Cunha BA. Fever in the intensive care unit. Infectious Disease Clinics of North America 10:185-210, 1996.

Tsang KW. Solutions for difficult diagnostic cases of acute exacerbations of chronic bronchitis. Chemotherapy 47 (Suppl) 4:28-38, 2001.

Wald ER. Diagnosis and management of sinusitis in children. Adv Pediatr Infect Dis 12:1-20, 1996.

Wellington K, Curran MP. Cefditoren pivoxil: a review of its use in the treatment of bacterial infections. Drugs 64:2597-618, 2004.

Wellington K, Curran MP. Spotlight on cefditoren pivoxil in bacterial infections. Treat Respir Med 4:149-52, 2005.

TEXTBOOKS

Brandstetter RD. Pulmonary Medicine. Oradell, NJ, Medical Economics Books, 1989.

Cunha BA (ed). Antibiotic Essentials, 7th Edition, Physicians' Press, Royal Oak, MI, 2008.

Fry DE. Surgical Infections. Boston, Little, Brown and Company, 1995.

Gorbach SL, Bartlett JG, Blacklow NR (eds). Infectious Diseases, 3rd Edition. Philadelphia, Lippincott, Williams & Wilkins, 2004.

Howard RJ, Simmons RL. Surgical Infectious Diseases, 2nd Edition. Norwalk, CT, Appleton & Lange, 1988.

Kucers A, Crowe S, Grayson ML (eds). The Use of Antibiotics: A Clinical Review of Antibacterial, Antifungal, and Antiviral Drugs, 5th Edition. Butterworth-Heinemann, Oxford, 1997.

Mandell GL, Bennett JE, Dolin R (eds). Mandell, Douglas and Bennett's Principles and Practice of Infectious Disease, 6th Edition. Philadelphia, Elsevier, 2005.

Schlossberg D. Current Therapy of Infectious Disease, 3rd Edition. Mosby-Yearbook, St. Louis, 2007.

Yoshikawa TT, Norman DC (eds). Antimicrobial Therapy in the Elderly. Marcel Dekker, New York, 1994.

Chapter 13

Prevention of Pneumonia:
Antibiotic Prophylaxis and Immunizations*

Pierce Gardner, MD
Burke A. Cunha, MD

* For prophylaxis of opportunistic infections in HIV/AIDS, see Chapter 9

POST-EXPOSURE MEDICAL PROPHYLAXIS (Table 13.1)

Some infectious diseases can be prevented by post-exposure prophylaxis (PEP). To be maximally effective, PEP should be administered within 24 hours of the exposure, since the effectiveness of prophylaxis > 24 hours after exposure decreases rapidly in most cases. PEP is usually reserved for persons with close face-to-face/intimate contact with an infected individual. Casual contact usually does not warrant PEP.

Table 13.1. Post-Exposure Prophylaxis

Exposure	Usual Organisms	Preferred Prophylaxis	Alternate Prophylaxis	Comments
Viral influenza	Influenza virus, type A or B	Oseltamivir (Tamiflu) 75 mg (PO) q24h for duration of outbreak (or at least 7 days after close contact to an infected person). For CrCl 10-30 cc/min, give 75 mg (PO) q48h	Rimantadine 100 mg (PO) q12h* for duration of outbreak (or at least 7-10 days after close contact to infected person) **or** Amantadine 200 mg (PO) q24h† for duration of outbreak (or at least 7-10 days after close contact to infected person)	Give to non-immunized contacts and high-risk contacts even if immunized. Begin at onset of outbreak or within 2 days of close contact to an infected person. Oseltamivir is active against both influenza A and B; rimantadine and amantadine are only active against influenza A
Avian influenza	Influenza A (H₅-N₁)	Oseltamivir (as for viral influenza, above)	Rimantadine **or** Amantadine (as for viral influenza, above)	Amantadine/Oseltamivir may be ineffective
Pertussis	B. pertussis	Erythromycin 500 mg (PO) q6h x 2 weeks	TMP-SMX 1 SS tablet (PO) q12h x 2 weeks **or** Levofloxacin 500 mg (PO) q24h x 2 weeks	Administer as soon as possible after exposure. Effectiveness is greatly reduced after 24 hours

*   For elderly, severe liver dysfunction, or CrCl < 10 cc/min, give 100 mg (PO) q24h

†   For age ≥65 years, give 100 mg (PO) q24h. For renal dysfunction, give 200 mg (PO) load followed by 100 mg q24h (CrCl 30-50 cc/min), 100 mg q48h (CrCl 15-29 cc/min), or 200 mg weekly (CrCl < 15 cc/min)

Table 13.1. Post-Exposure Prophylaxis

Exposure	Usual Organisms	Preferred Prophylaxis	Alternate Prophylaxis	Comments
TB	M. tuberculosis	INH 300 mg (PO) q24h x 9 months	Rifampin 600 mg (PO) q24h x 4 months	For INH, monitor SGOT/SGPT weekly x 4, then monthly x 3. Mild elevations are common and resolve spontaneously. INH should be stopped for SGOT/SGPT levels ≥ 5 x normal
Varicella (chicken-pox)	VZV	<u>Preferred</u>: For exposure < 72 hours, give varicella-zoster immune globulin (VZIG) 625 mcg (IM) x 1 dose to immuno-compromised hosts and pregnant women (esp. with respiratory conditions). For others or exposure > 72 hours, consider acyclovir 800 mg (PO) 5x/day x 5-10 days <u>Alternate</u>: Varicella vaccine 0.5 mL (SC) x 1 dose. Repeat in 4 weeks	Administer as soon as possible after exposure (< 72 hours). Varicella vaccine is a live attenuated vaccine and should not be given to immunocompromised or pregnant patients. If varicella develops, start acyclovir treatment immediately
BIOTERRORIST AGENTS				
Anthrax (inhalation)	B. anthracis	Doxycycline 100 mg (PO) q12h x 60 days **or** Quinolone* (PO) x 60 days	Amoxicillin 1 gm (PO) q8h x 60 days	Duration of anthrax PEP based on longest incubation period of inhaled spores in nares
Tularemia pneumonia	F. tularensis	Doxycycline 100 mg (PO) q12h x 2 weeks	Quinolone* (PO) x 2 weeks	Duration of PEP for tularemia is 2 weeks, not 1 week as for plague
Pneumonic plague	Y. pestis	Doxycycline 100 mg (PO) q12h x 7 days **or** Quinolone* (PO) x 7 days	Chloramphenicol 500 mg (PO) q6h x 7 days	Pneumonic plague should be considered bioterrorism since most natural cases of plague are bubonic plague

* Ciprofloxacin 500 mg (PO) q12h or levofloxacin 500 mg (PO) q24h

CHRONIC MEDICAL PROPHYLAXIS/SUPPRESSION (Table 13.2)

Some infectious diseases are prone to recurrence/relapse and may benefit from intermittent or chronic suppressive therapy. The goal of suppressive therapy is to minimize the frequency/severity of recurrent infectious episodes.

Table 13.2. Chronic Medical Prophylaxis/Suppression

Disorder	Usual Organisms	Preferred Prophylaxis	Alternate Prophylaxis	Comments
Asplenia	S. pneumoniae H. influenzae N. meningitidis	Amoxicillin 1 gm (PO) q24h indefinitely	Levofloxacin 500 mg (PO) q24h indefinitely **or** Moxifloxacin 400 mg (PO) q24h indefinitely	Chemoprophylaxis is uniformly effective but needs to be given long-term. Pneumococcal, H. influenzae, and meningococcal vaccines should be given if possible but are not always protective. Use amoxicillin in children, if possible
Prevention of CMV in organ transplants	CMV	Valganciclovir 900 mg (PO) q24h until CMV antigen levels ↓ to pre-flare levels		Begin pre-emptive therapy when semi-quantitative CMV antigen levels ↑. Pre-emptive therapy prevents CMV flare
Acute exacerbation of chronic bronchitis (AECB)	S. pneumoniae H. influenzae M. catarrhalis	Levofloxacin 500 mg *or* moxifloxacin 400 mg *or* gemifloxacin 320 mg (PO) q24h x 5 days **or** Doxycycline 100 mg (PO) q12h x 5 days **or** Telithromycin 800 mg (PO) q24h x 5 days **or** Amoxicillin/clavulanic acid XR 2 tablets (PO) q12h x 5 days **or** Clarithromycin XL 1 gm (PO) q24h x 5 days **or** Azithromycin 500 mg (PO) x 3 days, or 500 mg (PO) on day 1 followed by 250 mg (PO) q24h on days 2-5		Treat each episode individually

IMMUNIZATIONS (Tables 13.3-13.5)

Immunizations are designed to reduce infections in large populations, and may prevent/ decrease the severity of infection in non-immunized individuals. Compromised hosts with altered immune systems may not develop protective antibody titers to antigenic components of various vaccines. Immunizations are not fully protective, but are recommended (depending on the vaccine) for most normal hosts, since some protection is better than none.

Table 13.3. Adult Immunizations for the Prevention of Respiratory Infections

Vaccine	Indications	Dosage	Comments
Bacille Calmette Guérin (BCG)	Possibly beneficial for adults at high-risk of multiple-drug resistant tuberculosis	Primary: 1 dose (intradermal). Booster not recommended	Live attenuated vaccine. PPD remains positive for years/life. Contraindicated in immunocompromised hosts. Side effects include injection site infection or disseminated infection (rare)
Hemophilus influenzae (type B)	Patients with splenic dysfunction	Primary: 0.5 mL dose (IM). Booster not recommended	Capsular polysaccharide conjugated to diphtheria toxoid. Safety in pregnancy unknown. Mild local reaction in 10%
Influenza	Healthy persons ≥ 50 years, healthcare personnel, adults with high-risk conditions (e.g., heart disease, lung disease, diabetes, renal dysfunction, hemoglobinopathy, immunosuppression)	Annual vaccine. Single 0.5 mL dose (IM) between October and November (before flu season) is optimal, but can be given anytime during flu season	Trivalent inactivated whole and split virus. Contraindications include anaphylaxis to eggs or sensitivity to thimerosal. Mild local reaction in up to 30%. Occasional malaise/myalgia beginning 6-12 hours after vaccination. Neurologic and allergic reactions are rare. For pregnancy, administer in 2nd or 3rd trimester during flu season. A nasally-administered live attenuated influenza vaccine has been approved for healthy individuals aged 5-49 years

Table 13.3. Adult Immunizations for the Prevention of Respiratory Infections

Vaccine	Indications	Dosage	Comments
Pneumococcus (S. pneumoniae)	Immunocompetent hosts ≥ 65 years old, or > 2 years old with diabetes, CSF leaks, or chronic cardiac, pulmonary or liver disease. Also for immuno-compromised hosts > 2 years old with functional/ anatomic asplenia, leukemia, lymphoma, multiple myeloma, widespread malignancy, chronic renal failure, bone marrow/organ transplant, or on immunosuppressive /steroid therapy	Primary: 0.5 mL dose (SC or IM). A one-time booster at 5 years is recommended for immunocompromised hosts > 2 years old and for those who received the vaccine before age 65 for high-risk conditions	Polyvalent vaccine against 23 strains. Studies are inadequate to routinely recommend reimmunization

Adapted from: Recommended Adult Immunization Schedule United States, 2005-2006.

Table 13.4. Immunizations Before Organ Transplantation

Vaccine	Recommendation
Measles-mumps-rubella (MMR), polio, diphtheria-tetanus-pertussis (DPT), H. influenza (type b)	Complete series
Hepatitis A	Vaccinate, especially pre-liver transplant
Hepatitis B	Vaccinate; give 3rd dose ≥ 2 months after 2nd dose
Influenza	Vaccinate annually
Varicella	Vaccinate seronegative patients
Pneumococcal	Vaccinate high-risk patients with cardiac/ pulmonary disease
Meningococcal	Vaccinate young adults

Table 13.5. Immunizations in Pregnancy

Vaccine	Recommendation
Hepatitis A, Hepatitis B, influenza, tetanus/diphtheria, meningococcal, rabies, typhoid fever (ViCPS), polio (IPV), yellow fever*	Should be considered if otherwise indicated
Measles*, mumps*, rubella*, varicella*, BCG*, vaccinia*, typhoid (oral Ty21a*)	Contraindicated in pregnancy
Pneumococcal, cholera, Japanese encephalitis, plague	Inadequate information for recommendation

* Live attenuated vaccine

REFERENCES AND SUGGESTED READINGS

Batiuk TD, Bodziak KA, Goldman M. Infectious disease prophylaxis in renal transplant patients: a survey of US transplant centers. Clin Transplant 16:1-8, 2002.

Burroughs, MH. Immunization in transplant patients. Pediatr Infect Dis J 21:158-60, 2002.

Chattopadhyay B. Splenectomy pneumococcal vaccination and antibiotic prophylaxis. Br J Hosp Med 41:172-4, 1989.

Conte JE Jr. Antibiotic prophylaxis: non-abdominal surgery. Curr Clin Top Infect Dis 10:254-305, 1989.

Dennehy PH. Active immunization in the United States: developments over the past decade. Clin Microbiol Rev 14:872-908, 2001.

Faix, RG. Immunization during pregnancy. Clin Obstet Gynecol 45:42-58, 2002.

Gardner P, Eickhoff T. Immunization in adults in the 1990s. Curr Clin To Infect Dis 15:271-300, 1995.

Gardner P, Peter G. Recommended schedules for routine immunization of children and adults. Infect Dis Clin North Am 15:1-8, 2001.

Gardner P, Schaffner W. Immunization of adults. N Engl J Med 328:1252-8, 1993.

Gellin BG, Curlin GT, Rabinovich NR, et al. Adult immunization: principles and practice. Adv Intern Med 44:327-52, 1999.

Jackson LA, Neuzil KM, Yu O et al. Effectiveness of pneumococcal polysaccharide vaccine in older adults. N Engl J Med 348:1747-55, 2003.

McDonnell WM, Askari FK. Immunization. JAMA 278:2000-7, 1997.

Peter G, Gardner P. Standards for immunization practice for vaccines in children and adults. Infect Dis Clin North Am 15:9-19, 2001.

Vazquez M, LaRussa PS, Gershon AA, et al. The effectiveness of the varicella vaccine in clinical practice. N Engl J Med 344:955-60, 2001.

Whitney CG, Farley MM, Hadler J et al. Decline in invasive pneumococcal disease after the introduction of protein-polysaccharide conjugate vaccine. N Engl J Med 348:1737-46, 2003.

Wingard JR. Antifungal chemoprophylaxis after blood and marrow transplantation. Clin Infect Dis 34:1386-90, 2002.

Winston DJ, Busuttil RW. Randomized controlled trial of oral itraconazole solution versus intravenous/oral fluconazole for prevention of fungal infections in liver transplant recipients. Transplantation 74:688-95, 2002.

Wistrom J, Norrby R. Antibiotic prophylaxis of travellers' diarrhoea. Scand J Infect Dis Suppl 70:111-29, 1990.

GUIDELINES

Prevention and Control of Influenza: Recommendations of the Advisory Committee on Immunization Practices (ACIP). MMWR 55(RR-10):1-42, 2006.

Recommended Adult Immunization Schedule - United States, October 2007-September 2008. MMWR 56(41); October 19, 2007. Also available at www.cdc.gov/mmwr.

Recommended childhood & adolescent immunization schedule - United States. MMWR 55(51, 52); January 5, 2007. Also available at www.cdc.gov/mmwr.

TEXTBOOKS

Gorbach SL, Bartlett JG, Blacklow NR (eds). Infectious Diseases, 3rd Edition. Philadelphia, Lippincott, Williams & Wilkins, 2004.

Mandell GL, Bennett JE, Dolin R (eds). Mandell, Douglas, and Bennett's Principles and Practice of infectious Diseases, 6th Edition. Philadelphia, Elsevier, 2005.

Plotkin SA, Orenstein WA (eds). Vaccines 4th Edition. W.B. Saunders, Philadelphia, 2004.

Yu VL, Merigan Jr, TC, Barriere SL (eds). Antimicrobial Therapy and Vaccines. Williams & Wilkins, Baltimore, 1999.

Chapter 14

Collection Procedures, Stains, and Tests
for Pneumonia Pathogens

Paul E. Schoch, PhD
Burke A. Cunha, MD

*   For sputum Gram stain technique and interpretation, see Chapter 3.

Table 14.1. Culture Media, Collection, and Transport

Culture	Comments
Fungus	*Specimen*: Specimen types listed in the aerobic culture section may be cultured for fungi. When urine or sputum are cultured for fungi, a first morning specimen is usually preferred. *Minimum volume*: 1 mL or as specified for aerobic cultures under individual listing of specimens *Container*: Sterile container with tight-fitting cap *Collection*: Transport to the microbiology laboratory within 1 hour of collection. Avoid contamination with normal flora from the skin, rectum, vaginal tract, other body surfaces.
Mycobacterium (AFB culture)	*Specimen:* Sputum, tissue, urine, body fluids *Minimum volume:* 8-10 mL of fluid or small piece of tissue. Do not use swabs. *Container:* Sterile container with a tight-fitting cap *Other considerations:* Detection is improved by concentration techniques. Smears/cultures of pleural, peritoneal, pericardial fluids have low yields. Obtain multiple cultures from the same patient.
Legionella	*Specimen:* Pleural fluid, lung tissue (biopsy), bronchial lavage (BAL), bronchial biopsy, transbronchial biopsy. Rapid transport to the laboratory is required. *Minimum volume:* 1 mL of fluids; any size piece of tissue (0.5-gm sample when possible)
Anaerobes	*Specimen:* Aspirated specimens in capped syringes or other transport devices designed to limit oxygen exposure. Avoid contamination with normal microflora from the skin, rectum, vaginal vault, other body sites. Culture for obligate and facultative anaerobes. *Minimum volume:* At least 1 mL of aspirated fluid or two swabs in an anaerobic transport device. Collection containers for aerobic culture (e.g., dry swabs) and inappropriate specimens (e.g., refrigerated samples, expectorated sputum, stool, gastric aspirates, vaginal, throat, nose, rectal swabs) are unsuitable for culture.
Viral agents	*Specimen:* Respiratory secretions, wash aspirates from the respiratory tract, nasal swabs, blood samples (including buffy coats), vaginal and rectal swabs, and swab specimens from suspect skin lesions. Stool samples for some agents. Check with laboratory for other requirements before sending sample. In general, "culturette" devices kept on ice, but not frozen, are suitable. Plasma specimens/buffy coats in sterile collection tubes should be kept 4-8°C. If specimens are to be shipped/stored, freeze at –80°C to preserve viable replicating units. *Minimum volume:* 1 mL of fluid, one swab, or 1 gm of stool in appropriate transport medium *Other considerations:* Most samples for culture are transported to the laboratory in a holding medium containing antibiotics (prevents bacterial overgrowth and viral inactivation). Many specimens should be kept cool but not frozen. Procedures/transport media vary by viral agent and transport time.

Table 14.1. Culture Media, Collection, and Transport (cont'd)

Culture	Comments
Sputum	*Specimen:* Fresh sputum (not saliva) *Minimum volume:* 2 mL *Container:* Commercially available sputum collection system or similar sterile container with a screw top *Cause for rejection:* Care must be taken to ensure that the specimen is sputum, not saliva. Note number of epithelial cells/PMNs on Gram stain.
Blood culture, routine (aerobes, anaerobes, yeast)	*Specimen:* Whole blood *Minimum volume:* 10 mL, in each of two bottles for adults and children. *Containers:* For adults, two bottles (smaller sizes are available for pediatric patients), one with dextrose phosphate, tryptic soy, or other appropriate broth and the other with thioglycollate or other broth containing reducing agents appropriate for isolation of obligate anaerobes. For special situations (e.g., suspected fungal identification, culture-negative endocarditis, mycobacteremia) different blood collection systems may be used (Isolator systems). *Collection:* An appropriate disinfecting technique should be used on both the bottle septum and the patient. Do not allow air bubbles to get into anaerobic broth bottles. *Special considerations:* Bacteria may be present either continuously in blood (e.g., endocarditis, overwhelming sepsis, early stages of salmonellosis or brucellosis), or intermittently (most other bacterial infections in which bacteria are shed into the blood on a sporadic basis). Most blood culture systems employ two separate bottles containing broth medium, one that is vented in the laboratory for the growth of facultative and aerobic organisms and a second bottle that is maintained under anaerobic conditions. For suspected continuous bacteremia/fungemia, 2-3 samples should be drawn before the start of therapy, with additional sets obtained if fastidious organisms are suspected. For intermittent bacteremia, 2-3 sets should be obtained at least 1 hour apart during the first 24 hours.
Blood culture, (fungus/Mycobacterium sp.)	*Volume of specimen:* 10 mL in each bottle, as with routine blood cultures, or alternatively, request Isolator tube from the laboratory *Container:* See blood culture, routine. *Special instruction:* Be sure to specify "hold for extended incubation," since many fungal agents require 7-17 days to grow in standard blood culture bottles.
Blood culture, Isolator (lysis centrifugation)	*Specimen:* Blood *Container:* Isolator tubes *Note:* Used mainly for the isolation of fungi, Mycobacterium, or other fastidious aerobes, and for elimination of antibiotics from cultured blood in which organisms are concentrated by centrifugation.

Adapted from: Murray PR, Baron EJ, Jorgensen JH, et al. Manual of Clinical Microbiology, 8th Edition. Washington, D.C., ASM Press, 2003. Topley and Wilson's Principles of Bacteriology, Virology and Immunity, 10th edition. Baltimore, The Williams & Wilkins Company, 2006. Bottone EJ. An Atlas of the Clinical Microbiology of Infectious Diseases, Volume 1. Bacterial Agents. The Parthenon Publishing Group, Boca Raton, 2004. Bottone EJ. An Atlas of the Clinical Microbiology of Infectious Diseases, Volume 2. Viral, fungal, and parasitic agents. Taylor and Francis, 2006.

Table 14.2. Culture Media Used for Identification of Pneumonia Pathogens

Medium	Incubation	Purpose
Blood agar, 5% defibrinated sheep blood in enrichment agar base, chocolate agar with additives	CO_2 or anaerobic	Growth/amplification of bacterial pathogens, including obligate anaerobes
MacConkey agar, deoxycholate agar, eosin-methylene blue agar	O_2	Select for Enterobacteriaceae and other gram-negative rods; inhibits growth of most gram-positive organisms; differentiate Lac-positive from Lac-negative organisms
Phenylethyl alcohol agar, Columbia CNA agar	CO_2	Select for gram-positive species, particularly Staphylococcus and Streptolococcus; inhibits many gram-negative organisms
Brain-heart infusion, tryptic digest, thioglycollate, chopped-meat glucose	O_2, CO_2, anaerobic	General-purpose amplification broths

Adapted from: same as for Table 14.1.

Table 14.3. Primary Agar and Broth Media for Isolation of Infectious Agents

Source	Pathogen	Specimen	Growth media
Nasopharyngeal	Pertussis	Calcium alginate swab	Regan-Lowe, Bordet-Gengou
Sputum	Bacteria	Expectorated	BA, CA, Mac, CNA, BCYE[†]
Sputum	Mycobacteria	Expectorated, BAL	LJ, M–7H11, M–7H12 broth (BACTEC)
Lung biopsy	Bacteria and fungi	Tissue	BA, ABA, CA, Mac, BCYE[†]
Blood	Bacteria and fungi	Venipuncture	Broth, aerobic and anaerobic
Pleural and other body fluids	Bacteria and fungi	Aspirate in syringe	BA, ABA, CA, Mac, CNA, thio broth

ABA = anaerobic blood agar; BA = blood agar; BCYE = buffered charcoal yeast extract agar; CA = chocolate agar; CNA = Columbia nalidixic acid agar; LJ = Lowenstein Jensen agar; Mac = MacConkey agar; M-7H11/12 = Middlebrook 7H11/12 agar; ML = Martin-Lewis agar
† For detection of Legionella species on request (not routine)
Adapted from: same as for Table 14.1.

Table 14.4. Tests for Detection of Lower Respiratory Tract Pathogens

Pathogen	Specimen	Microscopy	Culture	Serology	Other
Bacteria					
Oral anaerobes	TTA, empyema fluid	Gram stain	X	—	—
Legionella	Sputum, pleural fluid TTA, bronch, blood	FA (L. Pneumophila)	X	IFA, EIA	Urinary antigen (L. pneumophila serogroup 1 only)*
Nocardia	Expectorated sputum, lung biopsy	Gram stain, modified carbolfuchsin stain	X	—	—
Chlamydia	Nasopharyngeal swab, sputum, BAL specimen	Negative	X*	CF for C. psittaci; MIF for C. pneumoniae*	PCR for C. pneumoniae*
Mycoplasma	Sputum, nasopharyngeal swab	Negative	X*	CF, EIA	PCR*, cold agglutinins (titer ≥ 1:64)
Mycobacteria	Expectorated or induced sputum, BAL specimen	Fluorochrome stain or carbolfuchsin stain	X	—	PPD skin test, PCR*
Endemic Mycoses					
Blastomyces	Expectorated or induced sputum, bronch, biopsy	KOH with phase contrast, calcofluor stain	X	—	—
Coccidioides	—	—	—	CF	—
Histoplasma	—	—	X	CF, ID	Antigen assay: BAL, blood, urine*
Opportunistic					
Pneumocystis (carinii) jiroveci	Induced sputum, BAL specimen, TBB	Giemsa, FA, or GMS stain	—	—	—
Aspergillus	Tissue biopsy	H&E, GMS stain	X	ID*	Galactomannan
Cryptococcus	Sputum, serum, tissue biopsy	H&E, GMS stain, calcofluor white	X	—	Serum, BAL antigen
Zygomycetes	tissue biopsy	H&E, GMS stain	X	—	—
Viruses					
Influenza virus, parainfluenza virus, RSV, CMV, adenoviruses	Nasal washings, nasopharyngeal aspirate, BAL specimen	FA: influenza and RSV	X*	CF, EIA, LA, FA	CMV PCR, FA stain of BAL, biopsy specimen, CMV Cowdry-type inclusion bodies
HSV-1	BAL cytology	Negative	X**	EIA	Cytology positive, for HSV inclusion bodies, PCR*

Table 14.4. Tests for Detection of Lower Respiratory Tract Pathogens

Pathogen	Specimen	Microscopy	Culture	Serology	Other
Hantavirus	Blood	Negative	—	EIA	PCR*, thrombo-cytopenia, > 10% immunoblasts
SARS	Blood	Negative	—	EIA	—

BAL = bronchoalveolar lavage; bronch = bronchoscopy specimen including aspirate, brushing, BAL, or biopsy; TTA = transtracheal aspirate or transthoracic aspirate; biopsy = transbronchial, transthoracic, or open lung biopsy; CF = complement fixation; EIA = enzyme immunoassay; FA = fluorescent antibody stain; GMS = Gomori methenamine-silver nitrate; H&E = hematoxylin and eosin; ID = immunodiffusion; IFA = indirect fluorescent antibody; LA = latex agglutination; MIF = microimmunofluorescence test; PCR = polymerase chain reaction; PPD = purified protein derivative; TBB = transbronchial biopsy
*   Available at few clinical microbiology laboratories
**   Culture of HSV-1 from respiratory secretions is not diagnostic or HSV-1 pneumonia
Adapted from: Bartlett JG. Approach to the Patient with Pneumonia. In Gorbach SL, Bartlett JG, Blacklow NE (eds). Infectious Diseases, 2nd edition. W. B. Saunders, Philadelphia, PA, 1998.

Table 14.5. Selected Microbiologic Stains Used for Pneumonia

Stain	Detection/Use	Expected Result
Acridine orange*	Bacteria/yeasts, WBCs	Bacteria/yeasts stain orange; WBCs are pale green
Auramine/rhodamine *	Mycobacterium spp.	Yellow fluorescence indicates Mycobacterium spp.
Calcofluor white*	Fungi	Fungal elements stain green
Gram's stain	Differentiation of bacteria into two groups	Gram-positive bacteria stain blue/purple; gram-negative bacteria stain red
Kinyoun acid-fast stain	Mycobacterium spp.	Acid-fast bacteria stain pink against a blue background.
Modified acid-fast stain	Weakly acid-fast organisms (Nocardia)	Weakly acid-fast organisms stain pink against a blue background
Giemsa stain	Chlamydias, malarial, other intracellular parasites	Varied, depending on agent
Methenamine-silver stain	Pneumocystis (carinii) jiroveci	Cell wall of PCP stains black against a light green background
Spore stain	Spores	Spores stain light green against a pink/red background; bacteria stain red
Toluidine blue	Pneumocystis (carinii) jiroveci	Cysts stain light purple/lavender
Wet mount India ink	Cryptococcus neoformans	Cryptococcus capsules are clear halos around yeasts
Lactophenol cotton blue	Fungal structures	Fungal elements stain intense blue

*   Uses UV light

Table 14.6. Methods/Stains for Detection of Fungi in Clinical Specimens by Microscopic Examination*

Method	Use	Comments
Gram stain	Detection of bacteria and fungi	Rapid. Stains most yeast and hyphal elements. Cryptococcus may stain weakly
KOH	Clearing of specimen to make fungal elements more visible	Rapid; some specimens difficult to clear. May produce artifacts that are confusing. Most useful in combination with Calcofluor white stain
Calcofluor white	Detection of all fungi and Pneumocystis carinii	Rapid; detects fungi due to bright fluorescence. Useful in combination with KOH. Requires fluorescent microscope/special filters. Background fluorescence may make examination of some specimens difficult
India ink	Detection of encapsulated yeasts	Rapid but insensitive (40%) means of detecting C. neoformans in spinal fluid
Wright's stain	Examination of bone marrow, peripheral smears, and touch preparations	Useful for diagnosis of histoplasmosis
Giemsa stain	Examination of bone marrow, peripheral smears, touch preparations, and respiratory specimens	Useful for diagnosis of histoplasmosis and P. (carinii) jiroveci pneumonia (induced sputum)
Toluidine blue	Examination of respiratory specimens	Useful for diagnosis of P. (carinii) jiroveci pneumonia
Methenamine silver stain	Detection of fungi in histologic section and P. (carinii) jiroveci in respiratory specimens	Staining of tissue may require 1 hour, respiratory specimens 5-10 min. Best stain to detect fungi. Yeast cells and P. carinii may appear similar
Papanicolaou stain	Cytologic stain used primarily to detect malignant cells	Stains most fungal elements. Hyphae may stain weakly. Allows cytologist to detect fungal elements
Periodic acid-Schiff stain	Detection of fungi	Stains yeasts and hyphae well. Artifacts may be confused with yeast cells
Mucicarmine stain	Stains mucin	Demonstrates mucoid capsule of C. neoformans and differentiates it from other yeasts. May also stain cell walls of B. dermatitidis and Rhinosporidium seeberi

Table 14.6. Methods/Stains for Detection of Fungi in Clinical Specimens by Microscopic Examination* (cont'd)

Method	Use	Comments
Fontana-Masson	Melanin stain	Confirms the presence of melanin in lightly pigmented cells of dematiaceous fungi. Useful for staining the cell wall of C. neoformans
Hematoxylin-eosin (H&E)	General purpose histologic stain	Best stain to demonstrate host tissue reaction. Stains most fungi. Useful in demonstrating natural pigment in dematiaceous fungi

*   Uses UV light
Adapted from: same as for Table 14.1.

Table 14.7. Serologic Tests for Detection of Bacterial and Fungal Pathogens

Pathogen	Method	Positive Test
Streptococcus pyogenes	ASO, ADB, AH	4-fold titer rise
Legionella	Immunofluorescence	≥ 1:128 positive
Mycoplasma	CF, EIA	4-fold titer rise
Chlamydia pneumoniae	CF, IFA	↑ Igm, ↑ IgG ≥ 1:512 or 4-fold titer rise
Chlamydia psittaci	CF	4-fold titer rise
Q fever	EIA, CF	4-fold titer rise
Francisella tularensis	Tube agglutination	≥ 1:40
Yersinia pestis	Passive hemagglutination	4-fold titer rise
Histoplasma capsulatum	CF Skin test	4-fold titer rise or ↑ IgG ≥ 1:32 Positive reaction
Coccidioides immitis	Tube precipitins; EIA Skin test	4-fold titer rise Positive reaction
Cryptococcus neoformans	Latex agglutination	Any titer
Blastomyces dermatitidis	CF, EIA	> 1:8 (CF); ≥ 1:32 (EIA)

ADB = anti-DNAse B; AH = anti-hyaluronidase; ASO = antistreptolysin O titer; CF = complement fixation; IFA = indirect immunofluorescent assay; EIA = enzyme immunoassay
Adapted from: Balows A, Hausler WJ, Jr., Ohashi M, Turano A (eds). Laboratory Diagnosis of Infectious Diseases. Principles and Practice (vol 1). New York, Springer-Verlag, 1988. Murray PR, Baron EJ, Jorgensen JH, et al. Manual of Clinical Microbiology, 8th Edition. Washington, D.C., ASM Press, 2003. Topley and Wilson's Principles of Bacteriology, Virology and Immunity, 10th edition. Baltimore, The Williams & Wilkins Company, 2006. Koneman EW, Allen SD, Janda WM, et al. Color Atlas and Textbook of Diagnostic Microbiology, 5th Edition. Philadelphia, Lippincott-Raven Publishers, 1997.

Table 14.8. DNA Probes for Culture Confirmation of Bacterial and Fungal Isolates

Organism	Sensitivity*	Specificity*	Comments
Mycobacterium avium	100	100	Can use with BACTEC pellet[†]
Mycobacterium avium complex	100	100	Can use with BACTEC pellet[†]
Mycobacterium gordonae	98.7	98.4	Can use with BACTEC pellet[†]
Mycobacterium intracellulare	97.5-100	100	Can use with BACTEC pellet[†]
Mycobacterium kansasii	100	100	Can use with BACTEC pellet[†]
Mycobacterium tuberculosis complex	93.4-100	96.6-100	Can use with BACTEC pellet[†]
Blastomyces dermatitidis	100	100	Hyphal growth
Coccidioides immitis	100	100	Hyphal growth
Histoplasma capsulatum	100	100	Hyphal growth

* Data from published studies
† DNA probes not yet approved for use with other commercial liquid mycobacterial growth systems
Adapted from: Murray PR, Baron EJ, Jorgensen JH, et al. Manual of Clinical Microbiology, 8th Edition. Washington, D.C., ASM Press, 2003. Topley and Wilson's Principles of Bacteriology, Virology and Immunity, 10th edition. Baltimore, The Williams & Wilkins Company, 2006.

Table 14.9. Rapid Tests for Detection of Respiratory Pathogens

Organism	Gram Stain	Acid-fast	KOH prep	DFA	Latex	EIA	DNA probe	PCR	TMA
Streptococcus pyogenes				x	x	x	x		
Bordetella pertussis				x				x	
Legionella				x					
Mycoplasma				x		x			
Nocardia	x	x							
Fungi			x						
Mycobacteria		x						x	x

DFA = direct fluorescent antibody test; EIA = enzyme immunoassay; KOH = potassium hydroxide mount; Latex = latex agglutination assay; PCR = polymerase chain reaction; TMA = transcription-mediated amplification
Adapted from: Murray PR, Baron EJ, Jorgensen JH, et al. Manual of Clinical Microbiology, 8th Edition. Washington, D.C., ASM Press, 2003. Topley and Wilson's Principles of Bacteriology, Virology and Immunity, 10th edition. Baltimore, The Williams & Wilkins Company, 2006.

REFERENCES AND SUGGESTED READINGS

TEXTBOOKS

Bottone EJ. An Atlas of the Clinical Microbiology of Infectious Diseases, Volume 1. Bacterial Agents. The Parthenon Publishing Group, Boca Raton, 2004.

Bottone EJ. An Atlas of the Clinical Microbiology of Infectious Diseases, Volume 2. Viral, fungal, and parasitic agents. Taylor and Francis, 2006.

Cimolai N. Laboratory Diagnosis of Bacterial Infections. New York, Marcel Dekker, Inc, 2001.

de la Maza, Pezzlo MT, Shigei JT, et al. Color Atlas of Medical Bacteriology. Washington, D.C., ASM Press, 2004.

Gorbach SL, Bartlett JG, Blacklow NR (eds). Infectious Diseases, 3rd Edition. Philadelphia, Lippincott, Williams & Wilkins, 2004.

Koneman EW, Allen SD, Janda WM, et al. Color Atlas and Textbook of Diagnostic Microbiology, 5th Edition. Philadelphia, Lippincott-Raven Publishers, 1997.

Madigan MT, Martinko JM, Parker J. Brock Biology of Microoganisms, 10th Edition. Upper Saddler River, NJ, Pearson Education, Inc., 2003.

Mandell GL, Bennett JE, Dolin R (eds). Mandell, Douglas and Bennett's Principles and Practice of Infectious Disease, 6th Edition. Philadelphia, Elsevier, 2005.

Murray PR, Baron EJ, Jorgensen JH, et al. Manual of Clinical Microbiology, 8th Edition. Washington, D.C., ASM Press, 2003.

Topley and Wilson's Principles of Bacteriology, Virology and Immunity, 10th Edition. Baltimore, The Williams & Wilkins Company, 2006.

Chapter 15

Pneumonia Pearls and Pitfalls

Burke A. Cunha, MD

Community-Acquired Pneumonia (CAP)

- The severity of CAP is primarily determined by host factors (i.e., cardiopulmonary and immune function) and to a lesser extent by pathogen virulence.

- Normal hosts with CAP do not present with hypotension/shock. CAP presenting with shock should prompt a search for underlying cardiopulmonary disease as an explanation for the hypotension.

- If no cardiopulmonary explanation cause is found for CAP with shock (e.g., exacerbation of severe COPD, acute pulmonary emboli, congestive heart failure), then adrenal insufficiency or an immunologic explanation should be sought.

- Recognize that P. aeruginosa is not a cause of CAP in normal hosts unless the patient has underlying chronic bronchiectasis or cystic fibrosis. Even neutropenic patients with frequent P. aeruginosa bacteremia do not present with P. aeruginosa CAP.

- Remember to consider PCP (Pneumocystis (carini) jiroveci) in the differential diagnosis of CAP. Unlike typical/atypical CAP, PCP presents with bilateral symmetrical infiltrates and progressive shortness of breath for up to a week prior to admission.

- The infiltrates in PCP, if present, are bilateral, peripheral and interstitial; they are rarely if ever focal. The exceptional case in which PCP presents with focal infiltrates occurs in HIV patients who have received pentamidine via inhalation; these patients may present with bilateral apical infiltrates.

- Consider PCP not only in patients with HIV but also in organ transplants and those on steroids.

- Recognize that patients on steroids present with CAP when the steroids are being *tapered*, which is when it is least expected.

Streptococcus pneumoniae

- CAP with cavitation on chest x-ray argues against the diagnosis of S. pneumoniae.

- Pleural effusion is unusual with S. pneumoniae CAP, but empyema is not uncommon.

- Do not assume that upper lobe CAP with a "bulging fissure sign" on chest x-ray is diagnostic of K. pneumoniae; it may also occur with S. pneumoniae.

- Do not overlook meningitis or endocarditis in alcoholics with S. pneumoniae CAP. The new appearance of a murmur/recrudescence of fever indicating S. pneumoniae ABE is easily overlooked during therapy.

- Remember that infiltrates on chest x-ray may persist for up to 14 weeks after clinical improvement/defervescence with S. pneumoniae CAP.

- Do not be overly concerned with S. pneumoniae bacteremia accompanying S. pneumoniae CAP; it is not, per se, a bad prognostic factor.

- Avoid using macrolides as monotherapy for S. pneumoniae CAP since 30% of S. pneumoniae strains are intrinsically or naturally resistant to all macrolides. In addition to intrinsic S. pneumoniae resistance, macrolide use is also associated with acquired resistance.

- Macrolide and TMP-SMX monotherapy for S. pneumoniae CAP predispose to PRSP and multi-drug resistant strains of S. pneumoniae (MDRSP). In contrast, "respiratory" quinolones are highly effective against PRSP and MDRSP strains and do not predispose to S. pneumoniae resistance.

- Vancomycin does not penetrate the CSF well and is unnecessary to prevent "seeding" of the CSF from pneumococcal bacteremia.

- Therapy with a beta-lactam that penetrates the CSF in high concentration (e.g., ceftriaxone) is effective against both PRSP and MDRSP in serum and CSF.

- S. pneumoniae susceptibility to tetracycline and doxycycline are not the same. Unlike tetracycline, doxycycline is effective against most strains of PRSP.

- Doxycycline is useful in penicillin-allergic patients and as a "quinolone sparing" antibiotic and provides both typical and atypical CAP coverage.

- Beta-lactam/beta-lactamase inhibitor combinations are effective against ampicillin-resistant H. influenzae (beta-lactamase mediated) but not against penicillin-resistant S. pneumoniae (penicillin-binding proteins [PBPs] mediated).

Hemophilus influenzae

- Obtain blood cultures on all patients where typical CAP is likely. H. influenzae is second only to S. pneumoniae in bacteremic potential.

- Treat all strains of H. influenzae as ampicillin-resistant since most current strains of H. influenzae produce beta-lactamase.

- Penicillin and first-generation cephalosporins are ineffective against H. influenza, and macrolides have only modest anti-H. influenzae activity.

- Be careful in assuming that all right lower lobe (RLL) CAP's are due to S. pneumoniae. H. influenzae also commonly presents as a RLL focal/segmental infiltrate with a small-to-moderate pleural effusion.

- The diagnosis of H. influenzae CAP should be questioned if either a pleural effusion is absent or a very large pleural effusion is present.

- Not all gram-negative pneumonias are necrotizing. H. influenzae is an example of a gram-negative pneumonia that is not associated with cavitation.

- Although H. influenzae colonizes the oropharynx and causes sinusitis, otitis, chronic bronchitis and CAP, it does not cause pharyngitis.

Moraxella catarrhalis

- M. catarrhalis is common in patients with COPD and is the most common cause of CAP in patients with COPD requiring hospitalization.

- M. catarrhalis is the only typical CAP pathogen not associated with bacteremia.

- Always question the diagnosis of M. catarrhalis CAP if cavitation or pleural effusion is present; these are not features of M. catarrhalis CAP.

- Remember to treat M. catarrhalis as ampicillin-resistant H. influenzae CAP since all current strains of M. catarrhalis produce beta-lactamase.

- Unlike S. pneumoniae or H. influenzae CAP, M. catarrhalis CAP has no lobar predilection.

Group A Streptococcus

- Although Group A streptococcal pneumonia is an uncommon cause of CAP, it should be suspected when CAP is accompanied by a large pleural effusion.

- Although the pleural effusion in Group A streptococcal CAP is serosanguineous, be sure not to miss an underlying bronchogenic carcinoma.

- Group A streptococcal CAP not infrequently is a complication of closed chest trauma.

Klebsiella pneumoniae

- Klebsiella pneumoniae CAP usually presents as an upper lobe infiltrate that typically cavitates in 3-5 days. A "shaggy border" within a thick-walled cavity on chest x-ray is a clue to the presence of Klebsiella pneumoniae.

- K. pneumoniae CAP is rare in normal hosts and occurs virtually only in chronic alcoholics and in those with splenic dysfunction.

- Empyema is not uncommon with K. pneumoniae CAP, but pleural effusion is rare.

- K. pneumoniae is readily recognizable on sputum gram stain by its unique appearance. K. pneumoniae is the only cause of gram-negative bacillus CAP that is plump, encapsulated, and has blunt ends on sputum gram stain. H. influenzae is smaller/thinner and has a less pronounced capsule.

- Do not confuse E. coli with K. pneumoniae on Gram stain. Both appear as gram-negative bacilli, but K. pneumoniae is plumper and encapsulated.

- Do not confuse the "red currant jelly" sputum typical of K. pneumoniae CAP with hemoptysis, which may accompany reactivation TB.

- Do not assume that K. pneumoniae CAP requires "double-drug therapy." With potent anti-Klebsiella agents, monotherapy is the preferred approach.

Viral Influenza

- An important clue to distinguish viral influenza from influenza like illnesses (ILI's) is the suddenness of onset. Patients with viral influenza can often recall the precise time when they became profoundly ill.

- Profound weakness is an often overlooked clue to influenza; malaise rapidly overtakes the patient making them quickly bedridden.

- Influenza pneumonia is virtually always accompanied by a severe headache and myalgias.

- Conjunctival suffusion is an easily missed clue in viral influenza. Among viral causes of pneumonia, only adenovirus and influenza are associated with conjunctival suffusion.

- Shortness of breath out of proportion to auscultatory or chest x-ray findings is an important early clue to influenza CAP.

- Although the chest x-ray is unremarkable or has minimal infiltrates early in influenza pneumonia, bilateral interstitial patchy infiltrates usually appear within 24 hours.

- Another important clue to influenza pneumonia is profound hypoxemia accompanied by an elevated A-a gradient (> 35). This is due to involvement of the lung interstitium causing a diffusion defect/hypoxemia.

- Always question the diagnosis of influenza in the absence of leukopenia, which almost always accompanies influenza pneumonia and is an important diagnostic clue.

- Lymphopenia is also an important diagnostic and prognostic indicator in influenza. Severe, prolonged leukopenia/relative lymphopenia are poor prognostic signs.

- Atypical lymphocytes are usually not present with viral influenza.

- Viral pneumonias are typically not accompanied by pleuritic chest pain or pleural effusions since they are interstitial rather than pleural processes. The chest pain of influenza pneumonia, which can be mistaken for pleuritic chest pain, represents influenza involvement of the intercostal muscles.

- Consider viral influenza in patients with headache, myalgias, and severe hypoxemia out of proportion to auscultatory or chest x-ray findings. SARS or HPS are also possibilities.

- Remember to add amantadine to influenza antivirals as soon as possible. Amantadine increases peripheral airway dilatation and may improve the profound hypoxemia of influenza pneumonia, the primary cause of death in severe cases.

- Patients with viral influenza and a focal/segmental infiltrate on chest x-ray also have superimposed bacterial pneumonia, most likely due to S. aureus. (The infiltrates of viral influenza are bilateral and patchy.) In these cases, S. aureus (MSSA/MRSA) requires urgent therapy.

- Do not overlook secondary bacterial pneumonia in patients with viral influenza who improve clinically but *subsequently* develop a new focal/segmental infiltrate after approximately one week. These patients have secondary bacterial pneumonia usually due to S. pneumoniae or H. influenzae, not MSSA/MRSA.

- Patients with non-fatal viral influenza usually recover rapidly after 3 days, but post-viral influenza malaise may persist for months.

Staphylococcus aureus (MSSA/MRSA)

- Be wary of diagnosing S. aureus (MSSA/MRSA) CAP in patients without viral influenza. S. aureus is not a cause of primary CAP.

- MSSA/MRSA CAP does not even occur in diabetics, the patient subset most frequently colonized by MSSA/MRSA.

- Rarely, community-acquired (CA) MRSA presents as a necrotizing hemorrhagic pneumonia, seen virtually only in patients with influenza/ILI's.

Mycoplasma pneumoniae

- Be wary of diagnosing M. pneumoniae CAP if consolidation or mild/moderate pleural effusions are present; these features argue against the diagnosis of M. pneumoniae.

- Loose stools/watery diarrhea occur in 50% of patients with M. pneumoniae CAP. The only other cause of CAP commonly associated with loose stools/diarrhea is Legionella.

- Be wary of diagnosing M. pneumoniae CAP if elevated serum transaminases are present, as M. pneumoniae does not involve the liver.

- Markedly elevated cold agglutinin titers (> 1:64) with CAP is diagnostic of M. pneumoniae CAP, although 25% of patients with M. pneumoniae CAP but do not have increased cold agglutinins titers.

- Order cold agglutinin titers on admission and daily x 3 days if M. pneumoniae CAP is suspected since cold agglutinin elevations occur early and transiently.

- Do not diagnosis M. pneumoniae CAP on the basis of elevated IgG titers — this indicates past exposure/infection. The serological diagnosis of active/current M. pneumoniae infection requires the presence of elevated IgM titers.

- Although meningoencephalitis is a rare manifestation of M. pneumoniae CAP, markedly elevated cold agglutinin titers (≥ 1:1024) is a clue to CNS involvement.

- In a patient with CAP and encephalopathy, Legionella or Q fever is the most likely diagnosis, not M. pneumoniae.

- Do not overlook the cutaneous manifestations of M. pneumoniae. CAP with otherwise unexplained E. multiforme suggests M. pneumoniae until proven otherwise.

- In a patient with CAP and a sore throat/pharyngitis, M. pneumoniae CAP is the most likely diagnosis. M. pneumoniae is an important cause of non-exudative pharyngitis in CAP and non-CAP patients. It is also the most likely diagnosis in a patient with CAP and otitis media or bullous myringitis.

- Relative bradycardia is not a sign of M. pneumoniae CAP and is a good way to differentiate M. pneumoniae (no relative bradycardia) from Legionnaires' disease (with relative bradycardia). CAP with relative bradycardia effectively rules out the diagnosis of M. pneumoniae CAP.

- In a patient with CAP and a prolonged non-productive/dry cough and minimal systemic symptoms, M. pneumoniae is the most likely diagnosis.

- Antibiotic therapy of M. pneumonia CAP decreases the patient's temperature and other systemic symptoms but does not affect the dry cough, which may last for weeks.

- M. pneumoniae should not be excluded as the cause of CAP based solely on a patient's age. Although most cases of M. pneumoniae CAP occur in young adults, the very young and the very old may also develop M. pneumoniae CAP.

- Treat M. pneumoniae CAP even if it is a mild/moderate infection in normal hosts. Antibiotics will reduce spread/prevent chronic sequelae (e.g., asthma).

- Remember, M. pneumoniae CAP can be a severe/fatal infection in compromised hosts.

- Unilateral, ill-defined, lower lobe infiltrates are typical for M. pneumoniae CAP; consolidation or large pleural effusion effectively rules out M. pneumoniae.

Chlamydophila (Chlamydia) pneumoniae

- Patients presenting with a "Mycoplasma-like" CAP have either M. pneumoniae CAP or C. pneumoniae CAP. C. pneumoniae CAP is often mistaken for M. pneumoniae CAP since the two conditions present with many of the same clinical features.

- Hoarseness is an easily overlooked clue to C. pneumoniae CAP. Hoarseness in a patient with CAP indicates C. pneumoniae until proven otherwise. Respiratory viruses are associated with hoarseness, but these viruses do not cause CAP.

- Do not diagnose C. pneumoniae CAP on the basis of elevated "chlamydia titers" —

these usually represent exposure to C. trachomatis, not C. pneumoniae. Always specifically order C. pneumoniae titers (IgM, IgG). Elevated C. pneumoniae IgM titers are diagnostic of current infection; elevated IgG titers only indicate past exposure/infection.

- Elevated cold agglutinin titers are a feature of M. pneumoniae, not C. pneumoniae CAP.

- Loose stools/diarrhea may occur with C. pneumoniae CAP but are much more common with M. pneumoniae CAP.

Legionella sp. (Legionnaires' disease)

- Do not overlook the diagnostic importance of relative bradycardia in CAP, the most consistent physical finding in Legionnaires' disease.

- Encephalopathy is an easily overlooked manifestation of Legionella CAP. Encephalitis/ meningoencephalitis occur less commonly with Q fever and only rarely with M. pneumoniae. The presence of one or more CNS abnormalities — mental status changes, headache, mental confusion, lethargy — is an important clue to Legionella in patients with CAP.

- Always inquire about loose stools/diarrhea in a patient with CAP, findings suggestive of Legionnaires' disease or M. pneumoniae CAP.

- Do not assume that patients with CAP and hyponatremia have Legionnaires' disease. Although hyponatremia is common with Legionnaires' disease, it is a nonspecific finding. Hyponatremia secondary to SIADH may occur with any cause of CAP or other pulmonary abnormalities.

- Do not overlook early/transient hypophosphatemia in CAP, the most specific and overlooked laboratory clue in the diagnosis of Legionella CAP. No other cause of CAP is associated with otherwise unexplained hypophosphatemia.

- Remember to order serial serum phosphorous levels (on admission and daily x 3) to avoid missing the important clue of hypophosphatemia in Legionella CAP. Hypophosphatemia is more likely to be present early, not late; is usually mild-to-moderate in severity; and usually resolves within 72 hours.

- Otherwise unexplained microscopic hematuria in a patient with CAP is an often overlooked Legionella clue.

- CAP in patients with upper respiratory findings (pharyngitis/ear findings) should suggest C. pneumoniae or M. pneumoniae, not Legionella. Although Legionella resides in the secretions of the oropharynx, it does not cause upper respiratory tract infections.

- Always order serum transaminases on admission and daily x 3 days in patients with atypical pneumonias. Mild/transiently elevated serum transaminases are associated with Legionnaires' disease (most common), psittacosis and Q fever, but not with M. pneumoniae CAP.

- Avoid erythromycin and tetracycline to treat Legionnaires' disease. Instead use doxycycline, a second generation macrolide, or a "respiratory" quinolone.

- In a patient with CAP, even mildly elevated cold agglutinin titers effectively rules out Legionella.

- Remember, Legionella titers are usually negative at clinical presentation. Like other titers, Legionella titers usually take 2 weeks to increase and peak at 4-6 weeks after clinical presentation.

- Recognize that a negative Legionella urinary antigen test does not exclude the diagnosis of Legionnaires' disease. The urinary Legionella antigen test is only diagnostic of Legionella pneumophila (serogroup 01), not other serotypes or species of Legionella. Also, do not assume that an initial negative Legionella urinary antigen test rules out Legionnaires' disease since Legionella urinary antigenemia begins 1-2 weeks into the illness.

- Although the Legionella urinary antigen test may be negative initially, when positive, it remains positive for weeks/months after infection.

- Remember to suspect Legionnaires' disease in patients presenting with severe CAP but without severe cardiopulmonary disease or a host defense defect.

- There is no pathognomonic chest x-ray appearance with Legionella CAP. Legionella may present with consolidation, pleural effusion, or rarely with cavitation.

- Although no radiographic feature is pathognomonic of Legionella CAP, rapidly progressive, asymmetrical, bilateral infiltrates are characteristic.

- Do not assume that anti-Legionella antimicrobial therapy is ineffective just because the chest x-ray infiltrates are progressing during therapy. The infiltrates of Legionella CAP typically progress during appropriate anti-Legionella therapy.

- Do not dismiss marked elevations of C-reactive protein CRP (> 35) in CAP as being solely a nonspecific manifestation of acute infection. CRP elevations > 35 in a patient with CAP point to the diagnosis of Legionella CAP.

- Do not overlook elevated CPK levels in CAP. Although Legionnaires' disease is associated with rhabdomyolysis, more commonly Legionella CAP is accompanied by mild/moderate increases in CPK, a clue to the diagnosis. No other cause of typical/atypical CAP is associated with CPK elevations.

- Treat Legionella CAP for at least two weeks to prevent relapse.

Coxiella burnetti (Q fever)

- In a patient with CAP and otherwise unexplained splenomegaly, Q fever is the most likely diagnosis.

- Otherwise unexplained relative bradycardia in a patient CAP should suggest Q fever after Legionnaires' disease. Psittacosis is another diagnostic possibility.

- Do not dismiss early mild/transient transaminase elevations as a clue to Q fever CAP. Like Legionnaires' disease and psittacosis, this finding is an important clue to liver involvement in zoonotic atypical pneumonias.

- Consider Q fever in the differential diagnosis of CAP in patients with a prominent headache; psittacosis and Legionnaires' should be considered as well. In contrast, encephalopathy (mental confusion) argues against the diagnosis of Q fever.

- Q fever CAP may be complicated by chronic Q fever manifest as Q fever endocarditis.

- Do not miss cat contact, an easily/often overlooked clue to the zoonotic vector in Q fever CAP. Coxiella burnetii, the organism of Q fever, is easily carried via aerosol from the afterbirth of parturient cats to nearby humans.

- If a history of recent/proximate contact with a parturient cat is negative after direct/repeated questioning, inquire about animal contact. Close contact with sheep may suggest Q fever in patients with otherwise unexplained obscure pneumonia.

- "Ovoid densities" on chest x-ray in a patient with atypical CAP suggests Q fever or Legionella micdadei.

- There is little experience using macrolides to treat Q fever CAP. The preferred antibiotics are doxycycline or a quinolone.

Chlamydia psittaci (Psittacosis)

- Psittacosis can be excluded from the differential diagnosis of CAP in the absence of exposure to parrots/psittacine birds.

- Like Q fever, psittacosis CAP is typically accompanied by a severe headache, not encephalopathy.

- Splenomegaly in a patient with CAP may suggest the possibility of psittacosis but is more common in Q fever.

- Relative bradycardia in a patient with CAP should include psittacosis in the differential diagnosis along with Legionnaires' disease and Q fever.

- Look for Horder's spots (maculopapular spots resembling the Rose spots of typhoid fever) on the face (but not the trunk) as a sign of psittacosis. Horder's spots are not always present with psittacosis but are an important and easily overlooked clue.

- Otherwise unexplained epistaxis in a patient with CAP should suggest the diagnosis of psittacosis.

- A retrospective clue to psittacosis CAP is obscure thrombophlebitis during convalescence.

- Pleuritic chest pain or pleural effusions are not a clinical feature of psittacosis CAP.

- Macrolides are less active against C. psittaci than against C. pneumoniae. In the treatment of psittacosis CAP, doxycycline or a quinolone are preferred.

Francisella tularensis (Tularemia)

- Be sure to obtain a detailed zoonotic contact history in patients with suspected tularemia. Specifically ask for recent contact with deer flies or rabbit/deer contact. Patients with tularemia typically are hunters who have recently skinned/cleaned rabbits or deer.

- In a patient with atypical CAP, the presence of bradycardia or mild/transiently elevated transaminases argues against the diagnosis of tularemia.

- The key radiographic clue to tularemia CAP is unilateral or bilateral hilar adenopathy, which is not present in any other typical/atypical CAP.

- Otherwise unexplained bloody pleural effusion in a patient with an atypical CAP points to the diagnosis of tularemia CAP. Be sure to exclude underlying bronchogenic carcinoma.

- Severe headache and myalgias that accompany tularemia CAP can mimic anthrax hemorrhagic mediastinitis in its early stages.

- Be careful not to miss tularemia pneumonia as a complication of the other forms of tularemia (glandular, oculoglandular, ulceroglandular, typhoidal).

- Do not miss the important cutaneous clue of a purple nodule or ulcer in rabbit/deer hunters. This represents ulceroglandular tularemia, which precedes tularemia CAP.

- Except for tularemia, the preferred therapy for zoonotic atypical CAP's is doxycycline. For tularemic CAP, even though doxycycline is effective, streptomycin is preferred.

Aspiration Pneumonia

- Remember, if community-acquired aspiration pneumonia is severe, the patient may develop anaerobic pneumonitis and anaerobic lung abscess.

- Community-acquired aspiration pneumonia is caused by anaerobes from the aspiration of oropharyngeal flora. All anaerobes above the waist are sensitive to penicillin and virtually all other antibiotics used to treat CAP.

- It is not necessary to treat community-acquired aspiration pneumonia with clindamycin or other anti-Bacteroides fragilis antibiotics. All anaerobes above the waist are effectively treated by macrolides, tetracyclines, β-lactams, or quinolones.

- After 1 week, the oropharyngeal flora of hospitalized patients is colonized by aerobic gram-negative bacilli. Treat nosocomial aspiration pneumonia the same as hospital-acquired (nosocomial) pneumonia or ventilator-associated pneumonia.

- Avoid adding anti-anaerobic (B. fragilis) coverage to patients with nosocomial aspiration pneumonia since anaerobes are not important pathogens in this setting.

- Anaerobic lung abscesses rarely need to be drained. Treat with prolonged antimicrobial therapy (IV/PO) until the abscess resolves.

Nursing Home Acquired Pneumonia (NHAP)

- NHAP is caused predominantly by the same pathogens that cause CAP, not by nosocomial pneumonia (NP) or ventilator-associated pneumonia (VAP) pathogens. Patients with NHAP have the same length of stay (LOS) as those with CAP, and patients with NHAP do not have P. aeruginosa, the hallmark pathogen of NP/VAP.

- Begin empiric antimicrobial therapy of NHAP as early as possible, which may prevent the need for hospital treatment.

- Do not assume that all outbreaks of pneumonia in nursing home/chronic care facilities are due to viral influenza. Not uncommonly, outbreaks of NHAP are caused by Legionella sp. or C. pneumoniae.

Nosocomial Pneumonia (NP)

- Nosocomial pneumonia (NP) is synonymous with hospital-acquired pneumonia (HAP) and ventilator-associated pneumonia (VAP) in terms of pathogen distribution and clinical presentation.

- Respiratory secretion cultures in intubated patients are not indicative of VAP pathogens. There is little correlation between isolates recovered from respiratory secretions and isolates recovered from distant lung parenchyma in ventilated patients.

- There is no need to "cover" all patients with NP/HAP/VAP for S. aureus.

- S. aureus (MSSA/MRSA) may be cultured from up to 30% of patients with VAP, but bona fide MSSA/MRSA VAP remains very rare.

- S. aureus (MSSA/MRSA) NP/HAP or VAP is a readily recognizable and distinctive clinical syndrome characterized by high spiking fevers, cyanosis, hypotension and rapid cavitation within 72 hours after the appearance of chest x-ray infiltrate.

- Remember that fever, leukocytosis and pulmonary infiltrates in ventilated patients are often due to non-infectious causes such as congestive heart failure, pulmonary emboli, pulmonary drug reactions, ARDS, pre-existing interstitial fibrosis, etc.

- Antimicrobial therapy against NP/HAP or VAP should be directed primarily against P. aeruginosa, the most virulent (but not the most common) cause of pneumonia.

- If effective anti-P. aeruginosa coverage is used for NP/HAP or VAP, then other aerobic gram-negative bacilli (GNB) pathogens will also be effectively treated. However, the converse is not necessarily true: aerobic GNB coverage does not necessarily assure a high degree of activity against P. aeruginosa.

- The culture of P. aeruginosa from respiratory secretions in ventilated patients is not diagnostic of P. aeruginosa pneumonia.

- P. aeruginosa NP/HAP/VAP, like S. aureus pneumonia, is a readily recognizable clinical syndrome. The hallmarks of P. aeruginosa pneumonia in ventilated patients are rapid cavitation on chest x-ray within 72 hours and a fulminant course that is frequently fatal. This is very different from the stable ventilated patient with P. aeruginosa in respiratory secretion cultures.

- Patients with fever, leukocytosis, and pulmonary infiltrates for days-to-weeks with P. aeruginosa cultured from respiratory secretions do not have P. aeruginosa pneumonia.

- P. aeruginosa NP/HAP or VAP acquired by inhalation typically presents with a focal segmental/lobar infiltrate. In contrast, hematogenously-acquired P. aeruginosa presents with bilateral, symmetrical, perihilar infiltrates resembling CHF.

- Avoid needlessly "covering" organisms cultured from respiratory secretions in ventilated patients that do not cause NP/HAP or VAP (e.g., Stenotrophomonas maltophilia, Enterobacter species, Burkholderia cepacia). These organisms are colonizers rather than pathogens in this setting.

- Avoid prolonged treatment for "presumed" NP (fever, leukocytosis, no change in pulmonary infiltrates) after 2 weeks of appropriate antimicrobial therapy. Patients appropriately treated for nosocomial pneumonia will show some degree of clinical/chest x-ray improvement within 3-5 days and certainly by 7-10 days.

- No change in infiltrates after 2 weeks of appropriate antimicrobial therapy in ventilated patients suggests a non-infectious process. Diagnostic bronchoscopy is required to make a definitive diagnosis.

- Do not assume persistent/unresponsive infiltrates are due to a "resistant organism" or an unusual pathogen. Changes in antimicrobial regimens and protracted courses of antimicrobial therapy in this setting should be avoided.

- Avoid "covering" Acinetobacter baumannii isolates from the secretions of ventilated patients, even those with pulmonary infiltrates. Acinetobacter is a common "colonizer" of respiratory secretions in ventilated patients but an infrequent pulmonary pathogen. Acinetobacter baumannii VAP primarily occurs in clusters or outbreaks and is associated with respiratory support equipment.

- For most strains of multi-drug resistant (MDR) P. aeruginosa, meropenem provides optimum empiric anti-P. aeruginosa therapy. For meropenem-resistant strains of MDR P. aeruginosa, use colistin or polymyxin B.

Chapter 16

Overview of Antimicrobial Therapy

Burke A. Cunha, MD
Paul E. Schoch, PhD

FACTORS IN ANTIBIOTIC SELECTION

A. **Spectrum.** Antibiotic spectrum refers to the range of microorganisms an antibiotic is usually effective against, and is the basis for empiric antibiotic therapy.

B. **Tissue Penetration**. Antibiotics that are effective against a microorganism in-vitro but unable to reach the site of infection are of little or no benefit to the host. Antibiotic tissue penetration depends on properties of the antibiotic (e.g., lipid solubility, molecular size) and tissue (e.g, adequacy of blood supply, presence of inflammation). Antibiotic tissue penetration is rarely problematic in acute infections due to increased microvascular permeability from local release of chemical inflammatory mediators. In contrast, chronic infections (e.g., chronic pyelonephritis, chronic prostatitis, chronic osteomyelitis) and infections caused by intracellular pathogens often rely on chemical properties of an antibiotic (e.g., high lipid solubility, small molecular size) for adequate tissue penetration. Antibiotics cannot be expected to eradicate organisms from areas that are difficult to penetrate or have impaired blood supply, such as abscesses, which usually require surgical drainage for cure. In addition, implanted foreign materials associated with infection usually need to be removed for cure, since microbes causing infections associated with prosthetic joints, shunts, and intravenous lines produce a slime glycocalyx on plastic and metal surfaces that permits organisms to survive despite antimicrobial therapy.

C. **Antibiotic Resistance**. Bacterial resistance to antimicrobial therapy can be natural or acquired, and relative or absolute. Pathogens not covered by the usual spectrum of an antibiotic are *naturally* resistant (e.g., 25% of S. pneumoniae are naturally resistant to macrolides); *acquired* resistance occurs when a previously sensitive pathogen is no longer as sensitive to an antibiotic (e.g., ampicillin-resistant H. influenzae). Organisms with *intermediate level (relative)* resistance manifest increases in minimum inhibitory concentrations (MICs), but they remain susceptible to the antibiotic at achievable serum/tissue concentrations (e.g., penicillin-resistant S. pneumoniae). In contrast, organisms with *high level (absolute)* resistance manifest a sudden increase in MICs during therapy, and cannot be overcome by higher-than-usual antibiotic doses (e.g., gentamicin-resistant P. aeruginosa).

Most acquired antibiotic resistance is *agent-specific*, not a class phenomenon, and is usually limited to one or two species. Resistance is *not* related, per se, to volume or duration of use. Some antibiotics have little resistance potential even when used in high volume; other antibiotics can induce resistance with little use. Successful antibiotic resistance control strategies include eliminating antibiotics from animal feeds, microbial surveillance to detect resistance problems early, infection control precautions to limit/contain spread of clonal resistance, restricted hospital formulary (i.e., controlled use of high resistance potential antibiotics), and preferential use of low resistance potential antibiotics by clinicians. Unsuccessful strategies include rotating formularies, restricted use of certain antibiotic classes (e.g., 3rd generation cephalosporins, fluoroquinolones), and use of combination therapy. In choosing between similar antibiotics, try to select an antibiotic with low resistance potential. Some antibiotics (e.g., ceftazidime) are associated with increased prevalence of methicillin-resistant S. aureus (MRSA); other antibiotics (e.g., vancomycin) are associated with increased prevalence of vancomycin-resistant enterococci (VRE).

D. Safety Profile. Whenever possible, avoid antibiotics with serious or frequent side effects.

E. Cost. Switching early from IV to PO antibiotics is the single most important cost saving strategy in hospitalized patients, as the institutional cost of IV administration (~$10/dose) may exceed the cost of the antibiotic itself. Antibiotic costs can also be minimized by using antibiotics with long half-lives and by choosing monotherapy over combination therapy. Other factors adding to the cost of antimicrobial therapy include the need for an obligatory second antimicrobial agent, antibiotic side effects (e.g., diarrhea, cutaneous reactions, seizures, phlebitis), and outbreaks of resistant organisms, which require cohorting and prolonged hospitalization.

FACTORS IN ANTIBIOTIC DOSING

Usual antibiotic dosing assumes normal renal and hepatic function. Patients with significant renal insufficiency and/or hepatic dysfunction may require dosage reduction in antibiotics metabolized/eliminated by these organs (Table 16.1). Specific dosing recommendations based on the degree of renal and hepatic insufficiency are detailed in Chapter 16.

A. Renal Insufficiency. Since most antibiotics eliminated by the kidneys have a wide "toxic-to-therapeutic ratio," dosing strategies are frequently based on formula-derived estimates of creatinine clearance (Table 16.1), rather than precise quantitation of glomerular filtration rates. Dosage adjustments are especially important for antibiotics with narrow toxic-to-therapeutic ratios (e.g., aminoglycosides), and for patients who are receiving other nephrotoxic medications or have preexisting renal disease.

   1. Loading and Maintenance Dosing in Renal Insufficiency. For drugs eliminated by the kidneys, the loading dose (if required) is left unchanged, and the maintenance dose and dosing interval are modified in proportion to the degree of renal insufficiency. For moderate renal insufficiency (CrCl ~ 40-60 mL/min), the maintenance dose is usually cut in half and the dosing interval is left unchanged. For severe renal insufficiency (CrCl ~ 10-40 mL/min), the maintenance dose is usually cut in half and the dosing interval is doubled. Dosing adjustment problems in renal insufficiency can be circumvented by selecting an antibiotic with a similar spectrum eliminated by the hepatic route.

   2. Aminoglycoside Dosing. Aminoglycosides have a narrow toxic-to-therapeutic ratio and high nephrotoxic potential and are of particular concern for patients with renal insufficiency. Single daily dosing—adjusted for the degree of renal insufficiency after the loading dose is administered—has virtually eliminated the nephrotoxic potential of aminoglycoside and is recommended for all patients, including the critically ill. (A possible exception is enterococcal endocarditis, where gentamicin dosing every 8 hours may be preferable.) Aminoglycoside-induced tubular dysfunction is best assessed by quantitative renal tubular cast counts in urine, which more accurately reflect aminoglycoside nephrotoxicity than serum creatinine.

B. Hepatic Insufficiency. Antibiotic dosing for patients with hepatic dysfunction is problematic, since there is no hepatic counterpart to the serum creatinine to accurately assess liver function. In practice, antibiotic dosing is based on clinical assessment of the severity of liver disease. For practical purposes, dosing adjustments are usually not required for mild or moderate hepatic insufficiency. For severe hepatic insufficiency, dosing adjustments are usually made for antibiotics with hepatotoxic potential. Relatively few antibiotics depend solely on hepatic inactivation/elimination, and dosing adjustment problems in these cases can be circumvented by selecting an appropriate antibiotic eliminated by the renal route.

C. Combined Renal and Hepatic Insufficiency. There are no good dosing adjustment guidelines for patients with hepatorenal insufficiency. If renal insufficiency is worse than hepatic insufficiency, antibiotics eliminated by the liver are often administered at half the total daily dose. If hepatic insufficiency is worse than renal insufficiency, antibiotics eliminated by the kidneys are usually administered and dosed in proportion to renal function.

Table 16.1. Dosing Strategies in Hepatic/Renal Insufficiency*

Hepatic Insufficiency
* Decrease total daily dose of hepatically-eliminated antibiotic by 50% in presence of clinically severe liver disease
* Alternative: Use antibiotic eliminated/inactivated by the renal route in usual dose

Renal Insufficiency
* If creatinine clearance ~ 40-60 mL/min, decrease dose of renally-eliminated antibiotic by 50% and maintain the usual dosing interval
* If creatinine clearance ~10-40 mL/min, decrease dose of renally-eliminated antibiotic by 50% and double the dosing interval
* Alternative: Use antibiotic eliminated/inactivated by the hepatic route in usual dose

Major Route of Elimination			
Hepatobiliary		**Renal**	
Chloramphenicol	Nafcillin	Most β-lactams	Gemifloxacin
Cefoperazone	Linezolid	Aminoglycosides	Vancomycin
Doxycycline	INH/EMB/RIF	TMP-SMX	Nitrofurantoin
Minocycline	Pyrazinamide	Monobactams	Fluconazole
Moxifloxacin	Itraconazole	Carbapenems	Acyclovir
Macrolides	Caspofungin	Polymyxin B	Valacyclovir
Telithromycin	Micafungin	Colistin	Famciclovir
Clindamycin	Anidulafungin	Ciprofloxacin	Tetracycline
Metronidazole	Ketoconazole	Ofloxacin	Flucytosine
Tigecycline	Voriconazole	Levofloxacin	Daptomycin
Quinupristin/dalfopristin	Posaconazole	Gatifloxacin	

* See individual drug summaries in Chapter 16 for specific dosing recommendations
Creatinine clearance (CrCl) is used to assess renal function, and can be estimated by the following formula: CrCl (mL/min) = [(140 − age) x weight (kg)] / [72 x serum creatinine (mg/dL)]. Multiply by 0.85 if female. It is important to recognize that due to age-dependent declines in renal function, elderly patients with "normal" serum creatinines may have CrCls requiring dosage adjustment. For example, a 70-year-old, 50-kg female with a serum creatinine of 1.2 mg/dL has an estimated CrCl of 34 mL/min

MICROBIOLOGY AND SUSCEPTIBILITY TESTING

A. **Overview.** In-vitro susceptibility testing provides information about microbial sensitivities of a pathogen to various antibiotics and is useful in guiding therapy. Proper application of microbiology and susceptibility data requires careful assessment of the in-vitro results to determine if they are consistent with the clinical context; if not, the clinical impression usually should take precedence.

B. **Limitations of Microbiology Susceptibility Testing**
   1. **In-vitro data do not differentiate between colonizers and pathogens.** Before treating a culture report from the microbiology laboratory, it is important

to determine whether the organism is a pathogen or a colonizer in the clinical context. As a rule, colonization should not be treated.

2. **In-vitro data do not necessarily translate into in-vivo efficacy**. Reports which indicate an organism is "sensitive" or "resistant" to a given antibiotic in-vitro do not necessarily reflect in-vivo activity. Table 16.2 lists antibiotic-microorganism combinations for which susceptibility testing is usually unreliable.

3. **In-vitro susceptibility testing is dependent on the microbe, methodology, and antibiotic concentration**. In-vitro susceptibility testing by the microbiology laboratory *assumes* the isolate was recovered from *blood* and is being exposed to *serum* concentrations of an antibiotic given in the *usual* dose. Since some body sites (e.g., bladder, urine) contain higher antibiotic concentrations than found in serum, and other body sites (e.g., CSF) contain lower antibiotic concentrations than found in serum, in-vitro data may be misleading for non-bloodstream infections. For example, a Klebsiella pneumoniae isolate obtained from the CSF may be reported as "sensitive" to cefazolin even though cefazolin does not penetrate the CSF. Likewise, E. coli and Klebsiella urinary isolates are often reported as "resistant" to ampicillin/sulbactam despite in-vivo efficacy, due to high antibiotic concentrations in the urinary tract. Antibiotics should be prescribed at the usual recommended doses; attempts to lower cost by reducing dosage may decrease antibiotic efficacy (e.g., cefoxitin 2 gm IV inhibits ~ 85% of B. fragilis isolates, whereas 1 gm IV inhibits only ~ 20% of strains).

4. **Unusual susceptibility patterns**. Organisms have predictable susceptibility patterns to antibiotics. When an isolate has an unusual susceptibility pattern (i.e., isolate of a species demonstrates the reverse of the usual susceptibility pattern) (Table 16.3), further testing should be performed by the microbiology laboratory to verify the identity of the isolate and characterize the mechanism of resistance. Expanded susceptibility testing is also warranted.

5. **Screening for extended-spectrum beta-lactamase (ESBL) activity (Table 16.4).**

C. **Susceptibility Breakpoints for Streptococcus pneumoniae**. Because antibiotic susceptibility is, in part, concentration related, the Clinical and Laboratory Standards Institute (CLSI) has revised its breakpoints for S. pneumoniae susceptibility testing, which differentiate between meningeal and non-meningeal sites of pneumococcal infection (Table 16.5).

Table 16.2. Antibiotic-Organism Combinations for Which In-Vitro Susceptibility Testing Is Unreliable*

Antibiotic	"Sensitive" Organism
Penicillin	H. influenzae, Yersinia pestis
TMP-SMX	Klebsiella, Enterococci, Bartonella
Polymyxin B	Proteus, Salmonella
Imipenem	Stenotrophomonas† maltophilia
Gentamicin	Mycobacterium tuberculosis
Vancomycin	Erysipelothrix rhusiopathiae
Aminoglycosides	Streptococci, Salmonella, Shigella
Clindamycin	Fusobacteria, Clostridia, enterococci, Listeria
Macrolides	P. multocida
1st, 2nd generation cephalosporins	Salmonella, Shigella, Bartonella
3rd, 4th generation cephalosporins§	Enterococci, Listeria, Bartonella
All antibiotics except vancomycin, minocycline, quinupristin/dalfopristin, linezolid, daptomycin, tigecycline	MRSA‡

* In-vitro susceptibility *does not* predict in-vivo activity; susceptibility data cannot be relied upon to guide therapy for antibiotic-organism combinations in this table
† Formerly Pseudomonas
‡ In spite of apparent in-vitro susceptibility of many antibiotics against MRSA, only vancomycin, quinupristin/dalfopristin, linezolid, daptomycin, and minocycline are effective in-vivo
§ Cefoperazone is the only cephalosporin with clinically useful anti-enterococcal activity (E. faecalis, not E. faecium [VRE])

D. **Summary.** In-vitro susceptibility testing is useful in most situations, but should not be followed blindly. Many factors need to be considered when interpreting in-vitro microbiologic data, and infectious disease consultation is recommended for all but the most straightforward susceptibility interpretation problems. Since susceptibility is concentration-dependent, IV-to-PO switch changes using antibiotics of the same class is best made when the oral antibiotic can achieve similar blood/tissue levels as the IV antibiotic. For example, IV-to-PO switch from cefazolin 1 gm (IV) to cephalexin 500 mg (PO) may not be effective against all pathogens at all sites, since cephalexin 500 mg (PO) achieves much lower serum concentrations compared to cefazolin 1 gm (IV) (16 mcg/mL vs. 200 mcg/mL).

Table 16.3. Unusual Susceptibility Patterns Requiring Further Testing

Organism	Unusual Susceptibility Patterns	Usual Susceptibility Patterns
Streptococcus pneumoniae	Vancomycin intermediate/resistant	Vancomycin susceptible
E. coli, P. mirabilis, Klebsiella	Cefoxitin/cefotetan resistant	2nd generation cephalosporin susceptible
Enterobacter, Serratia	Ampicillin/cefazolin susceptible	Ampicillin/cefazolin resistant
E. coli, Enterobacter, Klebsiella	Tobramycin susceptible; gentamicin/amikacin/imipenem resistant	Ceftazidime/cefepime/aztreonam/imipenem susceptible
Morganella, Providencia	Ampicillin/cefazolin susceptible	Ampicillin/cefazolin resistant
Klebsiella	Cefotetan susceptible; ceftazidime resistant	Cefotetan resistant; ceftazidime susceptible
Pseudomonas aeruginosa	Amikacin resistant; gentamicin/tobramycin susceptible	Amikacin susceptible; gentamicin/tobramycin resistant
Stenotrophomonas maltophilia	TMP-SMX resistant; imipenem susceptible	TMP-SMX susceptible

Isolates with unusual susceptibility patterns require further testing by the microbiology laboratory to verify the identity of the isolate and characterize resistance mechanism. Expanded susceptibility testing is indicated.

Table 16.4. Screening for Extended-Spectrum Beta-Lactamase (ESBL) Activity*

Pathogen	Positive Screening Result (MIC)
K. pneumoniae K. oxytoca E. coli	Cefpodoxime ≥ 4 mcg/mL Ceftazidime ≥ 1 mcg/mL Aztreonam ≥ 1 mcg/mL Cefotaxime ≥ 1 mcg/mL Ceftriaxone ≥ 1 mcg/mL
P. mirabilis	Cefpodoxime ≥ 1 mcg/mL Ceftazidime ≥ 1 mcg/mL Cefotaxime ≥ 1 mcg/mL

* The presence of an ESBL-producing isolate has important therapeutic implications and should be suspected based on positive screening results from susceptibility testing. Confirmation of ESBL activity requires a 2-fold or more decrease in MIC for either (ceftazidime + clavulanic acid) or (cefotaxime + clavulanic acid).

Table 16.5. CLSI Susceptibility Breakpoints for Streptococcus pneumoniae*

Antibiotic	MIC (mcg/mL)		
	Sensitive	Intermediate	Resistant
Amoxicillin (non-meningitis)	≤ 2	4	≥ 8
Amoxicillin-clavulanic acid (non-meningitis)	≤ 2/1	4/2	≥ 8/4
Penicillin	≤ 0.06	0.12-1	≥ 2
Azithromycin	≤ 0.5	1	≥ 2
Clarithromycin/erythromycin	≤ 0.25	0.5	≥ 1
Doxycycline/tetracycline	≤ 2	4	≥ 8
Telithromycin	≤ 1	2	≥ 4
Cefaclor	≤ 1	2	≥ 4
Cefdinir/cefpodoxime	≤ 0.5	1	≥ 2
Cefprozil	≤ 2	4	≥ 8
Cefuroxime axetil (oral)	≤ 1	2	≥ 4
Loracarbef	≤ 2	4	≥ 8
Cefepime (non-meningitis)	≤ 1	2	≥ 4
Cefepime (meningitis)	≤ 0.5	1	≥ 2
Cefotaxime (non-meningitis)	≤ 1	2	≥ 4
Cefotaxime (meningitis)	≤ 0.5	1	≥ 2
Ceftriaxone (non-meningitis)	≤ 1	2	≥ 4
Ceftriaxone (meningitis)	≤ 0.5	1	≥ 2
Imipenem	≤ 0.12	0.25–0.5	≥ 1
Meropenem	≤ 0.25	0.5	≥ 1
Ertapenem	≤ 1	2	> 4
Vancomycin	≤ 1	–	–
Gatifloxacin/moxifloxacin	≤ 1	2	≥ 4
Levofloxacin	≤ 2	4	≥ 8
TMP-SMX	≤ 0.5/9.5	1/19 – 2/38	≥ 4/78
Chloramphenicol	≤ 4	–	≥ 8
Clindamycin	≤ 0.25	0.5	≥ 1
Linezolid	≤ 2	–	–
Rifampin	≤ 1	2	≥ 4

CLSI = Clinical and Laboratory Standards Institute (formerly NCCLS = National Committee for Clinical Laboratory Standards) (2006)
* *Testing Conditions:* Medium: Mueller-Hinton broth with 2.5% lysed horse blood (cation-adjusted). Inoculum: colony suspension. Incubation: 35°C (20-24 hours)

OTHER CONSIDERATIONS IN ANTIMICROBIAL THERAPY

A. **Bactericidal vs. Bacteriostatic Therapy.** For most infections, bacteriostatic and bactericidal antibiotics inhibit/kill organisms at the same rate, and should not be a factor in antibiotic selection. Bactericidal antibiotics have an advantage in certain infections, such endocarditis, meningitis, and febrile leukopenia, but there are exceptions even in these cases.

B. **Monotherapy vs. Combination Therapy**. Monotherapy is preferred to combination therapy, and is possible for most infections. In addition to cost savings, monotherapy results in less chance of medication error and fewer missed doses/drug interactions. Combination therapy may be useful for drug synergy or for extending spectrum beyond what can be obtained with a single drug. However, since drug synergy is difficult to assess and the possibility of antagonism always exists, antibiotics should be combined for synergy only if synergy is likely based on experience or actual testing. Combination therapy is not effective in preventing antibiotic resistance, except in very few situations (Table 16.6).

C. **Intravenous vs. Oral Switch Therapy.** Patients admitted to the hospital are usually started on IV antibiotic therapy, then switched to equivalent oral therapy after clinical improvement/defervescence (usually within 72 hours). Advantages of early IV-to-PO switch programs include reduced cost, early hospital discharge, less need for home IV therapy, and virtual elimination of IV line infections. Drugs well-suited for IV-to-PO switch or for treatment entirely by the oral route include doxycycline, minocycline, clindamycin, quinolones, metronidazole, chloramphenicol, amoxicillin, trimethoprim-sulfamethoxazole, and linezolid. Only some penicillins and cephalosporins are useful for IV-to-PO switch programs due to limited bioavailability. Most infectious diseases should be treated orally unless the patient is critically ill, cannot take antibiotics by mouth, or there is no equivalent oral antibiotic. If the patient is able to take/absorb oral antibiotics, there is no difference in clinical outcome using equivalent IV or PO antibiotics. It is more important to think in terms of antibiotic spectrum, bioavailability and tissue penetration, rather than route of administration. Nearly all non-critically ill patients should be treated in part or entirely with oral antibiotics. When switching from IV to PO therapy, the oral antibiotic chosen ideally should achieve the same blood and tissue levels as the equivalent IV antibiotic (Table 16.7).

Table 16.6. Combination Therapy and Antibiotic Resistance

Examples of Antibiotic Combinations That Prevent Resistance
   Anti-pseudomonal penicillin (carbenicillin) + aminoglycoside (gentamicin,
      tobramycin, amikacin)
   Rifampin + other TB drugs (INH, ethambutol, pyrazinamide)
   5-flucytosine + amphotericin B

Examples of Antibiotic Combinations That Do Not Prevent Resistance*
   TMP-SMX
   Most other antibiotic combinations

* These combinations are often prescribed to prevent resistance when, in actuality, they do
not

D. Duration of Therapy. Most bacterial infections in normal hosts are treated with
antibiotics for 1-2 weeks. The duration of therapy may need to be extended in
patients with impaired immunity (e.g., diabetes, SLE, alcoholic liver disease,
neutropenia, diminished splenic function, etc.), chronic bacterial infections (e.g.,
endocarditis, osteomyelitis), chronic viral and fungal infections, or certain bacterial
intracellular pathogens (Table 16.8). Infections such as HIV and CMV in
compromised hosts usually require life-long suppressive therapy. Antibiotic therapy
should ordinarily not be continued for more than 2 weeks, even if low-grade fevers
persist. Prolonged therapy offers no benefit, and increases the risk of adverse side
effects, drug interactions, and superinfections.

Table 16.7. Bioavailability of Oral Antimicrobials

Bioavailability	Antimicrobials		
Excellent*	Amoxicillin	TMP	Minocycline
	Clindamycin	TMP-SMX	Linezolid
	Quinolones	Doxycycline	Fluconazole
	5-Flucytosine	Chloramphenicol	Voriconazole
	Rifampin	Metronidazole	Posaconazole
Good†	Most beta-lactams	Acyclovir	Itraconazole
	Most 1st,2nd,3rd gen.	Valacyclovir	
	oral cephalosporins	Famciclovir	
	Macrolides	Telithromycin	
Inadequate‡	Vancomycin		

* Oral administration results in equivalent blood/tissue levels as the same dose given IV (PO = IV)
† Oral administration results in lower blood/tissue levels than the same dose given IV (PO < IV)
‡ Oral administration results in inadequate blood/tissue levels

Table 16.8. Infectious Diseases Requiring Prolonged Antimicrobial Therapy

Therapy	Infectious Diseases
4 weeks	Chronic otitis media, chronic sinusitis, Legionella
6 weeks	Acute bacterial endocarditis (S. aureus)
3 months	Lung abscess*
6 months	Pulmonary TB, extrapulmonary TB, Actinomycosis[†], Nocardia[†], invasive pulmonary aspergillosis[†]
> 12 months	Chronic suppressive therapy for Pneumocystis (carinii) jiroveci pneumonia (PCP), cytomegalovirus (CMV), HIV

* Treat until resolved or until chest x-ray is normal/nearly normal and remains unchanged
† May require longer treatment

EMPIRIC ANTIBIOTIC THERAPY

Microbiology susceptibility data are not ordinarily available prior to initial treatment with antibiotics. Empiric therapy is based on directing coverage against the most likely pathogens, and takes into consideration drug allergy history, hepatic/renal function, possible antibiotic side effects, resistance potential, and cost. If a patient is moderately or severely ill, empiric therapy is usually initiated intravenously. Patients who are mildly ill, whether hospitalized or ambulatory, may be started on oral antibiotics with high bioavailability. Cultures of appropriate clinical specimens (e.g., sputum) should be obtained prior to starting empiric therapy to provide bacterial isolates for in-vitro susceptibility testing.

ANTIBIOTIC FAILURE

There are many possible causes of *apparent* antibiotic failure, including drug fever, antibiotic-unresponsive infections, and febrile non-infectious diseases. The most common error in the management of apparent antibiotic failure is changing/adding additional antibiotics instead of determining the cause (Tables 16.9, 16.10).

Table 16.9. Causes of Apparent/Actual Antibiotic Failure

In-vitro susceptibility but inactive in-vivo
Antibiotic tolerance with gram-positive cocci
Inadequate coverage/spectrum
Inadequate antibiotic blood levels
Inadequate antibiotic tissue levels
    Undrained abscess
    Foreign body-related infection
    Protected focus (e.g., cerebrospinal fluid)
    Organ hypoperfusion/diminished blood supply (e.g., chronic osteomyelitis in diabetics)
Drug-induced interactions
    Antibiotic inactivation
    Antibiotic antagonism
Decreased antibiotic activity in tissue
Fungal superinfection
Treating colonization, not infection
Non-infectious diseases
    Medical disorders mimicking infection (e.g., SLE)
    Drug fever (Table 16.10)
Antibiotic-unresponsive infectious diseases
    Most viral infections

Adapted from: Cunha BA, Ortega A. Antibiotic failure. Medical Clinics of North America 79:663-672, 1995.

Table 16.10. Clinical Features of Drug Fever

History
 Many but not all individuals are atopic
 Patients have been on a sensitizing medication for days or years "without a problem"

Physical exam
 Fevers may be low- or high-grade, but usually range between 102°-104°F and may exceed 106°F
 Relative bradycardia*
 Patient appears "inappropriately well" for degree of fever

Laboratory tests
 Elevated WBC count (usually with left shift)
 Eosinophils almost always present, but eosinophilia is uncommon
 Elevated erythrocyte sedimentation rate in majority of cases
 Early, transient, mild elevations of serum transaminases (common)
 Negative blood cultures (excluding contaminants)

---

* Relative bradycardia refers to heart rates that are inappropriately slow relative to body temperature (pulse must be taken simultaneously with temperature elevation). Applies to adult patients with temperature ≥ 102°F; does not apply to patients with second/third-degree heart block, pacemaker-induced rhythms, or those taking beta-blockers, verapamil, or diltiazem.
Appropriate Temperature-Pulse Relationships

Pulse (beats/min)	Temperature
150	41.1°C (106°F)
140	40.6°C (105°F)
130	40.7°C (104°F)
120	39.4°C (103°F)
110	38.9°C (102°F)

PITFALLS IN ANTIBIOTIC PRESCRIBING

- Use of antibiotics to treat non-infectious or antibiotic-unresponsive infectious diseases (e.g., viral infections) or colonization
- Overuse of combination therapy. Monotherapy is preferred over combination therapy unless compelling reasons prevail, such as drug synergy or extended spectrum beyond what can be obtained with a single drug. Monotherapy reduces the risk of drug interactions and side effects, and is usually less expensive
- Use of antibiotics for persistent fevers. For patients with persistent fevers on an antimicrobial regimens that appears to be failing, it is important to reassess the patient rather than add additional antibiotics. Causes of prolonged fevers include undrained septic foci, non-infectious medical disorders, and drug fevers. Undiagnosed causes of leukocytosis/low-grade fevers should not be treated with prolonged courses of antibiotics
- Inadequate surgical therapy. Infections involving infected prosthetic materials or fluid collections (e.g., abscesses) often require surgical therapy for cure. For infections such as chronic osteomyelitis, surgery is the only way to cure the infection; antibiotics are useful only for suppression or to prevent local infectious complications

REFERENCES AND SUGGESTED READINGS

Cunha BA. Antibiotic pharmacokinetic considerations in pulmonary infections. Sem Respir Infect 6:168-182, 1991.

Cunha BA. Antimicrobial side effects. Medical Clinics of North America 85:149-185, 2001.

Cunha BA. Clinical relevance of penicillin-resistant Streptococcus pneumoniae. Semin Respir Infect 17:204-14, 2002.

Cunha BA. Community-acquired pneumonia-Pearls. Infections in Medicine 20:27-30, 2003.

Cunha BA. Drug fever. Postgraduate Medicine 80:123-129, 1986.

Cunha BA. Effective antibiotic resistance and control strategies. Lancet 357:1307-1308, 2001.

Cunha BA. Factors in Antibiotic selection for hospital formularies (part I). Hospital Formulary 33:558-572, 1998.

Cunha BA. Factors in antibiotic selection for hospital formularies (part II). Hospital Formulary 33:659-662, 1998.

Cunha BA. Intravenous to oral antibiotic switch therapy. Drugs for Today 37:311-319, 2001.

Cunha BA, Ortega A. Antibiotic failure. Medical Clinics of North America 79:663-672, 1995.

Cunha BA. Penicillin resistant streptococcus pneumoniae. Drugs for Today 31:31-35, 1998.

Cunha BA. Pseudomonas aeruginosa: Resistance and therapy. Semin Respir Infect 17:231-9, 2002.

Cunha BA. Strategies to control the emergence of resistant organisms. Sem Respir Infect 17:250-258, 2002.

Cunha BA. The significance of antibiotic false sensitivity testing with in vitro testing. J Chemother 9:25-33, 1997.

Empey KM, Rapp RP, Evans ME. The effect of an antimicrobial formulary change on hospital resistance patterns. Pharmacotherapy 22:81-7, 2002.

Johnson DH, Cunha BA. Drug fever. Infectious Disease Clinics of North America 10:85-91, 1996.

TEXTBOOKS

Amabile-Cuevas CF (ed). Antibiotic Resistance From Molecular Basics to Therapeutic Options. R.G. Landes Company, Austin, 1996.

Ambrose P, Nightingale AT (eds). Principles of Pharmacodynamics. Marcel Dekker, Inc., New York, 2001.

Anaissie EJ, McGinnis MR, Pfaller MA (eds). Clinical Mycology. Churchill Livingstone, New York, 2003.

Chadwick DJ, Goode J (eds). Antibiotic Resistance: Origins, Evolution, Selection and Spread. John Wiley & Sons, New York, 1997.

Cunha BA (ed). Medical Clinics of North America Antimicrobial Therapy. W.B. Saunders Company, Philadelphia, PA,1982.

Cunha BA (ed). Medical Clinics of North America Antimicrobial Therapy I. W.B. Saunders Company, Philadelphia, PA,1995.

Cunha BA (ed). Medical Clinics of North America Antimicrobial Therapy II. W.B. Saunders Company, Philadelphia, PA,1995.

Cunha BA (ed). Medical Clinics of North America Antimicrobial Therapy I. W.B. Saunders Company, Philadelphia, PA, 2000.

Cunha BA (ed). Medical Clinics of North America Antimicrobial Therapy II. W.B. Saunders Company, Philadelphia, PA, 2001.

Cunha BA (ed). Medical Clinics of North America, Antimicrobial Therapy. Elsevier, New York, 2006.

Cunha BA (ed). Anitbiotic Essentials, 7th Edition. Physicians Press, Royal Oak, MI, 2008.

Finch RG, Greenwood D, Norrby SR, Whitley RJ (eds). Antibiotic and chemotherapy anti-infective agents and their use in therapy, 8th Edition. Edinburgh, Churchill Livingstone, 2003.

Gorbach SL, Bartlett JG, Blacklow NR (eds). Infectious Diseases, 3rd Edition. Philadelphia, Lippincott, Williams & Wilkins, 2004.

Kaye D (ed). Infectious Disease Clinics of North America Pharmacology, New Agents. W.B. Saunders Company, Philadelphia, PA,1997.

Kaye D (ed). Infectious Disease Clinics of North America Pharmacology, New Agents. W.B. Saunders Company, Philadelphia, PA, 2000.

Lorian V, (ed). Antibiotics in Laboratory Medicine, 5th Edition. Philadelphia, Lippincott Williams & Wilkins, 2005.

Mandell GL, Bennett JE, Dolin R (eds). Mandell, Douglas, and Bennett's Principles and Practice of infectious Diseases, 6th Edition. Philadelphia, Elsevier Churchill Livingstone, 2005.

Scholar EM Pratt WB (eds). The Antimicrobial Drugs, 2nd Edition. Oxford University Press, New York, 2000.

Chapter 17

Antimicrobial Drug Summaries

Burke A. Cunha, MD
Demary C. Torres, PharmD
John H. Rex, MD

This section contains prescribing information pertinent to the clinical use of antimicrobial agents in adults, as compiled from a variety of sources (pp. 347-348). Antimicrobial agents for pediatric infectious diseases are described in Chapter 10. The information provided is not exhaustive, and the reader is referred to other drug information references and the manufacturer's product literature for further information. Clinical use of the information provided and any consequences that may arise from its use are the responsibilities of the prescribing physician. The authors, editors, and publisher do not warrant or guarantee the information contained in this section, and do not assume and expressly disclaim any liability for errors or omissions or any consequences that may occur from such. The use of any drug should be preceded by careful review of the package insert, which provides indications and dosing approved by the U.S. Food and Drug Administration.

Drugs are listed alphabetically by generic name; trade names follow in parentheses. To search by trade name, consult the index. Each drug summary contains the following information:

Usual dose. Represents the usual dose to treat most susceptible infections in adult patients with normal hepatic and renal function. Dosing for special situations is listed under the comments section; additional information can be found in Chapters 4-10 and the manufacturer's product literature. Loading doses for doxycycline, fluconazole, itraconazole, voriconazole, caspofungin, ganciclovir, and valganciclovir are described in either the usual dose or comments section. Meningeal doses of antimicrobials used for CNS infection are described at the end of the comments section.

Peak serum level. Refers to the peak serum concentration (mcg/ml) after the usual dose is administered. Peak serum level is useful in calculating the "kill ratios," the ratio of peak serum level to minimum inhibitory concentration (MIC) of the organism. The higher the "kill ratio," the more effective the antimicrobial is likely to be against a particular organism.

Bioavailability. Refers to the percentage of the dose reaching the systemic circulation from the site of administration (PO or IM). For PO antibiotics, bioavailability refers to the percentage of dose adsorbed from the GI tract. For IV antibiotics, "not applicable" appears next to bioavailability, since the entire dose reaches the systemic circulation. Antibiotics with high bioavailability (> 90%) are ideal for IV-to-PO switch therapy. Antibiotics with low bioavailability are effective if their "kill ratios" are favorable.

Excreted unchanged. Refers to the percentage of drug excreted unchanged, and provides an indirect measure of drug concentration in the urine/feces. Antibiotics excreted unchanged in the urine in low percentage are unlikely to be useful for urinary tract infections.

Serum half-life (normal/ESRD). The serum half-life ($T_{1/2}$) is the time (in hours) in which serum concentration falls by 50%. Serum half-life is useful in determining dosing interval. If the half-life of drugs eliminated by the kidneys is prolonged in end-stage renal disease (ESRD), then the total daily dose is reduced in proportion to the degree of renal dysfunction. If the half-life in ESRD is similar to the normal half-life, then the total daily dose does not change.

Plasma protein binding. Expressed as the percentage of drug reversibly bound to serum albumin. It is the unbound (free) portion of a drug that equilibrates with tissues and imparts antimicrobial activity. Plasma protein binding is not typically a factor in antimicrobial effectiveness unless binding exceeds 95%, and then only if the "kill ratio" is relatively low. Decreases in serum albumin (nephrotic syndrome, liver disease) or competition for protein binding from other drugs or endogenously produced substances (uremia, hyperbilirubinemia) will increase the percentage of free drug available for antimicrobial activity, and may require a decrease in dosage. Increases in serum binding proteins (trauma, surgery, critical illness) will decrease the percentage of free drug available for antimicrobial activity, and may require an increase in dosage.

Volume of distribution (V_d). Represents the apparent volume into which the drug is distributed, and is calculated as the amount of drug in the body divided by the serum concentration (in liters/kilogram). V_d is related to total body water distribution (V_d H_2O = 0.7 L/kg). Hydrophilic (water soluble) drugs are restricted to extracellular fluid and have a $V_d \leq 0.7$ L/kg. In contrast, hydrophobic (highly lipid soluble) drugs penetrate most fluids/tissues of the body and have a large V_d. Drugs that are concentrated in certain tissues (e.g., liver) can have a V_d greatly exceeding total body water. V_d is affected by organ profusion, membrane diffusion/permeability, lipid solubility, protein binding, and state of equilibrium between body compartments. For hydrophilic drugs, increases in V_d may occur with burns, heart failure, dialysis, sepsis, cirrhosis, or mechanical ventilation; decreases in V_d may occur with trauma, hemorrhage, pancreatitis (early), or GI fluid losses. Increases in V_d may require an increase in total daily drug dose for antimicrobial effectiveness; decreases in V_d may require a decrease in drug dose. In addition to drug distribution, V_d reflects binding avidity to cholesterol membranes and concentration within organ tissues (e.g., liver).

Mode of elimination. Refers to the primary route of inactivation/excretion of the antibiotic, which impacts dosing adjustments in renal/hepatic failure.

Dosage adjustments. Each grid provides dosing adjustments based on renal and hepatic function. Antimicrobial dosing for hemodialysis (HD)/peritoneal dialysis (PD) patients is the same as indicated for patients with a CrCl < 10 mL/min. Some antimicrobial agents require a supplemental dose immediately after hemodialysis (post–HD)/peritoneal dialysis (post–PD); following the supplemental dose, antimicrobial dosing should once again resume as indicated for a CrCl < 10 mL/min. "No change" indicates no change from the usual dose. "Avoid" indicates the drug should be avoided in the setting described. "None" indicates no supplemental dose is required. "No information" indicates there are insufficient data from which to make a dosing recommendation. Dosing recommendations are based on data, experience, or pharmacokinetic parameters. CVVH dosing recommendations represent general guidelines, since antibiotic removal is dependent on area/type of filter, ultrafiltration rates, and sieving coefficients; replacement dosing should be individualized and guided by serum levels, if possible. Creatinine clearance (CrCl) is used to gauge the degree of renal insufficiency, and can be estimated by the following calculation: CrCl (mL/min) = [(140 – age) x weight (kg)] / [72 x serum creatinine (mg/dL)]. The calculated value is multiplied by 0.85 for females. It is important to recognize that due to age-dependent decline in renal function, elderly patients with "normal" serum creatinines may have low CrCls requiring dosage adjustments. (For example, a 70-year-old, 50-kg female with a serum creatinine of 1.2 mg/dL has an estimated CrCl of 34 mL/min.)

Drug interactions. Refers to common/important drug interactions, as compiled from various sources. If a specific drug interaction is well-documented (e.g, antibiotic X with lovastatin), than other drugs from the same drug class (e.g., atorvastatin) may also be listed, based on theoretical considerations. Drug interactions may occur as a consequence of altered absorption (e.g., metal ion chelation of tetracycline), altered distribution (e.g., sulfonamide displacement of barbiturates from serum albumin), altered metabolism (e.g., rifampin–induced hepatic P-450 metabolism of theophylline/warfarin; chloramphenicol inhibition of phenytoin metabolism), or altered excretion (e.g., probenecid competition with penicillin for active transport in the kidney).

Adverse side effects. Common/important side effects are indicated.

Allergic potential. Described as low or high. Refers to the likelihood of a hypersensitivity reaction to a particular antimicrobial.

Safety in pregnancy. Designated by the U.S. Food and Drug Administration's (USFDA) use-in-pregnancy letter code (Table 17.1).

Comments. Includes various useful information for each antimicrobial agent.

Cerebrospinal fluid penetration. Indicated as a percentage relative to peak serum concentration. If an antimicrobial is used for CNS infections, then its meningeal dose is indicated directly above CSF penetration. No meningeal dose is given if CSF penetration is inadequate for treatment of meningitis due to susceptible organisms.

Biliary tract penetration. Indicated as a percentage relative to peak serum concentrations. Percentages > 100% reflect concentration within the biliary system. This information is useful for the treatment of biliary tract infections.

Selected references. These references are classic, important, or recent. When available, the website containing the manufacturer's prescribing information/package insert is provided. (The use of any drug should be preceded by careful review of the package insert, which provides indications and dosing approved by the U.S. Food and Drug Administration.) Additional references, guidelines, and textbooks relating to antimicrobial therapy are listed at the back of each chapter.

Table 17.1. USFDA Use-in-Pregnancy Letter Code

Category	Interpretation
A	**Controlled studies show no risk.** Adequate, well-controlled studies in pregnant women have not shown a risk to the fetus in any trimester of pregnancy
B	**No evidence of risk in humans.** Adequate, well-controlled studies in pregnant women have not shown increased risk of fetal abnormalities despite adverse findings in animals, or, in the absence of adequate human studies, animal studies show no fetal risk. The chance of fetal harm is remote, but remains a possibility
C	**Risk cannot be ruled out.** Adequate, well-controlled human studies are lacking, and animal studies have shown a risk to the fetus or are lacking. There is a chance of fetal harm if the drug is administered during pregnancy, but potential benefit from use of the drug may outweigh potential risk
D	**Positive evidence of risk.** Studies in humans or investigational or post-marketing data have demonstrated fetal risk. Nevertheless, potential benefit from use of the drug may outweigh potential risk. For example, the drug may be acceptable if needed in a life-threatening situation or serious disease for which safer drugs cannot be used or are ineffective
X	**Contraindicated in pregnancy.** Studies in animals or humans or investigational or post-marketing reports have demonstrated positive evidence of fetal abnormalities or risk which clearly outweigh any possible benefit to the patient

Lipid-Associated Formulations of Amphotericin B. There are 3 licensed lipid-associated formulations of amphotericin B (LFAB) (Table 17.2). Although closely related in some ways, these formulations have distinct properties and must be understood separately. The principal advantage of the LFAB over amphotericin B deoxycholate (AMBD) is greater safety. In general, the rates of both acute infection-related toxicities (fever, chills, etc.) and chronic therapy-associated toxicities (principally nephrotoxicity) are reduced with LFAB. However, the LFAB can produce all of the toxicities of AMBD (and in selected patients, LFAB have been more toxic than AMBD). Overall, LAMB (AmBisome) and ABLC (Abelcet) appear to be safer than ABCD (Amphotec, Amphocil). Whichever formulation is selected for therapy, it is important to specify its name carefully when prescribing. The phrase "lipid amphotericin B" should be avoided due to its imprecision. Patients who are tolerating one formulation may develop all the standard infusion-related toxicities if switched inadvertently to a new formulation. In general (and in contrast to the usual preference for generic names), use of trade names is the clearest way to specify the choice of drug in this category. In this handbook, the phrase "lipid-associated formulation of amphotericin B" suggests use of any of the 3 formulations. The issues surrounding the selection of an LFAB for an individual patient are summarized in Table 17.2.

Table 17.2. Lipid-Associated Formulations of Amphotericin B

Generic name (abbreviation)	Trade names	Licensed (IV) dosages in the United States	Comments
Amphotericin B lipid complex (ABLC)	Abelcet	5 mg/kg/d	Reliable choice; long history of use
Liposomal amphotericin B (LAMB)	AmBisome	3 mg/kg/d (empiric therapy) 3-5 mg/kg/d (systemic fungal infections) 6 mg/kg/d (cryptococcal meningitis in HIV patients)	Reliable choice; best studied LFAB; well-supported dosing recommendations by indication; probably the least nephrotoxic; good data to support increasing the dose safely
Amphotericin B colloidal dispersion, amphotericin B cholesteryl sulfate complex (ABCD)	Amphotec, Amphocil	3-4 mg/kg/d	Infusion-related toxicities have limited its use

Arikan S, Rex JH. Lipid-based antifungal agents: Current status. Curr Pharm Design 7:393-415, 2001.
  Groll AH, Walsh TJ. Antifungal drugs. Side Effects of Drugs Annual 26:302-314, 2003.
Ostrosky-Zeichner L, Marr KA, Rex JH, Cohen SH. Amphotericin B: Time for a new "gold standard." Clin Infect Dis 37:415-425, 2003.

Acyclovir (Zovirax)

Drug Class: Antiviral
Usual Dose: Topical cream 5%. Apply 5 times/day for 4 days not systemic
HSV ½: Herpes labialis: 400 mg (PO) 5x/day x 5 days. Genital herpes: *Initial therapy*: 200 mg (PO) 5x/day x 10 days. *Recurrent/intermittent therapy* (< 6 episodes/year): 200 mg (PO) 5x/day x 5 days. *Chronic suppressive therapy* (> 6 episodes/year): 400 mg (PO) q12h x 1 year. Mucosal/genital herpes: 5 mg/kg (IV) q8h x 7 days or 400 mg (PO) 5x/day x 7 days. Encephalitis: 10 mg/kg (IV) q8h x 10 days or 800 mg (PO) 5x/day x 10 days
VZV: Chickenpox: 800 mg (PO) q6h x 5 days. Herpes zoster (shingles): *Dermatomal/localized*: 800 mg (PO) 5x/day x 7-10 days. *Disseminated*: 10 mg/kg (IV) q8h x 7-10 days
Pharmacokinetic Parameters:
Peak serum level: 1.21 mcg/mL
Bioavailability: 10-20%
Excreted unchanged (urine): 62-91%
Serum half-life (normal/ESRD): 3/5 hrs
Plasma protein binding: 9-33%
Volume of distribution (V_d): 0.8 L/kg
Primary Mode of Elimination: Renal
Dosage Adjustments* for HSV/VZV

CrCl 10-25 mL/min	No change/ 800 mg (PO) q8h
CrCl < 10 mL/min	200 mg (PO) q12h/ 800 mg (PO) q12h
Post–HD dose	200 mg (IV/PO)/ 800 mg (IV/PO)
Post–PD dose	None
CVVH dose	See CrCl 10-25 mL/min
Moderate or severe hepatic insufficiency	No change

Drug Interactions: Probenecid, meperidine (↑ meperidine metabolic levels, phenytoin (↓ phenytoin levels), valproic acid (↓ valproic levels), varicellovirus vaccine (↓ vaccine etteoticness), theophylline (↑ acyclovir levels); nephrotoxic drugs (↑ nephrotoxicity); zidovudine (lethargy); theophylline (↑ levels)
Adverse Effects: Seizures/tremors (dose related), crystalluria. Base dose on ideal body weight in the elderly to minimize adverse effects
Allergic Potential: Low
Safety in Pregnancy: C
Comments: Na^+ content = 4 mEq/g. CSF levels may be increased with probenecid. Meningeal dose = VZV/HSV encephalitis dose
Cerebrospinal Fluid Penetration: 50%

REFERENCES:
De Clercq E. Antiviral drugs in current clinical use. J Clin Virol 30:115-33, 2004.
Keating MR. Antiviral Agents. Mayo Clin Proc 67:160-78, 1992.
Owens RC, Ambrose PG. Acyclovir. Antibiotics for Clinicians 1:85-93, 1997.
Whitley RJ, Gnann JW Jr. Acyclovir: a decade later. N Engl J Med 327:782-3, 1992
Website: www.pdr.net.

Amantadine (Symmetrel)

Drug Class: Antiviral
Usual Dose: 200 mg (PO) q24h or 100 mg bid
Pharmacokinetic Parameters:
Peak serum level: 0.22 mcg/mL
Bioavailability: 90%
Excreted unchanged (urine): 90%
Serum half-life (normal/ESRD): 17/145 hrs
Plasma protein binding: 67%
Volume of distribution (V_d): 4.8 L/kg
Primary Mode of Elimination: Renal
Dosage Adjustments*

CrCl 30-50 mL/min	100 mg (PO) q24h
CrCl 15–30 mL/min	100 mg (PO) q48h
CrCl < 15 mL/min	200 mg (PO) qweek
Post–HD	200 mg (PO) qweek
Post–PD	None
CVVH dose	100 mg (PO) q48h

"Usual dose" assumes normal renal/hepatic function. * For renal insufficiency, give usual dose x 1 followed by maintenance dose per CrCl. For dialysis patients, dose the same as for CrCl < 10 mL/min and give supplemental (post-HD/PD dose) immediately after dialysis. CrCl = creatinine clearance; CVVH = continuous veno-venous hemo-filtration; HD/PD = hemodialysis/peritoneal dialysis. See pp. 275-278 for explanations, p. 1 for abbreviations

Moderate or severe hepatic insufficiency	No change

Drug Interactions: Alcohol (↑ CNS effects); benztropine, trihexyphenidyl (↑ interacting drug effect: dry mouth, ataxia); CNS stimulants (additive stimulation); digoxin (↑ digoxin levels); trimethoprim (↑ amantadine and trimethoprim levels); scopolamine (↑ scopolamine effect: blurred vision, slurred speech, toxic psychosis)
Adverse Effects: Confusion/delusions, dysarthria, ataxia, anticholinergic effects (blurry vision, dry mouth, orthostatic hypotension, urinary retention, constipation, livedo reticularis, may ↑ QT$_c$ interval
Allergic Potential: Low
Safety in Pregnancy: C
Comments: May precipitate heart failure. Avoid co-administration with anticholinergics, MAO inhibitors, or antihistamines. May improve peripheral airway function/oxygenation in influenza A
Cerebrospinal Fluid Penetration:
Non-inflamed meninges = 15%
Inflamed meninges = 20%

REFERENCES:
Douglas RG, Jr. Prophylaxis and treatment of influenza. N Engl J Med 322:443-50, 1990.
Geskey JM, Thomas NJ. Amantadine penetration into cerebrospinal fluid of a child with influenza A encephalitis. Pediatr Infect Dis J 23:270-2, 2004.
Gubareva LV, Kaiser L, Hayden FG. Influenza virus neuraminidase inhibitors. Lancet 355:827-5, 2000.
Keyers LA, Karl M, Nafziger AN, et al. Comparison of central nervous system adverse effects of amantadine and rimantadine used as sequential prophylaxis of influenza A in elderly nursing home patients. Arch Intern Med 160:1485-8, 2000.
Kawai N, Ikematsu H, Iwaki N, et al. Factors influencing the effectiveness of oseltamivir and amantadine for the treatment of influenza: A multicenter study from Japan of the 2002-2003 influenza season. Clin Infect Dis 40:1309-16, 2005.
Website: www.pdr.net

Amikacin (Amikin)

Drug Class: Aminoglycoside
Usual Dose: 15 mg/kg or 1 gm (IV) q24h (preferred to q12h dosing)

Pharmacokinetic Parameters:
Peak serum level: 20-30 mcg/mL (q12h dosing); 65-75 mcg/mL (q24h dosing)
Bioavailability: Not applicable
Excreted unchanged (urine): 95%
Serum half-life (normal/ESRD): 2/50 hrs
Plasma protein binding: < 5%
Volume of distribution (V$_d$): 0.25 L/kg
Primary Mode of Elimination: Renal
Dosage Adjustments*

CrCl 50–80 mL/min	7.5 mg/kg (IV) q24h or 500 mg (IV) q24h
CrCl 10–50 mL/min	7.5 mg/kg (IV) q48h or 500 mg (IV) q48h
CrCl < 10 mL/min	3.75 mg/kg (IV) q48h or 250 mg (IV) q48h
Post–HD dose	7.5 mg/kg (IV) or 500 mg (IV)
Post–PD dose	3.75 mg/kg (IV) or 250 mg (IV)
CVVH dose	7.5 mg/kg (IV) or 500 mg (IV) q12h
Moderate or severe hepatic insufficiency	No change

Drug Interactions: Amphotericin B, cephalothin, cyclosporine, enflurane, methoxyflurane, NSAIDs, polymyxin B, radiographic contrast, vancomycin (↑ nephrotoxicity); cis-platinum (↑ nephrotoxicity, ↑ ototoxicity); loop diuretics (↑ ototoxicity); neuromuscular blocking agents (↑ apnea, prolonged paralysis); non-polarizing muscle relaxants (↑ apnea)
Adverse Effects: Neuromuscular blockade with rapid infusion/absorption. Nephrotoxicity only with prolonged/extremely high serum trough levels; may cause reversible non–oliguric renal failure (ATN). Ototoxicity associated with prolonged/extremely high peak serum levels (usually irreversible): Cochlear toxicity (1/3 of ototoxicity) manifests as decreased high frequency hearing, but deafness is unusual.

"Usual dose" assumes normal renal/hepatic function. * For renal insufficiency, give usual dose x 1 followed by maintenance dose per CrCl. For dialysis patients, dose the same as for CrCl < 10 mL/min and give supplemental (post-HD/PD dose) immediately after dialysis. CrCl = creatinine clearance; CVVH = continuous veno-venous hemofiltration; HD/PD = hemodialysis/peritoneal dialysis. See pp. 275-278 for explanations, p. 1 for abbreviations

Vestibular toxicity (2/3 of ototoxicity) develops before ototoxicity (typically manifests as tinnitus)
Allergic Potential: Low
Safety in Pregnancy: D
Comments: Dose for synergy = 7.5 mg/kg (IV) q24h or 500 mg (IV) q24h. Single daily dosing virtually eliminates nephrotoxic/ototoxic potential. Incompatible with solutions containing β–lactams, erythromycin, chloramphenicol, furosemide, sodium bicarbonate. IV infusion should be given slowly over 30 minutes. May be given IM. Intraperitoneal infusion ↑ risk of neuromuscular blockade. Avoid intratracheal/aerosolized intrapulmonary instillation, which may predispose to antibiotic resistance. V_d increases with edema/ascites, trauma, burns, cystic fibrosis; may require ↑ dose. V_d decreases with dehydration, obesity; may require ↓ dose. Renal cast counts are the best indicator of aminoglycoside nephrotoxicity, not serum creatinine. Dialysis removes ~ 50% of amikacin from serum. Na^+ content = 1.3 mEq/g
CAPD dose: 10-20 mg/L in dialysate (I.P.) with each exchange
Therapeutic Serum Concentrations (for therapeutic efficacy, not toxicity):
Peak (q24h/q12h dosing): 65-75/20-30 mcg/mL
Trough (q24h/q12h dosing): 0/4-8 mcg/mL
Intrathecal (IT) dose = 10–40 mg (IT) q24h
Cerebrospinal Fluid Penetration:
Non-inflamed meninges = 15%
Inflamed meninges = 20%
Bile Penetration: 30%

REFERENCES:
Bacopoulou F, Markantonis SL, Pavlou E, et al. A study of once-daily amikacin with low peak target concentrations in intensive care unit patients: pharmacokinetics and associated outcomes. J Crit Care. 18:107-13, 2003.
Cunha BA. Aminoglycosides: Current role in antimicrobial therapy. Pharmacotherapy 8: 334-50,1988.
Cunha BA. Pseudomonas aeruginosa: Resistance and therapy. Semin Respir Infect 17:231-9, 2002.
Edson RS, Terrel CL. The Aminoglycosides. Mayo Clin Proc 74:519-28, 1999.
Fulnecky E, Wright D, Scheld WM, et al. Amikacin and colistin for treatment of Acinetobacter baumanni meningitis. Journal of Infection 51;e249-e251, 2005.

Giamarellos-Bourboulis E, Kentepozidis N, Antonopoulou A, et al. Postantibiotic effect of antimicrobial combinations on multidrug-resistant Pseudomonas aeruginosa. Diagnostic Microbiology and Infectious Disease 51:113-117, 2005.
Karakoc B, Gerceker AA. In-vitro activities of various antibiotics, alone and in combination with amikacin against Pseudomonas aeruginosa. Int J Antimicrob Agents 18:567-70, 2001.
Poole K. Aminoglycoside resistance in Pseudomonas aeruginosa. Antimicrobial Agents and Chemotherapy 49:479-487, 2005.

Amoxicillin (Amoxil, A-cillin, Polymox, Trimox, Wymox)

Drug Class: Aminopenicillin
Usual Dose: 1 gm (PO) q8h
Pharmacokinetic Parameters:
Peak serum level: 14 mcg/mL
Bioavailability: 90%
Excreted unchanged (urine): 60%
Serum half-life (normal/ESRD): 1.3/16 hrs
Plasma protein binding: 20%
Volume of distribution (V_d): 0.26 L/kg
Primary Mode of Elimination: Renal
Dosage Adjustments*

CrCl 50-80 mL/min	500 mg (PO) q8h
CrCl 10–50 mL/min	500 mg (PO) q12h
CrCl < 10 mL/min	500 mg (PO) q24h
Post–HD or post-PD	500 mg
CVVH dose	500 mg (PO) q12h
Moderate or severe hepatic insufficiency	No change

Drug Interactions: Allopurinol (↑ risk of rash)
Adverse Effects: Drug fever/rash, ↑SGOT/SGPT
Allergic Potential: High
Safety in Pregnancy: B
Comments: ↑ risk of rash with EBV infectious mononucleosis. No irritative diarrhea with 1 gm (PO) q8h dose due to nearly complete proximal GI absorption. Na^+ content = 2.7 mEq/g
Cerebrospinal Fluid Penetration:
Non-inflamed/inflamed meninges = 1%/8%

"Usual dose" assumes normal renal/hepatic function. * For renal insufficiency, give usual dose x 1 followed by maintenance dose per CrCl. For dialysis patients, dose the same as for CrCl < 10 mL/min and give supplemental (post-HD/PD dose) immediately after dialysis. CrCl = creatinine clearance; CVVH = continuous veno-venous hemo-filtration; HD/PD = hemodialysis/peritoneal dialysis. See pp. 275-278 for explanations, p. 1 for abbreviations

Bile Penetration: 3000%

REFERENCES:
[No authors listed]. Acute otitis media in children: amoxicillin remains the standard antibiotic, but justified in certain situations only. Prescrire Int. 12:184-9, 2003.

Addo-Yobo E, Chisaka N, Hassan M, et al. Oral amoxicillin versus injectable penicillin for severe pneumonia in children age 3 to 59 months: a randomized multicentre equivalency study. Lancet 364:1141-48, 2004.

Cunha BA. The aminopenicillins. Urology 40:186-190,1992.

Dhaon NA. Amoxicillin tablets for oral suspension in the treatment of acute otitis media: a new formulation with improved convenience. Adv Ther 21:87-95, 2004.

Donowitz GR, Mandell GL. Beta-lactam antibiotics. N Engl J Med 318:419-26 and 318:490-500, 1993.

Piglansky L, Leibovitz E, Raiz S, et al. Bacteriologic and clinical efficacy of high dose amoxicillin for therapy of acute otitis media in children. Pediatr Infect Dis J. 22:405-13, 2003.

Ready D, Lancaster H, Qureshi F, et al. Effect of amoxicillin use on oral microbiota in young children. Antimicrob Agents Chemother 48:2883-7, 2004.

Website: www.pdr.net

Amoxicillin/Clavulanic Acid (Augmentin)

Drug Class: Aminopenicillin/β-lactamase inhibitor combination
Usual Dose: 500/125 mg (PO) q8h or 875/125 mg (PO) q12h for severe infections or respiratory tract infections
Pharmacokinetic Parameters:
Peak serum level: 10.0/2.2 mcg/mL
Bioavailability: 90/60%
Excreted unchanged (urine): 80/40%
Serum half-life (normal/ESRD): [1.3/16]/[½] hrs
Plasma protein binding: 18/25%
Volume of distribution (V_d): 0.26/0.3 L/kg
Primary Mode of Elimination: Renal
Dosage Adjustments* (based on 500 mg q8h)

CrCl 50–80 mL/min	500/125 mg (PO) q12h
CrCl 10–50 mL/min	500/125 mg (PO) q24h
CrCl < 10 mL/min	250/125 mg (PO) q24h

Post–HD dose	250/125 mg (PO)
Post–PD dose	None
CVVH dose	500/125 mg (PO) q24h
Moderate or severe hepatic insufficiency	No change

Drug Interactions: Allopurinol (↑ risk of rash)
Adverse Effects: Drug fever/rash, diarrhea, ↑ SGOT/SGPT. Rash potential same as ampicillin
Allergic Potential: High
Safety in Pregnancy: B
Comments: ↑ risk of rash with EBV infectious mononucleosis. 875/125 mg formulation should not be used in patients with CrCl < 30 mL/min
Cerebrospinal Fluid Penetration:
Non-inflamed meninges = 1%
Inflamed meninges = 1%
Bile Penetration: 3000%

REFERENCES:
Cunha BA. Amoxicillin/clavulanic acid in respiratory infections: microbiologic and pharmacokinetic considerations. Clinical Therapeutics 14:418-25, 1992.

Donowitz GR, Mandell GL. Beta-lactam antibiotics. N Engl J Med 318:419-26 and 318:490-500, 1993.

Easton J, Noble S, Perry CM. Amoxicillin/clavulanic acid: a review of its use in the management of paediatric patients with acute otitis media. Drugs. 63:311-40, 2003.

Fernandez-Sabe N, Carratala J, Dorca J, et al. Efficacy and safety of sequential amoxicillin-clavulanate in the treatment of anaerobic lung infections. Eur J Clin Microbiol Infect Dis. 22:185-7, 2003.

File TM Jr, Lode H, Kurz H, et al. Double-blind, randomized study of the efficacy and safety of oral pharmacokinetically enhanced amoxicillin-clavulanic (2,000/125 milligrams) versus those of amoxicillin-clavulanic (875/125 milligrams), both given twice daily for 7 days, in treatment of bacterial community-acquired pneumonia adults. Antimicrob Agents Chemother 48:3323-31, 2004.

Klein JO. Amoxicillin/clavulanate for infections in infants and children: past, present and future. Pediatr Infect Dis J. 22:S139-48, 2003.

Scaglione F, Caronzolo D, Pintucci JP, et al. Measurement of cefaclor and amoxicillin-clavulanic acid levels in middle-ear fluid in patients with acute otitis media. Antimicrob Agents Chemother. 47:2987-9, 2003.

"Usual dose" assumes normal renal/hepatic function. * For renal insufficiency, give usual dose x 1 followed by maintenance dose per CrCl. For dialysis patients, dose the same as for CrCl < 10 mL/min and give supplemental (post-HD/PD dose) immediately after dialysis. CrCl = creatinine clearance; CVVH = continuous veno-venous hemofiltration; HD/PD = hemodialysis/peritoneal dialysis. See pp. 275-278 for explanations, p. 1 for abbreviations

Wright AJ, Wilkowske CJ. The penicillins. Mayo Clin
   Proc 66:1047-63, 1991.
Website: www.augmentin.com

Amoxicillin/Clavulanic Acid ES-600 (Augmentin ES-600)

Drug Class: Aminopenicillin/β-lactamase inhibitor combination
Usual Dose: 90 mg/kg/day oral suspension in 2 divided doses (see comments)
Pharmacokinetic Parameters:
Peak serum level: 15.7/1.7 mcg/mL
Bioavailability: 90/60%
Excreted unchanged (urine): 70/40%
Serum half-life (normal/ESRD): [1.4/16]/[1.1/2] hrs
Plasma protein binding: 18%/25%
Volume of distribution (V$_d$): 0.26/0.3 L/kg
Primary Mode of Elimination: Renal
Dosage Adjustments*

CrCl < 30 mL/min	Avoid
Moderate or severe hepatic insufficiency	Use with caution

Drug Interactions: Allopurinol (↑ risk of rash)
Adverse Effects: Drug fever/rash, diarrhea, ↑ SGOT/SGPT. Rash potential same as ampicillin
Allergic Potential: High
Safety in Pregnancy: B
Comments: 5 mL contains 600 mg amoxicillin and 42.9 mg clavulanatic acid. Use in children > 3 months. Take at start of meal to minimize GI upset. Do not substitute 400 mg or 200 mg/5 mL formulation for ES-600. Not for children < 3 months or > 40 kg. Contains phenylalanine
Volume of ES-600 to provide 90 mg/kg/day:

Weight	Volume (q12h)	Weight	Volume (q12h)
8 kg	3.0 mL	24 kg	9.0 mL
12 kg	4.5 mL	28 kg	10.5 mL
16 kg	6.0 mL	32 kg	12.0 mL
20 kg	7.5 mL	36 kg	13.5 mL

Cerebrospinal Fluid Penetration:
Non-inflamed meninges = 1%
Inflamed meninges = 1%
Bile Penetration: 3000%

REFERENCES:
Dagan R, Hoberman A, Johnson C, et al. Bacteriologic
   and clinical efficacy of high dose
   amoxicillin/clavulanate in children with acute otitis
   media. Pediatr Infect Dis J 20:829-37, 2001.
Easton J, Noble S, Perry CM. Amoxicillin/clavulanic acid:
   a review of its use in the management of paediatric
   patients with acute otitis media. Drugs 63:311-40,
   2003.
Ghaffar F, Muniz LS, Katz K, et al. Effects of large
   dosages of amoxicillin/clavulanate or azithromycin on
   nasopharyngeal carriage of Streptococcus
   pneumoniae, Haemophilus influenzae,
   nonpneumococcal alpha-hemolytic streptococci, and
   Staphylococcus aureus in children with acute otitis
   media. Clin Infect Dis 34:1301-9, 2002.
Website: www.augmentin.com

Amoxicillin/Clavulanic Acid XR (Augmentin XR)

Drug Class: Aminopenicillin/β-lactamase inhibitor combination
Usual Dose: 2000/125 mg (2 tablets) (PO) q12h (see comments)
Pharmacokinetic Parameters:
Peak serum level: 17/2 mcg/mL
Bioavailability: 90/60%
Excreted unchanged (urine): 70/40%
Serum half-life (normal/ESRD): [1.3/16]/[½] hrs
Plasma protein binding: 18/25%
Volume of distribution (V$_d$): 0.26/0.3 L/kg
Primary Mode of Elimination: Renal
Dosage Adjustments*

CrCl > 30 mL/min	No change
CrCl < 30 mL/min	Avoid
Post–HD/PD dose	Avoid
CVVH dose	Avoid
Moderate or severe hepatic insufficiency	Use with caution

"Usual dose" assumes normal renal/hepatic function. * For renal insufficiency, give usual dose x 1 followed by maintenance dose per CrCl. For dialysis patients, dose the same as for CrCl < 10 mL/min and give supplemental (post-HD/PD dose) immediately after dialysis. CrCl = creatinine clearance; CVVH = continuous veno-venous hemo-filtration; HD/PD = hemodialysis/peritoneal dialysis. See pp. 275-278 for explanations, p. 1 for abbreviations

Drug Interactions: Allopurinol (↑ risk of rash); may ↓ effectiveness of oral contraceptives
Adverse Effects: Drug fever, rash, diarrhea, ↑ SGOT/SGPT, nausea, abdominal pain
Allergic Potential: High
Safety in Pregnancy: B
Comments: Amoxicillin/clavulanic acid XR is a time-released formulation. Do not crush tablets. XR formulation contains a different ratio of amoxicillin/clavulanic acid so other formulations cannot be interchanged. 2 tablets (1000/62.5 mg per tablet) = 2000/125 mg per dose. 2 gm amoxicillin effective against most strains of PRSP. Take with food (not high fat meal) to increase absorption
Cerebrospinal Fluid Penetration:
Non-inflamed meninges = 1%
Inflamed meninges = 1%
Bile Penetration: 3000%

REFERENCES:
[No authors listed]. Augmentin XR. Med Lett Drugs Ther. 45:5-6, 2003.
Benninger MS. Amoxicillin/clavulanate potassium extended release tablets: a new antimicrobial for the treatment of acute bacterial sinusitis and community-acquired pneumonia. Expert Opin Pharmacother. 4:1839-46, 2003.
File Jr TM, Jacobs M, Poole M, et al. Outcome of treatment of respiratory tract infections due to Streptococcus pneumoniae, including drug-resistant strains, with pharmacokinetically enhanced amoxicillin/clavulatate. International J Antimicrobial Agents 20:235-247, 2002.
Kaye C, Allen A, Perry S, et al. The clinical pharmacokinetics of a new pharmacokinetically enhanced formulation of amoxicillin/clavulatate. Clin Therapeutics 23:578-584, 2001.
Website: www.augmentin.com

Amphotericin B (Fungizone)

Drug Class: Antifungal
Usual Dose: 0.5-0.8 mg/kg (IV) q24h
Pharmacokinetic Parameters:
Peak serum level: 1-2 mcg/mL
Bioavailability: Not applicable
Excreted unchanged (urine): 5%
Serum half-life (normal/ESRD): 15/48 days
Plasma protein binding: 90%

Volume of distribution (V_d): 4 L/kg
Primary Mode of Elimination: Metabolized
Dosage Adjustments*

CrCl 50–80 mL/min	No change
CrCl 10–50 mL/min	No change
Post–HD or post-PD	None
CVVH dose	None
Moderate or severe hepatic insufficiency	No change

Drug Interactions: Adrenocorticoids (hypokalemia); aminoglycosides, cyclosporine, polymyxin B (↑ nephrotoxicity); digoxin (↑ digitalis toxicity due to hypokalemia); flucytosine (↑ flucytosine levels if amphotericin B produces renal dysfunction); neuromuscular blocking agents (↑ neuromuscular blockade due to hypokalemia)
Adverse Effects: Fevers/chills, flushing thrombophlebitis, bradycardia, seizures, hypotension, distal renal tubular acidosis (↓ K⁺/↓ Mg⁺⁺), anemia. If renal insufficiency is secondary to amphotericin, either ↓ daily dose by 50%, give dose every other day, or switch to an amphotericin lipid formulation
Allergic Potential: Low
Safety in Pregnancy: B
Comments: Higher doses (1-1.5 mg/kg q24h) may be needed in life-threatening situations but are very nephrotoxic and should only be administered under expert supervision. Reconstitute in sterile water, not in dextrose, saline, or bacteriostatic water. Do not co-administer in same IV with other drugs. Give by slow IV infusion over 2 hours initially. Aggressive hydration (1-2 liters/d) may reduce nephrotoxicity. Test dose unnecessary. Amphotericin B with granulocyte colony stimulating factor (GCSF) may result in ARDS. Amphotericin B with pentamidine may cause acute tubular necrosis in HIV/AIDS patients. Fevers/chills may be reduced by meperidine, aspirin, NSAIDs, hydrocortisone or acetaminophen, if given 30-60 minutes before infusion. For bladder irrigation, use 50 mg/L until cultures are negative.

"Usual dose" assumes normal renal/hepatic function. * For renal insufficiency, give usual dose x 1 followed by maintenance dose per CrCl. For dialysis patients, dose the same as for CrCl < 10 mL/min and give supplemental (post-HD/PD dose) immediately after dialysis. CrCl = creatinine clearance; CVVH = continuous veno-venous hemofiltration; HD/PD = hemodialysis/peritoneal dialysis. See pp. 275-278 for explanations, p. 1 for abbreviations

Meningeal dose = usual dose plus 0.5 mg
3-5x/week (IT) via Ommaya reservoir
Cerebrospinal Fluid Penetration: < 10%

REFERENCES:
Arikan S, Lozano-Chiu M, Paetznick V, et al. In vitro synergy of caspofungin and amphotericin B against Aspergillus and Fusarium spp. Antimicrob Agents Chemother 46:245-7, 2002.
Boucher HW, Groll AH, Chiou CC, et al. Newer systemic antifungal agents: pharmacokinetics, safety and efficacy. Drugs 64:1997-2020, 2004.
Deray G. Amphotericin B nephrotoxicity. J Antimicrob Chemother Suppl 1:37-41, 2002.
Dupont B. Overview of the lipid formulations of amphotericin B. J Antimicrob Chemother 49 Suppl 1:31-6, 2002.
Ellis D. Amphotericin B: spectrum and resistance. J Antimicrob Chemother Suppl 1:7-10, 2002.
Gallis HA, Drew RH, Pickard WW. Amphotericin B: 30 years of clinical experience. Rev Infect Dis 12:308-29, 1990.
Lewis, RE, Wiederhold NP, Klepser ME. In vitro pharmacodynamics amphotericin B, itraconazole, and voriconazole against aspergillus, fusarium, and scedosporium spp. Antimicrobial Agents and Chemotherapy 49:945-951, 2005.
Lyman CA, Walsh TJ. Systemically administered antifungal agents: A review of their clinical pharmacology and therapeutic applications. Drugs 44:9-35, 1992.
Menzies D, Goel K, Cunha BA. Amphotericin B. Antibiotics for Clinicians 2:73-6, 1998.
Moosa MY, Alangaden GJ, Manavathu E. Resistance to amphotericin B does not emerge during treatment for invasive aspergillosis. J Antimicrob Chemother 49:209-13, 2002.
Website: www.pdr.net

Amphotericin B Lipid Complex (Abelcet) ABLC

Drug Class: Antifungal (see p. 279)
Usual Dose: 5 mg/kg (IV) q24h
Pharmacokinetic Parameters:
Peak *serum level:* 1.7 mcg/mL
Bioavailability: Not applicable
Excreted unchanged (urine): 5%
Serum half-life (normal/ESRD): 173/173 hrs
Plasma protein binding: 90%
Volume of distribution (V_d): 131 L/kg
Primary Mode of Elimination: Metabolized

Dosage Adjustments*

CrCl 50–80 mL/min	No change
CrCl < 50 mL/min	No change
Post–HD/PD dose	None
CVVH dose	None
Moderate or severe hepatic insufficiency	No change

Drug Interactions: Adrenocorticoids (hypokalemia); aminoglycosides, cyclosporine, polymyxin B (↑ nephrotoxicity); digoxin (↑ digitalis toxicity due to hypokalemia); flucytosine (↑ flucytosine effect); neuromuscular blocking agents (↑ neuromuscular blockade due to hypokalemia)
Adverse Effects: Fevers/chills, flushing thrombophlebitis, bradycardia, seizures, hypotension, distal renal tubular acidosis (↓ K⁺/↓ Mg⁺⁺), anemia. Fewer/less severe side effects and less nephrotoxicity than amphotericin B. Renal toxicity is dose-dependent (use caution)
Allergic Potential: Low
Safety in Pregnancy: B
Comments: See p. 279. Useful in patients unable to tolerate amphotericin B or in patients with amphotericin B nephrotoxicity. Infuse at 2.5 mg/kg/hr
Cerebrospinal Fluid Penetration: < 10%

REFERENCES:
Arikan S, Rex JH. Lipid-based antifungal agents: current status. Curr Pharm Des 7:393-415, 2001.
Dupont B. Overview of the lipid formulations of amphotericin B. J Antimicrob Chemother 49 Suppl 1:31-6, 2002
Hiemenz JW, Walsh TJ. Lipid formulations of Amphotericin B: Recent progress and future directions. Clin Infect Dis 2:133-44, 1996.
Kauffman CA, Carver PL. Antifungal agents in the 1990s: Current status and future developments. Drugs 53:539-49, 1997.
Slain D. Lipid-based Amphotericin B for the treatment of fungal infections. Pharmacotherapy 19:306-23, 1999.
Trouet A. The amphotericin B lipid complex or abelcet: its Belgian connection, its mode of action and specificity: a review. Acta Clin Belg 57:53-7, 2002.

"Usual dose" assumes normal renal/hepatic function. * For renal insufficiency, give usual dose x 1 followed by maintenance dose per CrCl. For dialysis patients, dose the same as for CrCl < 10 mL/min and give supplemental (post-HD/PD dose) immediately after dialysis. CrCl = creatinine clearance; CVVH = continuous veno-venous hemofiltration; HD/PD = hemodialysis/peritoneal dialysis. See pp. 275-278 for explanations, p. 1 for abbreviations

Website: www.pdr.net

Amphotericin B Liposomal (AmBisome)

Drug Class: Antifungal (see p. 279)
Usual Dose: 3-6 mg/kg (IV) q24h (see comments)
Pharmacokinetic Parameters:
Peak serum level: 17-83 mcg/mL
Bioavailability: Not applicable
Excreted unchanged (urine): 5%
Serum half-life (normal/ESRD): 153 hrs/no data
Plasma protein binding: 90%
Volume of distribution (V_d): 131 L/kg
Primary Mode of Elimination: Metabolized
Dosage Adjustments*

CrCl 50–80 mL/min	No change
CrCl < 50 mL/min	No change
Post–HD/PD dose	None
CVVH dose	None
Moderate or severe hepatic insufficiency	No change

Drug Interactions: Adrenocorticoids (hypokalemia); aminoglycosides, cyclosporine, polymyxin B (↑ nephrotoxicity); digoxin (↑ digitalis toxicity due to hypokalemia); flucytosine (↑ flucytosine effect); neuromuscular blocking agents (↑ neuromuscular blockade due to hypokalemia)
Adverse Effects: Fevers/chills, flushing, thrombophlebitis, bradycardia, seizures, hypotension, distal renal tubular acidosis (↓ K⁺/↓ Mg⁺⁺), anemia
Allergic Potential: Low
Safety in Pregnancy: B
Comments: See p. 279. Less nephrotoxicity than amphotericin B and other amphotericin lipid preparations. For empiric therapy of fungemia, 3 mg/kg (IV) q24h can be used. For suspected/ known Aspergillus infection, use 5 mg/kg (IV) q24h. For cryptococcal meningitis in HIV, use 6 mg/kg (IV) q24h
Cerebrospinal Fluid Penetration: < 10%

REFERENCES:
Adler-Moore J, Proffitt RT. AmBisome: liposomal formulation, structure, mechanism of action and preclinical experience. J Antimicrob Chemother 49 Suppl 1:211-30, 2002.
Chopra R. AmBisome in the treatment of fungal infections: the UK experience. J Antimicrob Chemother 49 Suppl 1:43-7, 2002.
De Marie S. Clinical use of liposomal and lipid-complexed amphotericin-B. J Antimicrob Chemother 33:907-16, 1994.
Hiemenz JW, Walsh TJ. Lipid formulations of amphotericin B: Recent progress and future directions. Clin Infect Dis 2:133-44, 1996.
Lequaglie C. Liposomal amphotericin B (AmBisome): efficacy and safety of low-dose therapy in pulmonary fungal infections. J Antimicrob Chemother 49 Suppl 1:49-50, 2002.
Slain D. Lipid-based amphotericin B for the treatment of fungal infections. Pharmacotherapy 19:306-23, 1999.
Website: www.ambisome.com

Amphotericin B Cholesteryl Sulfate Complex (Amphotec), ABCD (amphotericin B colloidal dispersion)

Drug Class: Antifungal (see p. 279)
Usual Dose: 3-4 mg/kg (IV) q24h
Pharmacokinetic Parameters:
Peak serum level: 2.9 mcg/mL
Bioavailability: Not applicable
Excreted unchanged (urine): 5%
Serum half-life (normal/ESRD): 39/29 hrs
Plasma protein binding: 90%
Volume of distribution (V_d): 4 L/kg
Primary Mode of Elimination: Metabolized
Dosage Adjustments*

CrCl 50–80 mL/min	No change
CrCl < 50 mL/min	No change
Post–HD/PD dose	None
CVVH dose	None

"Usual dose" assumes normal renal/hepatic function. * For renal insufficiency, give usual dose x 1 followed by maintenance dose per CrCl. For dialysis patients, dose the same as for CrCl < 10 mL/min and give supplemental (post-HD/PD dose) immediately after dialysis. CrCl = creatinine clearance; CVVH = continuous veno-venous hemo-filtration; HD/PD = hemodialysis/peritoneal dialysis. See pp. 275-278 for explanations, p. 1 for abbreviations

Moderate or severe hepatic insufficiency	No change

Drug Interactions: Adrenocorticoids (hypokalemia); aminoglycosides, cyclosporine, polymyxin B (↑ nephrotoxicity); digoxin (↑ digitalis toxicity due to hypokalemia); flucytosine (↑ flucytosine effect); neuromuscular blocking agents (↑ neuromuscular blockade due to hypokalemia)
Adverse Effects: Fevers/chills, flushing, thrombophlebitis, bradycardia, seizures, hypotension, distal renal tubular acidosis (↓ K⁺/↓ Mg⁺⁺), anemia, Fewer/less severe side effects/less nephrotoxicity vs. amphotericin B
Allergic Potential: Low
Safety in Pregnancy: B
Comments: See p. 279. Reconstitute in sterile water, not dextrose, saline or bacteriostatic water. Do not co-administer with in same IV line with other drugs. Give by slow IV infusion over 2 hours (1 mg/kg/hr). Test dose unnecessary
Cerebrospinal Fluid Penetration: < 10%

REFERENCES:
De Marie S. Clinical use of liposomal and lipid-complexed amphotericin B. J Antimicrob Chemother 33:907-16, 1994.
Kline S, Larsen TA, Fieber L, et al. Limited toxicity of prolonged therapy with high doses of amphotericin B lipid complex. Clin Infect Dis 21:1154-8, 1995.
Rapp RP, Gubbins PO, Evans ME. Amphotericin B lipid complex. Ann Pharmacother 31:1174-86, 1997.
Website: www.pdr.net

Ampicillin (various)

Drug Class: Aminopenicillin
Usual Dose: 2 gm (IV) q4h, 500 mg (PO) q6h
Pharmacokinetic Parameters:
Peak serum level: 48 (IV) / 5 (PO) mcg/mL
Bioavailability: 50%
Excreted unchanged (urine): 90%
Serum half-life (normal/ESRD): 0.8/10 hrs
Plasma protein binding: 20%
Volume of distribution (V_d): 0.25 L/kg
Primary Mode of Elimination: Renal

Dosage Adjustments*

CrCl 50–80 mL/min	1 gm (IV) q4h 500 mg (PO) q6h
CrCl 10–50 mL/min	1 gm (IV) q8h 250 mg (PO) q8h
CrCl < 10 mL/min	1 gm (IV) q12h 250 mg (PO) q12h
Post–HD dose	1 gm (IV) 500 mg (PO)
Post–PD dose	250 mg (PO)
CVVH dose	1 gm (IV) q8h 250 mg (PO) q12h
Moderate or severe hepatic insufficiency	No change

Drug Interactions: Allopurinol (↑ frequency of rash); warfarin (↑ INR)
Adverse Effects: Drug fever/rash, nausea, GI upset, irritative diarrhea, ↑ SGOT/SGPT, ↑ incidence of rash vs. penicillin in patients with EBV, HIV, lymphocytic leukemias, or allopurinol, C. difficile diarrhea/colitis
Allergic Potential: High
Safety in Pregnancy: B
Comments: Incompatible in solutions containing amphotericin B, heparin, corticosteroids, erythromycin, aminoglycosides, or metronidazole. Na⁺ content = 2.9 mEq/g. Meningeal dose = 2 gm (IV) q4h
Cerebrospinal Fluid Penetration:
Non-inflamed meninges = 1%
Inflamed meninges = 10%
Bile Penetration: 3000%

REFERENCES:
Donowitz GR, Mandell GL. Beta-lactam antibiotics. N Engl J Med 318:419-26 and 318:490-500, 1993.
Wright AJ. The penicillins. Mayo Clin Proc 74:290-307, 1999.
Wright AJ, Wilkowske CJ. The penicillins. Mayo Clin Proc 66:1047-63, 1991.

Ampicillin/sulbactam (Unasyn)

Drug Class: Aminopenicillin/β-lactamase inhibitor combination
Usual Dose: 1.5-3 gm (IV) q6h (see comments)
Pharmacokinetic Parameters:
Peak serum level: 109-150/48-88 mcg/mL
Bioavailability: Not applicable
Excreted unchanged (urine): 80/80%
Serum half-life (normal/ESRD): [1/9]/[1/9] hrs
Plasma protein binding: 28/38%
Volume of distribution (V_d): 0.25/0.38 L/kg
Primary Mode of Elimination: Renal/hepatic
Dosage Adjustments* (based on 3 gm q6h):

CrCl 50–80 mL/min	1.5 gm (IV) q6h
CrCl 10–50 mL/min	1.5 gm (IV) q12h
CrCl < 10 mL/min	1.5 gm (IV) q24h
Post–HD dose	1.5 gm (IV)
Post–PD dose	None
CVVH dose	1.5 gm (IV) q12h
Moderate or severe hepatic insufficiency	No change

Drug Interactions: Probenecid (↑ ampicillin/sulbactam levels); allopurinol (↑ rash)
Adverse Effects: Drug fever/rash, ↑ SGOT/SGPT, C. difficile diarrhea/colitis
Allergic Potential: High
Safety in Pregnancy: B
Comments: For mild/moderate infection, 1.5 gm (IV) q6h may be used. Pseudoresistance with E. coli/Klebsiella (resistant in-vitro, not in-vivo). Na+ content = 4.2 mEq/g
Cerebrospinal Fluid Penetration: < 10%

REFERENCES:
Itokazu GS, Danziger LH. Ampicillin-sulbactam and ticarcillin-clavulanic acid: A comparison of their in vitro activity and review of their clinical efficacy. Pharmacotherapy 11:382-414, 1991.
Jain R, Danziger LH. Multidrug-resistant Acinetobacter infections: an emerging challenge to clinicians. Ann Pharmacother 38:1449-59, 2004.
Sensakovic JW, Smith LG. Beta-lactamase inhibitor combinations. Med Clin North Am 79:695-704, 1995.
Swenson JM, Killgore GE, Tenover FC. Antimicrobial susceptibility testing of Acinetobacter spp. by NCCLS broth microdilution and disk diffusion methods. J Clin Microbiol 42:5102-8, 2004.
Wood GC, Hanes SD, Croce MA, et al. Comparison of ampicillin-sulbactam and imipenem-cilastatin for the treatment of Acinetobacter ventilator-associated pneumonia. Clin Infect Dis 34:1425-30, 2002.
Wright AJ. The penicillins. Mayo Clin Proc 73:290-307,1999.
Website: www.pdr.net

Anidulafungin (Eraxis)

Drug Class: Echinocandin antifungal
Usual Dose: For invasive Candida or invasive Aspergillus 200 mg (IV) x 1 dose, then 100 mg (IV) q24h
Pharmacokinetic Parameters:
Peak serum level: 4.2 mg/L (100/50 mg dose)/7.2 mg/L (200/100 mg dose)
Bioavailability: Not applicable
Excreted unchanged (urine): < 10%
Serum half-life (normal/ESRD): 40-50 hours/40-50 hours
Plasma protein binding: 84%
Volume of distribution (V_d): 30-50L
Primary Mode of Elimination: Fecal (90% as metabolites)
Dosage Adjustments*

CrCl ≥ 50 mL/min	No change
CrCl ~ 30–49 mL/min	No change
CrCl ~ 15-29 mL/min	No change
CrCl < 15 mL/min	No change
Post–HD dose	No change
Post–PD dose	No change
CVVH dose	No change
Moderate or severe hepatic insufficiency	No change

Drug Interactions: No significant interactions

"Usual dose" assumes normal renal/hepatic function. * For renal insufficiency, give usual dose x 1 followed by maintenance dose per CrCl. For dialysis patients, dose the same as for CrCl < 10 mL/min and give supplemental (post-HD/PD dose) immediately after dialysis. CrCl = creatinine clearance; CVVH = continuous veno-venous hemo-filtration; HD/PD = hemodialysis/peritoneal dialysis. See pp. 275-278 for explanations, p. 1 for abbreviations

Adverse Effects: Diarrhea, dyspepsia, nausea, vomiting, ↑ AST/ALT/GGTP/alkaline phosphatase, hypokalemia, neutropenia, headache. Histamine-related reaction including rash, urticaria, pruritus, flushing, fever, dyspnea and hypotension when infusion > 1.1 mg/min
Allergic Potential: Histamine-related symptoms
Safety in Pregnancy: C
Comments: Not an inducer, inhibitor, or substrate of CYP450 system. Rate of infusion should not exceed 1.1 mg/min. Incompatible with other drugs. Use reconstituted vials within 24 hours. Good activity against Candida spp. (Including azole-resistant and amphotericin-resistant strains), Aspergillus spp., and Pneumocystis carinii. No activity against Cryptococcus neoformans, Fusarium spp., and Zygomycetes spp.
Cerebrospinal Fluid Penetration:

REFERENCES:
Eraxis [package insert], New York: Pfizer, Inc; 2006.
Morrison VA. Echinocandin antifungals: review and update. Expert Rev Anti Infect Ther 4:325-42, 2006.
Pfaller MA. Anidulafungin: an echinocandin antifungal. Expert Opin Investig Drugs 13:1183-97, 2005.
Raasch RH. Anidulafungin: review of a new echinocandin antifungal agent. Expert Rev Anti Infect Ther 2:499-508, 2004.
Theuretzbacher U. Pharmacokinetics/pharmacodynamics of echinocandins. Eur J Clin Microbiol Infect Dis 23:805-12, 2004.
Turner MS, Drew RH, Perfect JR. Emerging echinocandins for treatment of invasive fungal infections. Expert Opin Emerg Drugs 11:231-50, 2006.
Vazquez JA. Anidulafungin: a new echinocandin with a novel profile. Clin Ther 27:657-73, 2005.
Vazquez JA, Sobel JD. Anidulafungin: a novel echinocandin. Clin Infect Dis 43:215-22, 2006.
Wiederhold NP, Lewis RE. The echinocandin antifungals: an overview of the pharmacology, spectrum and clinical efficacy. Expert Opin Investig Drugs 12:1313-33, 2003.
Website: www.eraxisrx.com

Azithromycin (Zithromax)

Drug Class: Macrolide (Azolide)
Usual Dose: 500 mg (IV/PO) x 1 dose, then 250 mg (IV/PO) q24h
Pharmacokinetic Parameters:
Peak serum level: 1.1 (IV)/0.2 (PO) mcg/mL
Bioavailability: 35%
Excreted unchanged (urine): 6%
Serum half-life (normal/ESRD): 68/68 hrs
Plasma protein binding: 50%
Volume of distribution (V_d): 31 L/kg
Primary Mode of Elimination: Hepatic
Dosage Adjustments*

CrCl 10–80 mL/min	No change
CrCl < 10 mL/min	Use caution
Post–HD/PD dose	None
CVVH dose	None
Moderate or severe hepatic insufficiency	No change

Drug Interactions: Carbamazepine, cisapride, clozapine, corticosteroids, midazolam, triazolam, valproic acid (not studied/not reported); cyclosporine, digoxin (↑ interacting drug levels); pimozide (may ↑ QT interval, torsade de pointes)
Adverse Effects: Nausea, GI upset, diarrhea
Allergic Potential: Low
Safety in Pregnancy: B
Comments: May ↑ QT_c interval. Bioavailability is decreased by food. For MAI prophylaxis, use 1200 mg (PO) weekly. For MAI therapy, use 600 mg (PO) q24h
Cerebrospinal Fluid Penetration: < 10%
Bile/serum ratio: > 3000%

REFERENCES:
Alvarez-Elcoro S, Enzler MJ. The macrolides: Erythromycin, clarithromycin and azithromycin. Mayo Clin Proc 74:613-34, 1999.
Cunha BA. Macrolides, doxycycline, and fluoroquinolones in the treatment of Legionnaires' Disease. Antibiotics for Clinicians 2:117-8, 1998.
Ioannidis JP, Contopoulos-Ioannidis DG, Chew P, Lau J. Meta-analysis of randomized controlled trials on the comparative efficacy and safety of azithromycin

against other antibiotics for upper respiratory tract infections. J Antimicrob Chemother 48:677-89, 2001.

Jain R, Danzinger LH. The macrolide antibiotics: a pharmacokinetic and pharmacodynamic overview. Curr Pharm Des 10:3045-53, 2004.

Paradisi F, Corti G. Azithromycin. Antibiotics for Clinicians 3:1-8, 1999.

Phillips P, Chan K, Hogg R, et al. Azithromycin prophylaxis for Mycobacterium avium complex during the era of highly active antiretroviral therapy: evaluation of a provincial program. Clin Infect Dis 34:371-8, 2002.

Pichichero ME, Hoeger WJ, Casey JR. Azithromycin for the treatment of pertussis. Pediatr Infect Dis J. 22:847-9, 2003.

Plouffe JF, Breiman RF, Fields BS, et al. Azithromycin in the treatment of Legionella pneumonia requiring hospitalization. Clin Infect Dis. 37:1475-80, 2003.

Saiman L, Marshall BC, Mayer-Hamblett N, et al. Azithromycin in patients with cystic fibrosis chronically infected with Pseudomonas aeruginosa: a randomized controlled trial. JAMA. 290:1749-5, 2003..

Schlossberg D. Azithromycin and clarithromycin. Med Clin N Amer 79:803-816, 1995.

Southern KW, Barker PM. Azithromycin for cystic fibrosis. Eur Respir J 24:834-8, 2004.

Wolter J, Seeney S, Bell S, et al. Effect of long term treatment with azithromycin on disease parameters in cystic fibrosis: a randomised trial. Thorax 57:212-6, 2002.

Website: www.zithromax.com

Aztreonam (Azactam)

Drug Class: Monobactam
Usual Dose: 2 gm (IV) q8h (see comments)
Pharmacokinetic Parameters:
Peak serum level: 204 mcg/mL
Bioavailability: Not applicable
Excreted unchanged (urine): 60-70%
Serum half-life (normal/ESRD): 1.7/7 hrs
Plasma protein binding: 56%
Volume of distribution (V_d): 0.2 L/kg
Primary Mode of Elimination: Renal
Dosage Adjustments* (based on 2 gm IV q8h):

CrCl 50–80 mL/min	2 gm (IV) q8h
CrCl 10–50 mL/min	1 gm (IV) q8h
CrCl < 10 mL/min	500 mg (IV) q8h
Post–HD dose	250 mg (IV)
Post–PD dose	500 mg (IV)
CVVH dose	1 gm (IV) q8h
Moderate hepatic insufficiency	No change
Severe hepatic insufficiency	No change

Drug Interactions: None
Adverse Effects: None
Allergic Potential: Low
Safety in Pregnancy: B
Comments: Incompatible in solutions containing vancomycin or metronidazole. No cross allergenicity with penicillins, β–lactams; safe to use in penicillin allergic patients. CAPD dose: 1 gm (I.P.), then 250 mg/L of dialysate (I.P.) with each exchange.
Meningeal dose = 2 gm (IV) q6h
Cerebrospinal Fluid Penetration:
Non-inflamed meninges = 1%
Inflamed meninges = 40%
Bile Penetration: 300%

REFERENCES:
Brogden RN, Heal RC. Aztreonam: A review of its antibacterial activity, pharmacokinetic properties, and therapeutic use. Drugs 31:96-130, 1986.

Critchley IA, Sahm DF, Kelly LJ, et al. In vitro synergy studies using aztreonam and fluoroquinolone combinations against six species of Gram-negative bacilli. Chemotherapy. 49:44-8, 2003.

Cunha BA. Aztreonam: A review. Urology 41:249-58, 1993.

Cunha BA. Cross allergenicity of penicillin with carbapenems and monobactams. J Crit Illness 13:344, 1998.

Hellinger WC, Brewer NS. Carbapenems and monobactams: Imipenem, meropenem, and aztreonam. Mayo Clin Proc 74:420-34, 1999.

Johnson, Cunha BA. Aztreonam. Med Clin North Am 79:733-43, 1995.

Pendland SL, Messick CR, Jung R. In vitro synergy testing of levofloxacin, ofloxacin, and ciprofloxacin in combination with aztreonam, ceftazidime, or piperacillin against Pseudomonas aeruginosa. Diagn Microbiol Infect Dis 42:75-8, 2002.

Sader HS, Huynh HK, Jones RN. Contemporary in vitro synergy rates for aztreonam combined with newer

fluoroquinolones and beta-lactams tested against gram-negative bacilli. Diagn Microbiol Infect Dis 47(3): 547-50, 2003.
Website: www.elan.com/Products/

Iseman MD. Treatment of multidrug resistant tuberculosis. N Engl J Med 329:784-91, 1993.
Website: www.pdr.net

Capreomycin (Capastat)

Drug Class: Anti–TB drug
Usual Dose: 1 gm (IM) q24h
Pharmacokinetic Parameters:
Peak serum level: 30 mcg/mL
Bioavailability: Not applicable
Excreted unchanged (urine): 50%
Serum half-life (normal/ESRD): 5/30 hrs
Plasma protein binding: No data
Volume of distribution (V_d): 0.4 L/kg
Primary Mode of Elimination: Renal
Dosage Adjustments*

CrCl 50–80 mL/min	500 mg (IM) q24h
CrCl 10–50 mL/min	500 mg (IM) q48h
CrCl < 10 mL/min	500 mg (IM) q72h
Post–HD dose	500 mg (IM)
Post–PD dose	None
CVVH dose	500 mg (IM) q48h
Moderate hepatic insufficiency	No change
Severe hepatic insufficiency	No change

Drug Interactions: None
Adverse Effects: Eosinophilia, leukopenia, drug fever/rash, ototoxicity (vestibular), nephrotoxicity (glomerular/tubular)
Allergic Potential: Moderate
Safety in Pregnancy: C
Comments: Pain/phlebitis at IM injection site. Additive toxicity with aminoglycosides/viomycin
Cerebrospinal Fluid Penetration: < 10%

REFERENCES:
Davidson PT, Le HQ. Drug treatment of tuberculosis - 1992. Drugs 43:651-73, 1992.
Drugs for tuberculosis. Med Lett Drugs Ther 35:99-101, 1993.

Caspofungin (Cancidas)

Drug Class: Echinocandin antifungal
Usual Dose: 70 mg (IV) x 1 dose, then 50 mg (IV) q24h (see comments)
Pharmacokinetic Parameters:
Peak serum level:
70 mg: 12.1/14.83 mcg/mL (multiple dose)
50 mg: 7.6/8.7 mcg/mL (multiple dose)
Bioavailability: Not applicable
Excreted unchanged (urine): 1.4%
Serum half-life (normal/ESRD): 10/10 hrs
Plasma protein binding: 97%
Volume of distribution (V_d): No data
Primary Mode of Elimination: Hepatic
Dosage Adjustments*

CrCl 50-80 mL/min	No change
CrCl 10-50 mL/min	No change
CrCl < 10 mL/min	No change
Post–HD/PD dose	None
CVVH dose	None
Moderate hepatic insufficiency	35 mg (IV) q24h (maintenance dose)
Severe hepatic insufficiency	No information

Drug Interactions: Carbamazepine, rifampin, dexamethasone, efavirenz, nelfinavir, nevirapine, phenytoin (↓ caspofungin levels; ↑ caspofungin maintenance dose to 70 mg/day); cyclosporine (↑ caspofungin levels, ↑ SGOT/SGPT; co-administration is discouraged unless careful monitoring can be ensured and unless the benefit of caspofungin outweighs the risk of hepatotoxicity); tacrolimus (↓ tacrolimus levels, ↑ SGOT/SGPT)
Adverse Effects: Drug fever/rash
Allergic Potential: Low
Safety in Pregnancy: C

"Usual dose" assumes normal renal/hepatic function. * For renal insufficiency, give usual dose x 1 followed by maintenance dose per CrCl. For dialysis patients, dose the same as for CrCl < 10 mL/min and give supplemental (post-HD/PD dose) immediately after dialysis. CrCl = creatinine clearance; CVVH = continuous veno-venous hemo-filtration; HD/PD = hemodialysis/peritoneal dialysis. See pp. 275-278 for explanations, p. 1 for abbreviations

Comments: Administer by slow IV infusion over 1 hour; do not give IV bolus. Do not mix/co-infuse with glucose solutions. If co-administered with drugs that ↓ caspofungin levels or for highly-resistant organisms, then 70 mg (IV) q24h dosing may be used. For esophageal candidiasis, therapy is initiated with 50 mg (70 mg loading dose has not been studied)
Cerebrospinal Fluid Penetration: No data

REFERENCES:
Arathoon EG, Gotuzzo E, Noriega LM, et al. Randomized, double-blind, multicenter study of caspofungin versus amphotericin B for treatment of oropharyngeal and esophageal candidiasis. Antimicrob Agents Chemother 46:451-7, 2002.
Bachmann SP, VandeWalle K, Ramage G, et al. In vitro activity of caspofungin against Candida albicans biofilms. Antimicrob Agents Chemother 46:3591-3596, 2002.
Barchiesi F, Schimizzi AM, Fothergill AW, et al. In vitro activity of the new echinocandin antifungal against common and uncommon clinical isolates of Candida species. Eur J Clin Microbiol Infect Dis 18:302-4, 1999.
Deresinski SC, Stevens DA. Caspofungin. Clin Infect Dis 36:1445-57, 2003.
Gallagher JC, MacDougall C, Ashley ES, et al. Recent advances in antifungal pharmacotherapy for invasive fungal infections. Expert Rev Anti Infect Ther 2:253-68, 2004.
Grau S, Mateu-De Antonio J. Caspofungin acetate for treatment of invasive fungal infections. Ann Pharmacother. 37:1919, 2003.
Keating G, Figgitt D. Caspofungin: a review of its use in esophageal candidiasis, invasive candidiasis and invasive aspergillosis. Drugs 63:2235-63, 2003.
Lomaestro BM. Caspofungin. Hospital Formulary 36:527-36, 2001.
Maertens J, Raad I, Petrikkos G, et al. Efficacy and safety of caspofungin for treatment of invasive aspergillosis in patients refractory to or intolerant of conventional antifungal therapy. Clin Infect Dis. 39:1563-71, 2004.
Mora-Duarte J, Betts R, Rotstein C, et al. Comparison of caspofungin and amphotericin B for invasive candidiasis. N Engl J Med 347:2020-9, 2002.
Nevado J, De Alarcon A, Hernandez A. Caspofungin: a new therapeutic option for fungal endocarditis. Clin Microbiol Infect. 11:248, 2005.
Pacetti SA, Gelone SP. Caspofungin acetate for treatment of invasive fungal infections. Ann Pharmacother 37:90-8, 2003.
Pfaller MA, Messer SA, Boyken L, et al. Caspofungin activity against clinical isolates of fluconazole-resistant Candida. J Clin Microbiol 2003;41:5729-31.
Rubin MA, Carroll KC, Cahill BC. Caspofungin in combination with itraconazole for the treatment of invasive aspergillosis in humans. Clin Infect Dis 34:1160-1, 2002.
Stone EA, Fung HB, Hirschenbaum HL. Caspofungin: an echinocandin antifungal agent. Clin Ther 24:351-77, 2002.
Walsh TJ, Adamson PC, Seibel NL, et al. Pharmacokinetics, safety, and tolerability of caspofungin in children and adolescents. Antimicrobial Agents and Chemotherapy 49:4536-45, 2005.
Walsh TJ, Teppler H, Donowitz GR, et al. Caspofungin versus liposomal amphotericin B for empirical antifungal therapy in patients with persistent fever and neutropenia. N Engl J Med. 351:1391-402, 2004.
Website: www.cancidas.com

Cefadroxil (Duricef, Ultracef)

Drug Class: 1st generation oral cephalosporin
Usual Dose: 1000 mg (PO) q12h
Pharmacokinetic Parameters:
Peak serum level: 16 mcg/mL
Bioavailability: 99%
Excreted unchanged (urine): 85%
Serum half-life (normal/ESRD): 0.5/22 hrs
Plasma protein binding: 20%
Volume of distribution (V_d): 0.31 L/kg
Primary Mode of Elimination: Renal
Dosage Adjustments*

CrCl 50-80 mL/min	500 mg (PO) q12h
CrCl 10–50 mL/min	500 mg (PO) q24h
CrCl < 10 mL/min	500 mg (PO) q36h
Post–HD dose	500 mg (PO)
Post–PD dose	250 mg (PO)
CVVH dose	500 mg (PO) q24h
Moderate hepatic insufficiency	No change
Severe hepatic insufficiency	No change

Drug Interactions: None
Adverse Effects: Drug fever/rash

"Usual dose" assumes normal renal/hepatic function. * For renal insufficiency, give usual dose x 1 followed by maintenance dose per CrCl. For dialysis patients, dose the same as for CrCl < 10 mL/min and give supplemental (post-HD/PD dose) immediately after dialysis. CrCl = creatinine clearance; CVVH = continuous veno-venous hemofiltration; HD/PD = hemodialysis/peritoneal dialysis. See pp. 275-278 for explanations, p. 1 for abbreviations

Allergic Potential: High
Safety in Pregnancy: B
Comments: Penetrates oral/respiratory secretions well
Cerebrospinal Fluid Penetration: < 10%
Bile Penetration: 20%

REFERENCES:
Bucko AD, Hunt BJ, Kidd SL, et al. Randomized, double-blind, multicenter comparison of oral cefditoren 200 or 400 mg BID with either cefuroxime 250 mg BID or cefadroxil 500 mg BID for the treatment of uncomplicated skin and skin-structure infections. Clin Ther 24:1134-47, 2002.
Cunha BA. Antibiotics selection for the treatment of sinusitis, otitis media, and pharyngitis. Infect Dis Pract 7:S324-S326, 1998.
Gustaferro CA, Steckelberg JM. Cephalosporins: Antimicrobic agents and related compounds. Mayo Clin Proc 66:1064-73, 1991.
Smith GH. Oral cephalosporins in perspective. IDCP 24:45-51, 1990.
Website: www.pdr.net

Cefamandole (Mandol)

Drug Class: 2nd generation cephalosporin
Usual Dose: 2 gm (IV) q6h
Pharmacokinetic Parameters:
Peak serum level: 240 mcg/mL
Bioavailability: Not applicable
Excreted unchanged (urine): 85%
Serum half-life (normal/ESRD): 1/11 hrs
Plasma protein binding: 76%
Volume of distribution (V_d): 0.29 L/kg
Primary Mode of Elimination: Renal
Dosage Adjustments* (based on 2 gm q6h):

CrCl 50-80 mL/min	1 gm (IV) q6h
CrCl 10–50 mL/min	1 gm (IV) q6h
CrCl < 10 mL/min	1 gm (IV) q12h
Post–HD dose	1 gm (IV)
Post–PD dose	1 gm (IV)
CVVH dose	1 gm (IV) q6h
Moderate or severe hepatic insufficiency	No change

Drug Interactions: Alcohol (disulfiram-like reaction); antiplatelet agents, heparin, thrombolytics, warfarin (↑ risk of bleeding)
Adverse Effects: Drug fever/rash, ↑ INR
Allergic Potential: High
Safety in Pregnancy: B
Comments: Incompatible in solutions with Mg++ or Ca++. Contains MTT side chain, but no increase in clinical bleeding. Na+ content = 3.3 mEq/g
Cerebrospinal Fluid Penetration: < 10%
Bile Penetration: 300%

REFERENCES:
Cunha BA, Klimek JJ, Qunitiliani R. Cefamandole nafate in respiratory and urinary tract infections. Curr Ther Res 25:584-9, 1971.
Gentry LO, Zeluff BJ, Cooley DA. Antibiotic prophylaxis in open-heart surgery: A comparison of cefamandole, cefuroxime, and cefazolin. Ann Thorac Surg 46:167-71, 1988.
Peterson CD, Lake KD, Arom KV. Antibiotic prophylaxis in open-heart surgery patients: Comparison of cefamandole and cefuroxime. Drug Intell Clin Pharmacol 21:728-32, 1987.

Cefdinir (Omnicef)

Drug Class: 3rd generation oral cephalosporin
Usual Dose: 600 mg (PO) q24h
Pharmacokinetic Parameters:
Peak serum level: 2.9 mcg/mL
Bioavailability: 16% (tab) / 25% (suspension)
Excreted unchanged (urine): 11-18%
Serum half-life (normal/ESRD): 1.7/3 hrs
Plasma protein binding: 70%
Volume of distribution (V_d): 0.35 L/kg
Primary Mode of Elimination: Renal
Dosage Adjustments*

CrCl > 30 mL/min	No change
CrCl < 30 mL/min	300 mg (PO) q24h
Post–HD dose	300 mg (PO)
Post–PD dose	None
CVVH dose	600 mg (PO) q24h

"Usual dose" assumes normal renal/hepatic function. * For renal insufficiency, give usual dose x 1 followed by maintenance dose per CrCl. For dialysis patients, dose the same as for CrCl < 10 mL/min and give supplemental (post-HD/PD dose) immediately after dialysis. CrCl = creatinine clearance; CVVH = continuous veno-venous hemofiltration; HD/PD = hemodialysis/peritoneal dialysis. See pp. 275-278 for explanations, p. 1 for abbreviations

Moderate or severe hepatic insufficiency	No change

Drug Interactions: Probenecid (↑ cefdinir levels)
Adverse Effects: Drug fever/rash
Allergic Potential: High
Safety in Pregnancy: B
Comments: Good activity against bacterial respiratory pathogens. Available as capsules or suspension. Treat community-acquired pneumonia with 300 mg (PO) q12h; for other respiratory infections, use 600 mg (PO) q24h
Cerebrospinal Fluid Penetration: No data

REFERENCES:
Cefdinir: A new oral cephalosporin. Med Lett Drugs Therap 40:85-7, 1998.
Fogarty CM, Bettis RB, Griffin TJ, et al. Comparison of a 5 day regimen of cefdinir with a 10 day regimen of cefprozil for treatment of acute exacerbations of chronic bronchitis. J Antimicrob Chemother 45:851-8, 2000.
Guay DR. Cefdinir: an advanced-generation, broad-spectrum oral cephalosporin. Clin Ther 24:473-89, 2002.
Nemeth MA, Gooche WM 3rd, Hedrick J, et al. Comparison of cefdinir and penicillin for the treatment of pediatric streptococcal pharyngitis. Clin Ther 21:1525-32, 1999.
Perry CM, Scott LJ. Cefdinir: a review of its use in the management of mild-to-moderate bacterial infections. Drugs 64:1433-64, 2004.
Website: www.omnicef.com

Cefditoren (Spectracef)

Drug Class: 3rd generation oral cephalosporin
Usual Dose: 400 mg (PO) q12h
Pharmacokinetic Parameters:
Peak serum level: 1.8 mcg/mL
Bioavailability: 16%
Excreted unchanged (urine): 20%
Serum half-life (normal/ESRD): 1.5/5 hrs
Plasma protein binding: 88%
Volume of distribution (V_d): 0.13 L/kg
Primary Mode of Elimination: Renal

Dosage Adjustments*

CrCl 50–80 mL/min	No change
CrCl 30-50 mL/min	200 mg (PO) q12h
CrCl < 30 mL/min	200 mg (PO) q24h
Post–HD dose	200 mg (PO)
Post–PD dose	No information
CVVH dose	No information
Moderate or severe hepatic insufficiency	No change

Drug Interactions: H₂ receptor antagonists, Al⁺⁺, Mg⁺⁺ antacids (↓ absorption of cefditoren); Probenecid (↓ elimination of cefditoren)
Adverse Effects: Drug fever/rash
Allergic Potential: Low
Safety in Pregnancy: B
Comments: Serum concentrations increased ~ 50% if taken without food. ↑ elimination of carnitine; do not use in carnitine deficiency or hereditary carnitine metabolism disorder. Contains Na⁺ caseinate; avoid in patients with protein hypersensitivity
Cerebrospinal Fluid Penetration: No data

REFERENCES:
Balbisi EA. Cefditoren, a new aminothiazolyl cephalosporin. Pharmacotherapy 22:1278-93, 2002.
Chow J, Russel M, Bolk S. et al. Efficacy of cefditoren pivoxil vs. amoxicillin-clavulanic in acute maxillary sinusitis. Presented at the 40th Interscience Conference on Antimicrobial Agents and Chemotherapy; Abstract 835, Toronto, ON 2000.
Clark CL, Nagai K, Dewasse BE, et al. Activity of cefditoren against respiratory pathogens. J Antimicrob Chemother 50:33-41, 2002.
Darkes MJ, Plosker GL. Cefditoren pivoxil. Drugs 62:319-36, 2002.
Guay DR. Review of cefditoren, an advanced-generation, broad-spectrum oral cephalosporin. Clin Ther 23:1924-37, 2002.
Wellington K, Curran MP. Cefditoren pivoxil: a review of its use in the treatment of bacterial infections. Drugs 64:2597-618, 2004.
Website: www.pdr.net

Cefepime (Maxipime)

Drug Class: 4th generation cephalosporin
Usual Dose: 2 gm (IV) q12h (see comments)
Pharmacokinetic Parameters:
Peak serum level: 163 mcg/mL
Bioavailability: Not applicable
Excreted unchanged (urine): 80%
Serum half-life (normal/ESRD): 2.2/18 hrs
Plasma protein binding: 20%
Volume of distribution (V_d): 0.29 L/kg
Primary Mode of Elimination: Renal
Dosage Adjustments* (based on 2 gm q12h):

CrCl 50–80 mL/min	2 gm (IV) q24h
CrCl 10–50 mL/min	2 gm (IV) q48h
CrCl < 10 mL/min	500 mg (IV) q24h
Post-HD dose:	2 gm (IV)
Post-PD dose:	1 gm (IV)
CAPD	2 gm (IV) q48h
CVVH dose	1 gm (IV) q24h
Moderate or severe hepatic insufficiency	No change

Drug Interactions: None
Adverse Effects: Drug fever/rash
Allergic Potential: Moderate
Safety in Pregnancy: B
Comments: For proven serious systemic P. aeruginosa infections, febrile neutropenia, or cystic fibrosis, use 2 gm (IV) q8h. Effective against most strains of ceftazidime-resistant P. aeruginosa. Meningeal dose: 2 gm (IV) q8h
Cerebrospinal Fluid Penetration:
Non-inflamed meninges = 1%
Inflamed meninges = 15%
Bile Penetration: 10%

REFERENCES:
Ambrose PF, Owens RC Jr, Garvey MJ, et al. Pharmacodynamic considerations in the treatment of moderate to severe pseudomonal infections with cefepime. J Antimicrob Chemother 49:445-53, 2002.
Badaro R, Molinar F, Seas C, et al. A multicenter comparative study of cefepime versus broad-spectrum antibacterial therapy in moderate and severe bacterial infections. Braz J Infect Dis 6:206-18, 2002.
Boselli E, Breilh D, Duflo F, et al. Steady-state plasma and intrapulmonary concentrations of cefepime administered in continuous infusion in critically ill patients with severe nosocomial pneumonia. Crit Care Med 31: 2102-6, 2003.
Chapman TM, Perry CM. Cefepime: a review of its use in the management of hospitalized patients with pneumonia. Am J Respir Med 2: 75-107, 2003.
Cunha BA, Gill MV. Cefepime. Med Clin North Am 79:721-32, 1995.
Cunha BA. Pseudomonas aeruginosa: Resistance and therapy. Semin Respir Infect 17:231-9, 2002.
Fritsche TR, Sader HS, Jones RN. Comparative activity and spectrum of broad-spectrum beta-lactams (cefepime, ceftazidime, ceftriaxone, piperacillin/tazobactam) tested against 12,295 staphylococci and streptococci: report from the SENTRY antimicrobial surveillance program (North America: 2001-2002). Diagn Microbiol Infect Dis 47: 435-40, 2003.
Paradisi F, Corti G, Strohmeyer M. Cefepime. Antibiotics for Clinicians 3:41-50, 1999.
Tam VH, McKinnon PS, Akins RL, et al. Pharmacodynamics of cefepime in patients with gram-negative infections. J Antimicrob Chemother 50:425-8, 2002.
Tam VH, McKinnon PS, Akins RL, et al. Pharmacokinetics and pharmacodynamics of cefepime in patients with various degrees of renal function. Antimicrob Agents Chemother 47: 1853-61, 2003.
Toltzis P, Dul M, O'Riordan MA, et al. Cefepime use in a pediatric intensive care unit reduces colonization with resistant bacilli. Pediatr Infect Dis J. 22:109-14, 2003.
Website: www.elan.com/Products/

Cefixime (Suprax)

Drug Class: 3rd generation oral cephalosporin
Usual Dose: 400 mg (PO) q12h or 200 mg (PO) q12h
Pharmacokinetic Parameters:
Peak serum level: 3.7 mcg/mL
Bioavailability: 50%
Excreted unchanged (urine): 50%
Serum half-life (normal/ESRD): 3.1/11 hrs
Plasma protein binding: 65%
Volume of distribution (V_d): 0.1 L/kg
Primary Mode of Elimination: Renal

"Usual dose" assumes normal renal/hepatic function. * For renal insufficiency, give usual dose x 1 followed by maintenance dose per CrCl. For dialysis patients, dose the same as for CrCl < 10 mL/min and give supplemental (post-HD/PD dose) immediately after dialysis. CrCl = creatinine clearance; CVVH = continuous veno-venous hemo-filtration; HD/PD = hemodialysis/peritoneal dialysis. See pp. 275-278 for explanations, p. 1 for abbreviations

Dosage Adjustments*

CrCl 10–50 mL/min	300 mg (PO) q24h
CrCl < 10 mL/min	200 mg (PO) q24h
Post–HD dose	300 mg (PO)
Post–PD dose	200 mg (PO)
CVVH dose	200 mg (PO) q12h
Moderate hepatic insufficiency	No change
Severe hepatic insufficiency	No change

Drug Interactions: Carbamazepine (↑ carbamazepine levels)
Adverse Effects: Drug fever/rash, diarrhea
Allergic Potential: High
Safety in Pregnancy: B
Comments: PPNG dose: 400 mg (PO) x 1 dose. Little/no activity against S. aureus (MSSA)
Cerebrospinal Fluid Penetration: < 10%
Bile Penetration: 800%

REFERENCES:
Markham A, Brogden RN. Cefixime: A review of its therapeutic efficacy in lower respiratory tract infections. Drugs 49:1007-22, 1995.
Marshall WF, Blair JE. The cephalosporins. Mayo Clin Proc 74:187-95, 1999.
Quintiliani R. Cefixime in the treatment of patients with lower respiratory tract infections: Results of US clinical trials. Clinical Therapeutics 18:373-90, 1996.
Website: www.pdr.net

Cefoperazone (Cefobid)

Drug Class: 3rd generation cephalosporin
Usual Dose: 2 gm (IV) q12h
Pharmacokinetic Parameters:
Peak serum level: 240 mcg/mL
Bioavailability: Not applicable
Excreted unchanged (urine): 20%
Serum half-life (normal/ESRD): 2.4/2.4 hrs
Plasma protein binding: 90%
Volume of distribution (V_d): 0.17 L/kg
Primary Mode of Elimination: Hepatic

Dosage Adjustments*

CrCl 50–80 mL/min	No change
CrCl 10–50 mL/min	No change
CrCl < 10 mL/min	No change
Post–HD dose	None
Post–PD dose	None
CVVH dose	None
Moderate hepatic insufficiency	No change
Severe hepatic insufficiency	1 gm (IV) q12h

Drug Interactions: Alcohol (disulfiram-like reaction); antiplatelet agents, heparin, thrombolytics, warfarin (↑ risk of bleeding)
Adverse Effects: Drug fever/rash. ↑ INR due to MTT side chain, but no increase in clinical bleeding. Prophylactic vitamin K unnecessary
Allergic Potential: Low
Safety in Pregnancy: B
Comments: One of the few antibiotics to penetrate into an obstructed biliary tract. May be administered IM. Concentration dependent serum half life = 1.5 mEq/g. Na^+ content = 1.5 mEq/g. Meningeal dose = 2 gm (IV) q8h
Cerebrospinal Fluid Penetration:
Non-inflamed meninges = 1%
Inflamed meninges = 10%
Bile Penetration: 1200%

REFERENCES:
Cunha BA: 3rd generation cephalosporins: A review. Clin Ther 14:616-52, 1992.
Klein NC, Cunha BA. Third-generation cephalosporins. Med Clin North Am 79:705-19, 1995.
Marshall WF, Blair JE. The cephalosporins. Mayo Clin Proc 74:187-95, 1999.
Oie S, Uematsu T, Sawa A, et al. In vitro effects of combinations of antipseudomonal agents against seven strains of multidrug-resistant Pseudomonas aeruginosa. J Antimicrob Chemother 52:911-4, 2004.
Website: www.pdr.net

"Usual dose" assumes normal renal/hepatic function. * For renal insufficiency, give usual dose x 1 followed by maintenance dose per CrCl. For dialysis patients, dose the same as for CrCl < 10 mL/min and give supplemental (post-HD/PD dose) immediately after dialysis. CrCl = creatinine clearance; CVVH = continuous veno-venous hemo-filtration; HD/PD = hemodialysis/peritoneal dialysis. See pp. 275-278 for explanations, p. 1 for abbreviations

Cefotaxime (Claforan)

Drug Class: 3rd generation cephalosporin
Usual Dose: 2 gm (IV) q6h
Pharmacokinetic Parameters:
Peak serum level: 214 mcg/mL
Bioavailability: Not applicable
Excreted unchanged (urine): 20-36%; 15-25%
excreted as active metabolite
Serum half-life (normal/ESRD): 1/15 hrs
Plasma protein binding: 37%
Volume of distribution (V_d): 0.25 L/kg
Primary Mode of Elimination: Renal
Dosage Adjustments*

CrCl 50–80 mL/min	No change
CrCl 10–50 mL/min	1 gm (IV) q6h
CrCl < 10 mL/min	1 gm (IV) q12h
Post–HD dose	1 gm (IV)
Post–PD dose	1 gm (IV)
CVVH dose	2 gm (IV) q8h
Moderate hepatic insufficiency	No change
Severe hepatic insufficiency	No change

Drug Interactions: None
Adverse Effects: Drug fever/rash
Allergic Potential: Moderate
Safety in Pregnancy: B
Comments: Incompatible in solutions
containing sodium bicarbonate, metronidazole,
or aminoglycosides. Desacetyl metabolite (t_{1/2} =
1.5 hrs) synergistic with cefotaxime against
S. aureus/B. fragilis. Na+ content = 2.2 mEq/g.
Meningeal dose = 3 gm (IV) q6h
Cerebrospinal Fluid Penetration:
Non-inflamed meninges = 1%
Inflamed meninges = 10%
Bile Penetration: 75%

REFERENCES:
Brogden RN, Spencer CM. Cefotaxime: A reappraisal
    of its antibacterial activity and pharmacokinetic
properties and a review of its therapeutic efficacy
    when administered twice daily for the treatment of
    mild to moderate infections. Drugs 53:483-510,
    1987.
Klein NC, Cunha BA. Third-generation cephalosporins.
    Med Clin North Am 79:705-19, 1995.
Marshall WF, Blair JE. The cephalosporins. Mayo Clin
    Proc 74:187-95, 1999.
Patel KB, Nicolau DP, Nightingale CH, et al.
    Comparative serum bactericidal activities of
    ceftizoxime and cefotaxime against intermediately
    penicillin-resistant Streptococcus pneumoniae.
    Antimicrob Agents Chemother 40:2805-8, 1996.
Website: www.pdr.net

Cefprozil (Cefzil)

Drug Class: 2nd generation oral cephalosporin
Usual Dose: 500 mg (PO) q12h
Pharmacokinetic Parameters:
Peak serum level: 10 mcg/mL
Bioavailability: 95%
Excreted unchanged (urine): 60%
Serum half-life (normal/ESRD): 1.3/5.9 hrs
Plasma protein binding: 36%
Volume of distribution (V_d): 0.23 L/kg
Primary Mode of Elimination: Renal
Dosage Adjustments*

CrCl 50–80 mL/min	No change
CrCl 10–50 mL/min	250 mg (PO) q12h
CrCl < 10 mL/min	250 mg (PO) q12h
Post–HD dose	500 mg (PO)
Post–PD dose	250 mg (PO)
CVVH dose	500 mg (PO) q24h
Moderate hepatic insufficiency	No change
Severe hepatic insufficiency	No change

Drug Interactions: None
Adverse Effects: Drug fever/rash
Allergic Potential: Low
Safety in Pregnancy: B
Comments: Penetrates oral/respiratory
secretions well

"Usual dose" assumes normal renal/hepatic function. * For renal insufficiency, give usual dose x 1 followed by
maintenance dose per CrCl. For dialysis patients, dose the same as for CrCl < 10 mL/min and give supplemental
(post-HD/PD dose) immediately after dialysis. CrCl = creatinine clearance; CVVH = continuous veno-venous hemo-
filtration; HD/PD = hemodialysis/peritoneal dialysis. See pp. 275-278 for explanations, p. 1 for abbreviations

Cerebrospinal Fluid Penetration: < 10%

REFERENCES:
Cunha BA. New antibiotics for the treatment of acute exacerbations of chronic bronchitis. Adv Ther 13:313-23, 1996.
Gainer RB 2nd. Cefprozil: A new cephalosporin; its use in various clinical trials. South Med J 88:338-46, 1995.
Marshall WF Blair JE. The cephalosporins. Mayo Clin Proc 74:187-95, 1999.
Schatz BS, Karavokiros KT, Taeubel MA, et al. Comparison of cefprozil, cefpodoxime, proxetil, loracarbef, cefixime, and ceftibuten. Ann Pharmacother 30:258-68, 1996.
Website: www.pdr.net

Ceftazidime (Fortaz, Tazicef, Tazidime)

Drug Class: 3rd generation cephalosporin
Usual Dose: 2 gm (IV) q8h (see comments)
Pharmacokinetic Parameters:
Peak serum level: 170 mcg/mL
Bioavailability: Not applicable
Excreted unchanged (urine): 80-90%
Serum half-life (normal/ESRD): 1.9/21 hrs
Plasma protein binding: 10%
Volume of distribution (V_d): 0.36 L/kg
Primary Mode of Elimination: Renal
Dosage Adjustments*

CrCl 50–80 mL/min	1 gm (IV) q12h
CrCl 10–50 mL/min	1 gm (IV) q24h
CrCl < 10 mL/min	500 mg (IV) q24h
Post–HD dose	1 gm (IV)
Post–PD dose	500 mg (IV)
CVVH dose	1 gm (IV) q12h
Moderate hepatic insufficiency	No change
Severe hepatic insufficiency	No change

Drug Interactions: None
Adverse Effects: Phlebitis, Drug fever/rash
Allergic Potential: High

Safety in Pregnancy: B
Comments: Incompatible in solutions containing vancomycin or aminoglycosides. Use increases prevalence of MRSA. Inducer of E. coli/Klebsiella ESBLs. Na+ content = 2.3 mEq/g. CAPD dose: 125 mg/L of dialysate (I.P.) with each exchange. Meningeal dose = 2 gm (IV) q8h
Cerebrospinal Fluid Penetration:
Non-inflamed meninges = 1%
Inflamed meninges = 20%
Bile Penetration: 50%

REFERENCES:
Berkhout J, Visser LG, van den Broek PJ, et al. Clinical pharmacokinetics of cefamandole and ceftazidime administered by continuous intravenous infusion. Antimicrob Agents Chemother. 47:1862-6, 2003.
Briscoe-Dwyer L. Ceftazidime. Antibiotics for Clinicians 1:41-8, 1997.
Klein NC, Cunha BA. Third-generation cephalosporins. Med Clin North Am 79:705-19, 1995.
Marshall WF, Blair JE. The cephalosporins. Mayo Clin Proc 74:187-95, 1999.
Nicolau DP, Nightingale CH, Banevicius MA, et al. Serum bactericidal activity of ceftazidime: Continuous infusion versus intermittent injections. Antimicrob Agents Chemother 40:61-4, 1996.
Owens JC, Jr, Ambrose PG, Quintiliani R. Ceftazidime to cefepime formulary switch: Pharmacodynamic rationale. Conn Med 61:225-7, 1997.
Rains CP, Bryson HM, Peters DH. Ceftazidime: An update of its antibacterial activity, pharmacokinetic properties, and therapeutic efficacy. Drugs 49:577-617, 1995.
Website: www.pdr.net

Ceftizoxime (Cefizox)

Drug Class: 3rd generation cephalosporin
Usual Dose: 2 gm (IV) q8h (see comments)
Pharmacokinetic Parameters:
Peak serum level: 132 mcg/mL
Bioavailability: Not applicable
Excreted unchanged (urine): 90%
Serum half-life (normal/ESRD): 1.7/35 hrs
Plasma protein binding: 30%
Volume of distribution (V_d): 0.32 L/kg
Primary Mode of Elimination: Renal
Dosage Adjustments*

CrCl 50–80 mL/min	1 gm (IV) q8h

"Usual dose" assumes normal renal/hepatic function. * For renal insufficiency, give usual dose x 1 followed by maintenance dose per CrCl. For dialysis patients, dose the same as for CrCl < 10 mL/min and give supplemental (post-HD/PD dose) immediately after dialysis. CrCl = creatinine clearance; CVVH = continuous veno-venous hemofiltration; HD/PD = hemodialysis/peritoneal dialysis. See pp. 275-278 for explanations, p. 1 for abbreviations

CrCl 10–50 mL/min	1 gm (IV) q12h
CrCl < 10 mL/min	1 gm (IV) q24h
Post–HD dose	1 gm (IV)
Post–PD dose	1 gm (IV)
CVVH dose	1 gm (IV) q12h
Moderate hepatic insufficiency	No change
Severe hepatic insufficiency	No change

Drug Interactions: None
Adverse Effects: Drug fever/rash
Allergic Potential: High
Safety in Pregnancy: B
Comments: Na^+ content = 2.6 mEq/g. PPNG dose: 500 mg (IM) x 1 dose. Meningeal dose = 3 gm (IV) q6h
Cerebrospinal Fluid Penetration:
Non-inflamed meninges = 1%
Inflamed meninges = 10%
Bile Penetration: 50%

REFERENCES:
Klein NC, Cunha BA. Third-generation cephalosporins. Med Clin North Am 79:705-19, 1995.
Donowitz GR, Mandell GL. Beta-lactam antibiotics. N Engl J Med 318:419-26 and 318:490-500, 1993.
Marshall WF Blair JE. The cephalosporins. Mayo Clin Proc 74:187-95, 1999.
Website: www.pdr.net

Ceftriaxone (Rocephin)

Drug Class: 3rd generation cephalosporin
Usual Dose: 1-2 gm (IV) q24h (see comments)
Pharmacokinetic Parameters:
Peak serum level: 151-257 mcg/mL
Bioavailability: Not applicable
Excreted unchanged (urine/feces): 33-67%
Serum half-life (normal/ESRD): 8/16 hrs
Plasma protein binding: 90%
Volume of distribution (V_d): 0.08-0.3 L/kg
Primary Mode of Elimination: Renal/hepatic

Dosage Adjustments*

CrCl 50–80 mL/min	No change
CrCl 10–50 mL/min	No change
CrCl < 10 mL/min	No change
Post–HD dose	None
Post–PD dose	None
CVVH dose	No change
Moderate hepatic insufficiency	No change
Severe hepatic insufficiency	No change (max dose: 2 gm/d)

Drug Interactions: None
Adverse Effects: Drug fever/rash, irritative diarrhea, pseudo-biliary lithiasis, may interfere with platelet aggregation
Allergic Potential: High
Safety in Pregnancy: B. Avoid near term in 3rd trimester (↑ incidence of kernicterus in newborns)
Comments: Useful to treat penicillin-resistant S. pneumoniae in CAP/CNS. CSF breakpoints for ceftriaxone are S (sensitive) ≤ 0.5 mcg/mL, I (intermediate) = 1 mcg/mL, and R (resistant) ≥ 2 mcg/mL. Non-meningeal breakpoints are S ≤ 1 mcg/mL, I = 2 mcg/mL, and R ≥ 4 mcg/mL. Ceftriaxone 1-2 gm (IV) q24h is useful for intra-abdominal/pelvic sepsis in combination with metronidazole 1 gm (IV) q24h. Ceftriaxone also has excellent activity against Group A streptococci and S. aureus (MSSA), making it useful for skin/soft tissue infections. May be given IV or IM. Incompatible in solutions containing vancomycin. Na^+ content = 2.6 mEq/g. PPNG dose: 125 mg (IM) x 1 dose. Meningeal dose = 2 gm (IV) q12h
Cerebrospinal Fluid Penetration:
Non-inflamed meninges = 1%
Inflamed meninges = 10%
Bile Penetration: 500%

"Usual dose" assumes normal renal/hepatic function. * For renal insufficiency, give usual dose x 1 followed by maintenance dose per CrCl. For dialysis patients, dose the same as for CrCl < 10 mL/min and give supplemental (post-HD/PD dose) immediately after dialysis. CrCl = creatinine clearance; CVVH = continuous veno-venous hemo-filtration; HD/PD = hemodialysis/peritoneal dialysis. See pp. 275-278 for explanations, p. 1 for abbreviations

REFERENCES:
Cunha BA, Klein NC. The selection and use of cephalosporins: A review. Adv Ther 12:83-101, 1995.
Grassi C. Ceftriaxone. Antibiotics for Clinicians 2:49-57, 1998.
Karlowsky JA, Jones ME. Importance of using current NCCLS breakpoints to interpret cefotaxime and ceftriaxone MICs for Streptococcus pneumoniae. J Antimicrob Chemother. 51:467-8, 2003.
Klein NC, Cunha BA. Third -generation cephalosporins. Med Clin North Am 79:705-19, 1995.
Lamb HM, Ormrod D, Scott LJ, et al. Ceftriaxone: an update of its use in the management of community-acquired and nosocomial infections. Drugs 62:1041-89, 2002.
Marshall WF, Blair JE. The cephalosporins. Mayo Clin Proc 74:187-95, 1999.
Schaad UB, Suter S, Gianella-Borradori A, et al. A comparison of ceftriaxone and cefuroxime for the treatment of bacterial meningitis in children. N Engl J Med 322:141-7, 1990.
Website: www.rocheusa.com/products/rocephin

Ciprofloxacin (Cipro)

Drug Class: Fluoroquinolone
Usual Dose: 400 mg (IV) q8-12h; 500-750 mg (PO) q12h
Pharmacokinetic Parameters:
Peak serum level: 4.6 (IV)/2.9 (PO) mcg/mL
Bioavailability: 70%
Excreted unchanged (urine): 70%
Serum half-life (normal/ESRD): 4/8 hrs
Plasma protein binding: 20-40%
Volume of distribution (V_d): 2.5 L/kg
Primary Mode of Elimination: Renal
Dosage Adjustments*

CrCl 50–80 mL/min	No change
CrCl 10–50 mL/min	400 mg (IV) q12h 500 mg (PO) q12h
CrCl < 10 mL/min	400 mg (IV) q24h 500 mg (PO) q24h
Post–HD dose	200-400 mg (IV) 250-500 mg (PO)
Post–PD dose	200-400 mg (IV) 250-500 mg (PO)

CVVH dose	200 mg (IV) q12h 250 mg (PO) q12h
Moderate hepatic insufficiency	No change
Severe hepatic insufficiency	No change

Drug Interactions: Al^{++}, Ca^{++}, Fe^{++}, Mg^{++}, Zn^{++} antacids, citrate/citric acid, dairy products (↓ absorption of ciprofloxacin only if taken together); caffeine, cyclosporine, theophylline (↑ interacting drug levels); cimetidine (↑ ciprofloxacin levels); foscarnet (↑ risk of seizures); oral hypoglycemics (slight ↑ or ↓ in blood glucose); NSAIDs (may ↑ risk of seizures/CNS stimulation); phenytoin (↑ or ↓ phenytoin levels); probenecid (↑ ciprofloxacin levels); warfarin (↑ INR)
Adverse Effects: Drug fever/rash, headache, dizziness, insomnia, malaise, seizures, Achilles tendon rupture/tendinitis (class effect)
Allergic Potential: Low
Safety in Pregnancy: C
Comments: Enteral feeding decreases ciprofloxacin absorption ≥ 30%. Use with caution in patients with severe renal insufficiency or seizure disorder. Administer 2 hours before or after H_2 antagonists, omeprazole, sucralfate, calcium, iron, zinc, multivitamins, or aluminum/magnesium containing medications. Administer ciprofloxacin (IV) as an intravenous infusion over 1 hour. Dose for nosocomial pneumonia: 400 mg (IV) q8h
Cerebrospinal Fluid Penetration:
Non-inflamed meninges = 10%
Inflamed meninges = 26%
Bile Penetration: 3000%

REFERENCES:
Bellmann R, Egger P, Gritsch W, et al. Pharmacokinetics of ciprofloxacin in patients with acute renal failure undergoing continuous venovenous haemofiltration: influence of concomitant liver cirrhosis. Acta Med Austriaca 29:112-6, 2002.
Davis R, Markham A, Balfour JA. Ciprofloxacin: An updated review of its pharmacology, therapeutic efficacy, and tolerability. Drugs 51:1019-74, 1996.

"Usual dose" assumes normal renal/hepatic function. * For renal insufficiency, give usual dose x 1 followed by maintenance dose per CrCl. For dialysis patients, dose the same as for CrCl < 10 mL/min and give supplemental (post-HD/PD dose) immediately after dialysis. CrCl = creatinine clearance; CVVH = continuous veno-venous hemo-filtration; HD/PD = hemodialysis/peritoneal dialysis. See pp. 275-278 for explanations, p. 1 for abbreviations

Debon R, Breilh D, Boselli E, et al. Pharmacokinetic parameters of ciprofloxacin (500 mg/5mL) oral suspension in critically ill patients with severe bacterial pneumonia: a comparison of two dosages. J Chemother 14:175-80, 2002.

Pankey GA, Ashcraft DS. In vitro synergy of ciprofloxacin and gatifloxacin against ciprofloxacin-resistant pseudomonas aeruginosa. Antimicrobial Agents and Chemotherapy 49:2959-2964, 2005.

Sanders CC. Ciprofloxacin: In vitro activity, mechanism of action, resistance. Rev Infect Dis 10:516-27, 1998.

Walker RC, Wright AJ. The fluoroquinolones. Mayo Clin Proc 66:1249-59, 1991.

Website: www.cipro.com

Ciprofloxacin Extended-Release (Cipro XR)

Drug Class: Fluoroquinolone
Usual Dose: 500 mg or 1000 mg (PO) q24h (see comments)
Pharmacokinetic Parameters (500/1000 mg):
Peak serum level: 1.59/3.11 mcg/mL
Bioavailability: 70%
Excreted unchanged (urine): 50-70%; 22% excreted as active metabolite
Serum half-life: 6.6/6.3 hrs
Plasma protein binding: 20-40%
Volume of distribution (V_d): 2.5 L/kg
Primary Mode of Elimination: Renal
Dosage Adjustments*

CrCl > 30 mL/min	No change
CrCl < 30 mL/min	No change for 500 mg dose; reduce 1000 mg dose to 500 mg (PO) q24h
Post–HD/PD dose	500 mg (PO)
CVVH dose	see CrCl < 30 mL/min
Moderate or severe hepatic insufficiency	No change

Drug Interactions: Al^{++}, Ca^{++}, Fe^{++}, Mg^{++}, Zn^{++} antacids, citrate/citric acid, dairy products, didanosine (↓ absorption of ciprofloxacin only if taken together); caffeine, cyclosporine, theophylline (↑ interacting drug levels); cimetidine (↑ ciprofloxacin levels); foscarnet (↑

risk of seizures); insulin, oral hypoglycemics (slight ↑ or ↓ in blood glucose); NSAIDs (may ↑ risk of seizures/CNS stimulation); phenytoin (↑ or ↓ phenytoin levels); probenecid (↑ ciprofloxacin levels); warfarin (↑ INR)
Adverse Effects: Drug fever/rash, seizures, Achilles tendon rupture/tendinitis (class effect)
Allergic Potential: Low
Safety in Pregnancy: C
Comments: Use 500 mg (PO) q 24h to treat uncomplicated UTI (acute cystitis); use 1000 mg (PO) q24h to treat complicated UTI or acute uncomplicated pyelonephritis. May be administered with or without food. Administer at least 2 hours before or 6 hours after H_2 antagonists, omeprazole, sucralfate, calcium, iron, zinc, multivitamins, or aluminum/magnesium containing medications

REFERENCES:
Website: www.ciproxr.com

Clarithromycin (Biaxin)

Drug Class: Macrolide
Usual Dose: 500 mg (PO) q12h
Pharmacokinetic Parameters:
Peak serum level: 1-4 mcg/mL
Bioavailability: 50%
Excreted unchanged (urine): 20%
Serum half-life (normal/ESRD): 3-7/4 hrs
Plasma protein binding: 70%
Volume of distribution (V_d): 3 L/kg
Primary Mode of Elimination: Hepatic
Dosage Adjustments*

CrCl 10–80 mL/min	No change
CrCl < 10 mL/min	250 mg (PO) q12h
Post–HD dose	500 mg (PO)
Post–PD dose	None
CVVH dose	No change
Moderate hepatic insufficiency	No change

"Usual dose" assumes normal renal/hepatic function. * For renal insufficiency, give usual dose x 1 followed by maintenance dose per CrCl. For dialysis patients, dose the same as for CrCl < 10 mL/min and give supplemental (post-HD/PD dose) immediately after dialysis. CrCl = creatinine clearance; CVVH = continuous veno-venous hemo-filtration; HD/PD = hemodialysis/peritoneal dialysis. See pp. 275-278 for explanations, p. 1 for abbreviations

Severe hepatic insufficiency	No change

Drug Interactions: Amiodarone, procainamide, sotalol, astemizole, terfenadine, cisapride, pimozide (may ↑ QT interval, torsade de pointes); carbamazepine (↑ carbamazepine levels, nystagmus, nausea, vomiting, diarrhea); cimetidine, digoxin, ergot alkaloids, midazolam, triazolam, phenytoin, ritonavir, tacrolimus, valproic acid (↑ interacting drug levels); clozapine, corticosteroids (not studied); cyclosporine (↑ cyclosporine levels with toxicity); efavirenz (↓ clarithromycin levels); rifabutin, rifampin (↓ clarithromycin levels, ↑ interacting drug levels); statins (↑ risk of rhabdomyolysis); theophylline (↑ theophylline levels, nausea, vomiting, seizures, apnea); warfarin (↑ INR); zidovudine (↓ zidovudine levels)

Adverse Effects: Nausea, vomiting, GI upset, irritative diarrhea, abdominal pain. May ↑ QT$_c$; avoid with other medications that prolong the QT$_c$ interval and in patients with cardiac arrhythmias/heart block

Allergic Potential: Low

Safety in Pregnancy: C

Comments: Peculiar taste of "aluminum sand" sensation on swallowing

Cerebrospinal Fluid Penetration: < 10%

Bile Penetration: 7000%

REFERENCES:

Alcaide F, Calatayud L, Santin M, et al. Comparative in vitro activities of linezolid, telithromycin, clarithromycin, levofloxacin, moxifloxacin and four conventional antimycobacterial drugs against mycobacterium kansasii. Antimicrob Agents Chemother 48:4562-5, 2004.

Alvarez-Elcoro S, Enzler MJ. The macrolides: Erythromycin, clarithromycin and azithromycin. Mayo Clin Proc 4:613- 34, 1999.

Benson CA, Williams PL, Cohn DL, and the ACTG 196/CPCRA 009 Study Team. Clarithromycin or rifabutin alone or in combination for primary prophylaxis of Mycobacterium avium complex disease in patients with AIDS: A randomized, double-blinded, placebo-controlled trial. J Infect Dis 181:1289-97, 2000.

Berg HF, Tjhie JH, Scheffer GJ, et al. Emergence and persistence of macrolide resistance in oropharyngeal flora and elimination of nasal carriage of Staphylococcus aureus after therapy with slow-release clarithromycin: a randomized, double-blind, placebo-controlled study. Antimicrob Agents Chemother 48:4138-8, 2004.

Chaisson RE, Keiser P, Pierce M, et al. Clarithromycin and ethambutol with or without clofazimine for the treatment of bacteremic Mycobacterium avium complex disease in patients with HIV infection. AIDS 11:311-317, 1997.

Jain R, Danzinger LH. The macrolide antibiotics: a pharmacokinetic and pharmacodynamic overview. Curr Pharm Des 10:3045-53, 2004.

Kraft M, Cassell AGH, Jpak J, et al. Mycoplasma pneumoniae and Chlamydia pneumoniae in asthma: effect of clarithromycin. Chest 121:1782-8, 2002.

McConnell SA, Amsden GW. Review and comparison of advanced-generation macrolides clarithromycin and dirithromycin. Pharmacotherapy 19:404-15, 1999.

Periti P, Mazzei T. Clarithromycin: Pharmacokinetic and pharmacodynamic interrelationships and dosage regimen. J Chemother 11:11-27, 1999.

Portier H, Filipecki J, Weber P, et al Five day clarithromycin modified release versus 10 day penicillin V for group A streptococcal pharyngitis: a multi-centre, open-label, randomized study. J Antimicrob Chemother 49:337-44, 2002.

Rodvold KA. Clinical pharmacokinetics of clarithromycin. Clin Pharmacother 37:385-98, 1999.

Schlossberg D. Azithromycin and clarithromycin. Med Clin North Am 79:803-16, 1995.

Stein GE, Schooley S. Serum bactericidal activity of extended-release clarithromycin against macrolide-resistant strains of Streptococcus pneumoniae. Pharmacotherapy 22:593-6, 2002.

Tartaglione TA. Therapeutic options for the management and prevention of Mycobacterium avium complex infection in patients with acquired immunodeficiency syndrome. Pharmacotherapy 16:171-82, 1996.

Website: www.biaxin.com

Clarithromycin XL (Biaxin XL)

Drug Class: Macrolide

Usual Dose: 1 gm (PO) q24h

Pharmacokinetic Parameters:

Peak serum level: 3 mcg/mL

Bioavailability: 50%

Excreted unchanged (urine): 20%; 10-15% excreted as active metabolite

Serum half-life (normal/ESRD): 4/4 hrs

Plasma protein binding: 70%

Volume of distribution (V$_d$): 3 L/kg

"Usual dose" assumes normal renal/hepatic function. * For renal insufficiency, give usual dose x 1 followed by maintenance dose per CrCl. For dialysis patients, dose the same as for CrCl < 10 mL/min and give supplemental (post-HD/PD dose) immediately after dialysis. CrCl = creatinine clearance; CVVH = continuous veno-venous hemo-filtration; HD/PD = hemodialysis/peritoneal dialysis. See pp. 275-278 for explanations, p. 1 for abbreviations

Primary Mode of Elimination: Hepatic
Dosage Adjustments*

CrCl 30–60 mL/min	No change
CrCl < 30 mL/min	500 mg (PO) q24h
Post–HD dose	None
Post–PD dose	None
CVVH dose	No change
Moderate hepatic insufficiency	No change
Severe hepatic insufficiency	No change

Drug Interactions: Amiodarone, procainamide, sotalol, astemizole, terfenadine, cisapride, pimozide (may ↑ QT interval, torsade de pointes); carbamazepine (↑ carbamazepine levels, nystagmus, nausea, vomiting, diarrhea); cimetidine, digoxin, ergot alkaloids, midazolam, triazolam, phenytoin, ritonavir, tacrolimus, valproic acid (↑ interacting drug levels); clozapine, corticosteroids (not studied); cyclosporine (↑ cyclosporine levels with toxicity); efavirenz (↓ clarithromycin levels); rifabutin, rifampin (↓ clarithromycin levels, ↑ interacting drug levels); statins (↑ risk of rhabdomyolysis); theophylline (↑ theophylline levels, nausea, vomiting, seizures, apnea); warfarin (↑ INR); zidovudine (↓ zidovudine levels)
Adverse Effects: Few/no GI symptoms. May ↑ QT$_c$; avoid with other medications that prolong the QT$_c$ interval and in patients with cardiac arrhythmias/heart block
Allergic Potential: Low
Safety in Pregnancy: C
Comments: Two 500 mg tablets of XL preparation permits once daily dosing and decreases GI intolerance
Cerebrospinal Fluid Penetration: < 10%
Bile Penetration: 7000%

REFERENCES:
Adler JL, Jannetti W, Schneider D, et al. Phase III, randomized, double-blind study of clarithromycin extended-release and immediate-release formulations in the treatment of patients with acute exacerbation of chronic bronchitis. Clin Ther 22:1410-20, 2000.
Anzueto A, Fisher CL Jr, Busman T. Comparison of the efficacy of extended-release clarithromycin tablets and amoxicillin/clavulanate tablets in the treatment of acute exacerbation of chronic bronchitis. Clin Ther 23:72-86, 2000.
Gotfried HM. Clarithromycin (Biaxin) extended-release tablet: a therapeutic review. Expert Rev Anti Infect Ther 1:9-20, 2004.
Nalepa P, Dobryniewska M, Busman T, et al. Short-course therapy of acute bacterial exacerbation of chronic bronchitis: a double-blind, randomized, multicenter comparison of extended-release versus immediate-release clarithromycin. Curr Med Res Opin. 19:411-20, 2003.
Website: biaxinxl.com

Clindamycin (Cleocin)

Drug Class: Lincosamide
Usual Dose: 600-900 mg (IV) q8h; 150-450 mg (PO) q6h
Pharmacokinetic Parameters:
Peak serum level: 2.5-10 mcg/mL
Bioavailability: 90%
Excreted unchanged (urine): 10%; 3.6% excreted as active metabolite
Serum half-life (normal/ESRD): 2.4/4 hrs
Plasma protein binding: 90%
Volume of distribution (V_d): 1 L/kg
Primary Mode of Elimination: Hepatic
Dosage Adjustments*

CrCl < 10 mL/min	No change
Post–HD/PD dose	None
CVVH dose	No change
Moderate or severe hepatic insufficiency	No change

Drug Interactions: Muscle relaxants, neuromuscular blockers (↑ apnea, respiratory paralysis); kaolin (↓ clindamycin absorption); theophylline (↑ theophylline levels, seizures)
Adverse Effects: C. difficile diarrhea/colitis, neuromuscular blockade
Allergic Potential: Low
Safety in Pregnancy: B

"Usual dose" assumes normal renal/hepatic function. * For renal insufficiency, give usual dose x 1 followed by maintenance dose per CrCl. For dialysis patients, dose the same as for CrCl < 10 mL/min and give supplemental (post-HD/PD dose) immediately after dialysis. CrCl = creatinine clearance; CVVH = continuous veno-venous hemo-filtration; HD/PD = hemodialysis/peritoneal dialysis. See pp. 275-278 for explanations, p. 1 for abbreviations

Comments: C. difficile diarrhea more common with PO vs. IV clindamycin. Anti-spasmodics contraindicated in C. difficile diarrhea
Cerebrospinal Fluid Penetration: < 10%
Bile Penetration: 300%

REFERENCES:
Coyle EA, Cha R, Rybak MJ. Influences of linezolid, penicillin, and clindamycin, alone and in combination, on streptococcal pyrogenic exotoxin a release. Antimicrob Agents Chemother. 47:1752-5, 2003.
Falagas ME, Gorbach SL. Clindamycin and metronidazole. Med Clin North Am 79:845-67, 1995.
Kadowaki M, Demura Y, Mizuno S, et al. Reappraisal of clindamycin IV monotherapy for treatment of mild-to-moderate aspiration pneumonia in elderly patients. Chest 127:1276-1282, 2005.
Kasten MJ. Clindamycin, metronidazole, and chloramphenicol. Mayo Clin Proc 74:825-33, 1999.
Levin TP, Suh B, Axelrod P, et al. Potential clindamycin resistance in clindamycin-susceptible, erythromycin-resistant staphylococcus aureus: Report of a clinical failure. Antimicrobial Agents and Chemotherapy 49:1222-24, 2005

Colistin/ Colistin methanesulfonate (Coly-Mycin M)

Drug Class: Cell membrane altering antibiotic
Usual Dose: 1.7 mg/kg (IV) q8h (1 mg = 12,500 U)
Pharmacokinetic Parameters:
Peak serum level: 5 mcg/mL
Bioavailability: Not applicable
Excreted unchanged (urine): 90%
Serum half-life (normal/ESRD): 3.5/48-72 hrs
Plasma protein binding: < 10%
Volume of distribution (V_d): 15.8 L/kg
Primary Mode of Elimination: Renal
Dosage Adjustments*

CrCl 40–60 mL/min	2.5 mg/kg (IV) q12h
CrCl 10–40 mL/min	2.5 mg/kg (IV) q24h
CrCl < 10 mL/min	1.5 mg/kg (IV) q36h
Post–HD dose	None
Post–PD dose	None
CVVH dose	2.5 mg/kg (IV) q24h
Mild hepatic insufficiency	No change
Moderate or severe hepatic insufficiency	No change

Drug Interactions: Neuromuscular blocking agents (↑ neuromuscular blockade); nephrotoxic drugs (↑ nephrotoxic potential)
Adverse Effects: Dose dependent/reversible nephrotoxic potential (acute tubular necrosis). Paresthesias, vertigo, dizziness, slurred speech, blurry vision, respiratory arrest
Allergic Potential: Low
Safety in Pregnancy: B
Comments: Colistin (Polymyxin E) has less nephrotoxic potential than previously thought. Useful for multidrug resistant P. aeruginosa and Acinetobacter species. Colistin is more active against P. aeruginosa than polymixin B. For P. aeruginosa or Acinetobacter meningitis also give amikacin 10-40 mg (I.T.) q24h or colistin 10 mg (I.T.) q24h. Intrathecal colistin dose: 10 mg (I.T.) Q24h. Nebulizer dose: 80 mg in saline q8h; for recurrent infection use 160 mg q8h (freshly prepare solution and use within 24 hours). Continuous infusion dose: Give ½ of daily dose (IV) over 5-10 min, then give other ½ dose (in D5W or NS) 1 hour after initial dose over next 24 hours
Cerebrospinal Fluid Penetration: 25%

REFERENCES:
Berlana D, Llop JM, Fort E, et al. Use of colistin in the treatment of multidrug resistant gram-negative infections. Am J Health Syst Pharm 62:39-47, 2005.
Canton R, Cobos N, de Gracia J, et al. Antimicrobial therapy for pulmonary pathogenic colonization and infection by Pseudomonas aeruginosa in cystic fibrosis patients. Clin Microbiol Infect 11:690-703, 2005.
Evans ME, Feola DJ, Rapp RP. Polymyxin B sulfate and colistin: old antibiotics for emerging multiresistant gram-negative bacteria. Ann Pharmacother 33:960-7, 1999.
Falagas ME, Kasiakou SK. Colistin: The revival of polymyxins for the management of multidrug-

resistant gram-negative bacterial infections. Clin Infect Dis 40:1333-41, 2005.

Fulnecky EJ, Wright D, Scheld M, et al. Amikacin and colistin for treatment of Acinetobacter baumannii meningitis. J Infect 51:e249-e251, 2005.

Goodwin NJ, Friedman EA. The effects of renal impairment, peritoneal dialysis, and hemodialysis on serum sodium colistimethate levels. Ann Intern Med 68:984-94, 1968.

Gump WC, Walsh JW. Intrathecal colistin for treatment of highly resistant Pseudomonas ventriculitis. Case report and review of the literature. J Neurosurg 102:915-7, 2005.

Horton J, Pankey GA. Polymyxin B, colistin, and sodium colistimethate. Med Clin North Am 66:135-42, 1982.

Koch-Weser G, Sidel VW, Federman EB, et al. Adverse effects of sodium colistimethate. Ann Intern Med 72:857-68, 1970.

Levin AS, Baron AA, Penco J, et al. Intravenous colistin as therapy for nosocomial infections caused by multidrug resistant Pseudomonas aeruginosa and Acinetobacter baumannii. Clin Infect Dis 28:1008-11, 1999.

Li H, Turnidge J, Milne R, et al. In vitro pharmacodynamic properties of colistin and colistin methanesulfonate against Pseudomonas aeruginosa isolates from patients with cystic fibrosis. Antimicrob Agents Chemother 45:781-5, 2001.

Li J, Rayner CR, Nation RL, et al. Pharmacokinetics of colistin methanesulfonate and colistin in a critically ill patient receiving continuous venovenous hemodiafiltration. Antimicrob Agents Chemother 49:4814-5, 2005.

Linden PK, Kusne S, Coley K, et al. Use of parenteral colistin for the treatment of serious infection due to antimicrobial-resistant Pseudomonas aeruginosa. Clin Infect Dis 37:154-60, 2003.

Michalopoulos AS, Tsiodras S, Rellos K, et al. Colistin treatment in patients with ICU-acquired infections caused by multiresistant gram-negative bacteria: the renaissance of an old antibiotic. Clin Microbiol Infect 11:115-121, 2005.

Michalopoulos A, Kasiakou SK, Evangelos S, et al. Cure of multidrug-resistant Acinetobacter baumannii bacteraemia with continuous intravenous infusion of colistin. Clin Microbiol Infect 11:119-21, 2005.

Michalopoulos A, Kasiakou S, Rosmarakis E, et al. Cure of multidrug-resistance Acinetobacter baumannii bacteraemia with continuous intravenous infusion of colistin. Scand J Infect Dis 37:142-5, 2005.

Obritsch MD, Fish DN, MacLaren R, et al. Nosocomial infections due to multidrug-resistant Pseudomonas aeruginosa: epidemiology and treatment options. Pharmacotherapy 25:1353-64, 2005.

Reed MD, Stern RC, O'Riordan MA, et al. The pharmacokinetics of colistin in patients with cystic fibrosis. J Clin Pharmacol 41:645-54, 2001.

Rynn C, Wooton M, Bowker KE, et al. In vitro assessment of colistin's antipseudomonal antimicrobial interactions with other antibiotics. Clin Microbiol Infect 5:32-6, 1999.

Stein A, Raoult D. Colistin: an antimicrobial for the 21st century? Clin Infect Dis 35:901-2, 2002.

Cycloserine (Seromycin)

Drug Class: Anti–TB drug
Usual Dose: 250 mg (PO) q12h
Pharmacokinetic Parameters:
Peak serum level: 20 mcg/mL
Bioavailability: 90%
Excreted unchanged (urine): 65%
Serum half-life (normal/ESRD): 10-25 hrs/no data
Plasma protein binding: No data
Volume of distribution (V_d): 0.2 L/kg
Primary Mode of Elimination: Renal
Dosage Adjustments*

CrCl 50–80 mL/min	No change
CrCl 10–50 mL/min	250 mg (PO) q12-24h
CrCl < 10 mL/min	250 mg (PO) q24h
Post-HD dose	None
Post-PD dose	250 mg (PO)
CVVH dose	No change
Moderate or severe hepatic insufficiency	No change

Drug Interactions: Alcohol (seizures); ethambutol, ethionamide (drowsiness, dizziness); phenytoin (↑ phenytoin levels)
Adverse Effects: Peripheral neuropathy, seizures (dose related), psychosis/delirium
Allergic Potential: Low
Safety in Pregnancy: C
Comments: Avoid in patients with seizures. Ethambutol, ethionamide, or ethanol may increase CNS toxicity.
Meningeal dose = usual dose

"Usual dose" assumes normal renal/hepatic function. * For renal insufficiency, give usual dose x 1 followed by maintenance dose per CrCl. For dialysis patients, dose the same as for CrCl < 10 mL/min and give supplemental (post-HD/PD dose) immediately after dialysis. CrCl = creatinine clearance; CVVH = continuous veno-venous hemo-filtration; HD/PD = hemodialysis/peritoneal dialysis. See pp. 275-278 for explanations, p. 1 for abbreviations

Cerebrospinal Fluid Penetration:
Non-inflamed meninges = 90%
Inflamed meninges = 90%

REFERENCES:
Davidson PT, Le HQ. Drug treatment of tuberculosis - 1992. Drugs 43:651-73, 1992.
Drugs for tuberculosis. Med Lett Drugs Ther 35:99-101,1993.
Iseman MD. Treatment of multidrug resistant tuberculosis. N Engl J Med 329:784-91, 1993.

Dapsone

Drug Class: Antiparasitic (PABA antagonist)
Usual Dose: 100 mg (PO) q24h (see comments)
Pharmacokinetic Parameters:
Peak serum level: 1.8 mcg/mL
Bioavailability: 85%
Excreted unchanged (urine): 10%
Serum half-life (normal/ESRD): 25/30 hrs
Plasma protein binding: 80%
Volume of distribution (V_d): 1.2 L/kg
Primary Mode of Elimination: Hepatic/renal
Dosage Adjustments*

CrCl 50–80 mL/min	No change
CrCl 10–50 mL/min	No change
CrCl < 10 mL/min	No change
Post–HD dose	None
Post–PD dose	None
CVVH dose	No change
Moderate hepatic insufficiency	No change
Severe hepatic insufficiency	No information

Drug Interactions: Didanosine (↓ dapsone absorption); oral contraceptives (↓ oral contraceptive effect); pyrimethamine, zidovudine (↑ bone marrow suppression); rifabutin, rifampin (↓ dapsone levels); trimethoprim (↑ dapsone and trimethoprim levels, methemoglobinemia)

Adverse Effects: Drug fever/rash, nausea, vomiting, hemolytic anemia in G6PD deficiency, methemoglobinemia
Allergic Potential: High
Safety in Pregnancy: C
Comments: Useful in sulfa (SMX) allergic patients. Avoid, if possible, in G6PD deficiency or hemoglobin M deficiency. PCP prophylaxis dose: 100 mg (PO) q24h. PCP therapy dose: 100 mg (PO) q24h plus TMP or TMP-SMX 5mg/kg (IV/PO) q8h x 3 weeks

REFERENCES:
El-Sadr WM, Murphy Rl, Yurik TM, et al. Atovaquone compared with dapsone to the prevention of Pneumocystis carinii in patients with HIV infection who cannot tolerate trimethoprim, sulfonamides, or both. N Engl J Med 339:1889-95, 1998.
Medina I, Mills J, Leoung G, et al. Oral therapy for Pneumocystis carinii pneumonia in the acquired immunodeficiency syndrome. A controlled trial of trimethoprim-sulfamethoxazole versus trimethoprim-dapsone. N Engl J Med 323:776-82, 1990.
Podzamczer D, Salazar A, Jiminez J, et al. Intermittent trimethoprim-sulfamethoxazole compared with dapsone-pyrimethamine for the simultaneous primary prophylaxis of Pneumocystis pneumonia and toxoplasmosis in patients infected with HIV. Ann Intern Med 122:755-61, 1995.
Website: www.pdr.net

Doxycycline (Vibramycin, Vibra-tabs)

Drug Class: 2nd generation IV/PO tetracycline
Usual Dose: 100-200 mg (IV/PO) q12h or 200 mg (IV/PO) q24h. For serious systemic infection, begin therapy with a loading dose of 200 mg (IV/PO) q12h x 3 days, then continue at same dose or decrease to 100 mg (IV/PO) q12h to complete therapy (see comments)
Pharmacokinetic Parameters:
Peak serum level: 100/200 mg = 4/8 mcg/mL
Bioavailability: 93%
Excreted unchanged (urine): 40%
Serum half-life (normal/ESRD): 18-22/18-22 hrs
Plasma protein binding: 93%
Volume of distribution (V_d): 0.75 L/kg
Primary Mode of Elimination: Hepatic

"Usual dose" assumes normal renal/hepatic function. * For renal insufficiency, give usual dose x 1 followed by maintenance dose per CrCl. For dialysis patients, dose the same as for CrCl < 10 mL/min and give supplemental (post-HD/PD dose) immediately after dialysis. CrCl = creatinine clearance; CVVH = continuous veno-venous hemofiltration; HD/PD = hemodialysis/peritoneal dialysis. See pp. 275-278 for explanations, p. 1 for abbreviations

Dosage Adjustments*

CrCl < 10 mL/min	No change
Post–HD or PD dose	None
CVVH dose	No change
Moderate or severe hepatic insufficiency	No change

Drug Interactions: Antacids, Al^{++}, Ca^{++}, Fe^{++}, Mg^{++}, Zn^{++}, multivitamins, sucralfate (↓ doxycycline absorption); barbiturates, carbamazepine, phenytoin (↓ doxycycline half-life); bicarbonate (↓ doxycycline absorption, ↑ doxycycline clearance); warfarin (↑ INR)
Adverse Effects: Nausea if not taken with food. Phlebitis if given IV in inadequate volume. Avoid in pregnancy and children < 8 years
Allergic Potential: Low
Safety in Pregnancy: D
Comments: Minimal potential for Candida overgrowth/diarrhea. Photosensitivity rare. Tablets better tolerated than capsules. Absorption minimally effected by iron, bismuth, milk, or antacids containing Ca^{++}, Mg^{++}, or Al^{++}. Serum half-life increases with multiple doses. GC dose (not PPNG/TRNG): 100 mg (PO) q12h x 7 days. Meningeal dose = 200 mg (IV/PO) q12h
Cerebrospinal Fluid Penetration:
Non-inflamed meninges = 25%
Inflamed meninges = 25%
Bile Penetration: 3000%

REFERENCES:
Cunha BA. Doxycycline. Antibiotics for Clinicians 3:21-33, 1999.
Cunha BA. Doxycycline for community-acquired pneumonia. Clin Infect Dis. 37:870, 2003.
Cunha BA. Doxycycline re-revisited. Arch Intern Med 159:1006-7, 1999.
Cunha BA, Domenico PD, Cunha CB. Pharmacodynamics of doxycycline. Clin Micro Infect Dis 6:270-3, 2000.
Johnson JR. Doxycycline for treatment of community-acquired pneumonia. Clin Infect Dis 35:632, 2002.
Jones RN, Sader HS, Fritsche TR. Doxycycline use for community-acquired pneumonia: contemporary in vitro spectrum of activity against Streptococcus pneumoniae. Diagn Microbiol Infect Dis 49:147-9, 2004.
Shea KW, Ueno Y, Abumustafa F, et al. Doxycycline activity against Streptococcus pneumoniae. Chest 107:1775-6, 1995.

Ertapenem (Invanz)

Drug Class: Carbapenem
Usual Dose: 1 gm (IV/IM) q24h
Pharmacokinetic Parameters:
Peak serum level: 150 mcg/mL
Bioavailability: 90% (IM)
Excreted unchanged (urine): 40%; 40% excreted as active metabolite
Serum half-life (normal/ESRD): 4/14 hrs
Plasma protein binding: 95%
Volume of distribution (V_d): 8 L/kg
Primary Mode of Elimination: Renal
Dosage Adjustments*

CrCl 30–80 mL/min	No change
CrCl < 30 mL/min	500 mg (IV) q24h
Post–HD dose	500 mg (IV) if within 6h of HD
Post–PD dose	No information
CVVH dose	No information
Moderate hepatic insufficiency	No change
Severe hepatic insufficiency	No change

Drug Interactions: Not a substrate/inhibitor of cytochrome P-450 enzymes; probenecid (↓ clearance of ertapenem)
Adverse Effects: Mild headache, infrequent nausea or diarrhea. Low seizure potential. Probenecid (significant ↓ clearance of ertapenem)
Allergic Potential: Low
Safety in Pregnancy: B
Comments: Concentration-dependent protein binding. Compared to imipenem, ertapenem has little activity vs. enterococci, Acinetobacter or P. aeruginosa. No cross-allergenicity with penicillins, β–lactams. Safe to use in penicillin allergic patients. For deep muscle (IM) injection,

mix 1 gm with 3.2 mL of 1% lidocaine. Na^+
content = 6 mEq/g

REFERENCES:
Aldridge KE. Ertapenem (MK-0826), a new carbapenem: comparative in vitro activity against clinically significant anaerobes. Diagn Microbiol Infect Dis 44:181-6, 2002.
Curran M, Simpson D, Perry C. Ertapenem: a review of its use in the management of bacterial infections. Drugs 63:1855-78, 2003.
Decousser JW, Methlouthi I, Pina P, et al. In vitro activity of ertapenem against bacteremic pneumococci: report of a French multicentre study including 339 strains. Journal of Antimicrobial Chemotherapy 55: 396-8, 2005.
Livermore DM, Sefton AM, Scott GM. Properties and potential of ertapenem. J Antimicrob Chemother. 52:331-44, 2003.
Musson DG, Majumdar A, Holland S, et al. Pharmacokinetics of total and unbound ertapenem in healthy elderly subjects. Antimicrob Agents Chemother 48:521-4, 2004.
Shah PM, Isaacs RD. Ertapenem, the first of a new group of carbapenems. J Antimicrob Chemother. 52:538-42, 2003.
Teppler H, Gesser RM, Friedland Ir, et al. Safety and tolerability of ertapenem. J Antimicrob Chemother 53:75-81, 2004.
Vetter N, Cambronero-Hernandez E, Rohlf J, et al. A prospective, randomized, double-blind multicenter comparison of parenteral ertapenem and ceftriaxone for the treatment of hospitalized adults with community-acquired pneumonia. Clin Ther 24:1770-85, 2002.
Website: www.invanz.com

Erythromycin lactobionate, base (various)

Drug Class: Macrolide
Usual Dose: 1 gm (IV) q6h; 500 mg (PO) q6h
Pharmacokinetic Parameters:
Peak serum level: 12 (IV)/1.2 (PO) mcg/mL
Bioavailability: 50%
Excreted unchanged (urine): 5%; 5% exerted as active metabolite
Serum half-life (normal/ESRD): 1.4/5.4 hrs
Plasma protein binding: 80%
Volume of distribution (V_d): 0.5 L/kg
Primary Mode of Elimination: Hepatic

Dosage Adjustments*

CrCl 50–80 mL/min	No change
CrCl 10–50 mL/min	No change
CrCl < 10 mL/min	No change
Post–HD/PD dose	None
CVVH dose	No change
Moderate or severe hepatic insufficiency	No change

Drug Interactions: Amiodarone, procainamide, sotalol, astemizole, terfenadine, cisapride, pimozide (may ↑ QT interval, torsade de pointes); carbamazepine (↑ carbamazepine levels, nystagmus, nausea, vomiting, diarrhea; avoid combination); cimetidine, digoxin, ergot alkaloids, felodipine, midazolam, triazolam, phenytoin, ritonavir, tacrolimus, valproic acid (↑ interacting drug levels); clozapine (↑ clozapine levels; CNS toxicity); corticosteroids (↑ corticosteroid effect); cyclosporine (↑ cyclosporine levels with toxicity); efavirenz (↓ erythromycin levels); rifabutin, rifampin (↓ erythromycin levels, ↑ interacting drug levels); statins (↑ risk of rhabdomyolysis); theophylline (↑ theophylline levels, nausea, vomiting, seizures, apnea); warfarin (↑ INR); zidovudine (↓ zidovudine levels)
Adverse Effects: Nausea, vomiting, GI upset, irritative diarrhea, abdominal pain, phlebitis. May ↑ QT_c; avoid with other medications that prolong the QT_c interval and in patients with cardiac arrhythmias/heart block
Allergic Potential: Low
Safety in Pregnancy: B
Comments: Do not mix erythromycin with B/C vitamins, glucose solutions, cephalothin, tetracycline, chloramphenicol, heparin, or warfarin. Increases GI motility. Monitor potential hepatotoxicity with serial SGOTs/SGPTs
Cerebrospinal Fluid Penetration: < 10%

REFERENCES:
Alvarez-Elcoro S, Enzler MJ. The macrolides: Erythromycin, clarithromycin and azithromycin. Mayo Clin Proc 74:613-34, 1999.

"Usual dose" assumes normal renal/hepatic function. * For renal insufficiency, give usual dose x 1 followed by maintenance dose per CrCl. For dialysis patients, dose the same as for CrCl < 10 mL/min and give supplemental (post-HD/PD dose) immediately after dialysis. CrCl = creatinine clearance; CVVH = continuous veno-venous hemo-filtration; HD/PD = hemodialysis/peritoneal dialysis. See pp. 275-278 for explanations, p. 1 for abbreviations

Amsden GW. Erythromycin, clarithromycin, and azithromycin: Are the differences real? Clinical Therapeutics 18:572, 1996.

Cunha BA. The virtues of doxycycline and the evils of erythromycin. Adv Ther 14:172-80, 1997.

Jain R, Danzinger LH. The macrolide antibiotics: a pharmacokinetic and pharmacodynamic overview. Curr Pharm Des 10:3045-53, 2004.

Smilack JD, Wilson WE, Cocerill FR 3rd. Tetracycline, chloramphenicol, erythromycin, clindamycin, and metronidazole. Mayo Clin Proc 66:1270-80, 1991.

Website: www.pdr.net

Ethambutol (Myambutol) EMB

Drug Class: Anti–TB drug
Usual Dose: 15 mg/kg (PO) q24h (see comments)
Pharmacokinetic Parameters:
Peak serum level: 2-5 mcg/mL
Bioavailability: 80%
Excreted unchanged (urine): 50%
Serum half-life (normal/ESRD): 4/10 hrs
Plasma protein binding: 20%
Volume of distribution (V_d): 2 L/kg
Primary Mode of Elimination: Renal/hepatic
Dosage Adjustments*

CrCl > 40 mL/min	No change
CrCl < 40 mL/min	No change
Post–HD/PD dose	None
CVVH dose	No change
Moderate or severe hepatic insufficiency	No change

Drug Interactions: Aluminum salts, didanosine buffer (↓ ethambutol and interacting drug absorption)
Adverse Effects: Drug fever/rash, ↓ visual acuity, central scotomata, color blindness (red–green), metallic taste, mental confusion, peripheral neuropathy, ↑ uric acid
Allergic Potential: Low
Safety in Pregnancy: B
Comments: Optic neuritis may occur with high doses (≥ 15 mg/kg/day). TB D.O.T. dose: 4 gm

(PO) 2x/week or 3 gm (PO) 3x/week. MAI dose: 15 mg/kg (PO) q24h (with azithromycin 500 mg [PO] q24h)
Meningeal dose = 25 mg/kg (PO) q24h
Cerebrospinal Fluid Penetration:
Non-inflamed meninges = 1%
Inflamed meninges = 40%

REFERENCES:

Chaisson RE, Keiser P, Pierce M, et al. Clarithromycin and ethambutol with or without clofazimine for the treatment of bacteremic Mycobacterium avium complex disease in patients with HIV infection. AIDS 11:311-317, 1997.

Davidson PT, Le HQ. Drug treatment of tuberculosis 1992. Drugs 43:651-73, 1992.

Drugs for tuberculosis. Med Lett Drugs Ther 35:99-101,1993.

Perlman DC, Segal Y, Rosenkranz S, et al. The clinical pharmacokinetics of rifampin and ethambutol in HIV-infected persons with tuberculosis. Clinical Infectious Disease 41:1638-47, 2005.

Schlossberg D. Treatment of multi-drug resistant tuberculosis. Antibiotics for Clinicians 9:317-21, 2005.

Van Scoy RE, Wilkowske CJ. Antituberculous agents. Mayo Clin Proc 67:179-87, 1992.

Ethionamide (Trecator)

Drug Class: Anti–TB drug
Usual Dose: 500 mg (PO) q12h
Pharmacokinetic Parameters:
Peak serum level: 5 mcg/mL
Bioavailability: Complete
Excreted unchanged (urine): 1%
Serum half-life (normal/ESRD): 2/9 hrs
Plasma protein binding: 30%
Volume of distribution (V_d): No data
Primary Mode of Elimination: Renal/hepatic
Dosage Adjustments*

CrCl 40–60 mL/min	No change
CrCl < 40 mL/min	No change
Post–HD/PD dose	No information
CVVH dose	No information
Moderate hepatic insufficiency	No change

"Usual dose" assumes normal renal/hepatic function. * For renal insufficiency, give usual dose x 1 followed by maintenance dose per CrCl. For dialysis patients, dose the same as for CrCl < 10 mL/min and give supplemental (post-HD/PD dose) immediately after dialysis. CrCl = creatinine clearance; CVVH = continuous veno-venous hemofiltration; HD/PD = hemodialysis/peritoneal dialysis. See pp. 275-278 for explanations, p. 1 for abbreviations

Severe hepatic insufficiency	500 mg (PO) q24h

Drug Interactions: Cycloserine (↑ neurologic toxicity); ethambutol (↑ GI distress, neuritis, hepatotoxicity); INH (peripheral neuritis, hepatotoxicity); pyrazinamide, rifampin (hepatotoxicity)
Adverse Effects: ↑ SGOT/SGPT, headache, nausea/vomiting, abdominal pain, tremor, olfactory abnormalities, alopecia, gynecomastia, hypoglycemia, impotence, neurotoxicity (central/peripheral neuropathy)
Allergic Potential: Low
Safety in Pregnancy: C
Comments: Additive toxicity with thiacetazone
Cerebrospinal Fluid Penetration: 100%

REFERENCES:
Davidson PT, Le HQ. Drug treatment of tuberculosis 1992. Drugs 43:651-73, 1992.
Drugs for tuberculosis. Med Lett Drugs Ther 35:99-101,1993.
Iseman MD. Treatment of multidrug resistant tuberculosis. N Engl J Med 329:784-91, 1993.
Schlossberg D. Treatment of multi-drug resistant tuberculosis. Antibiotics for Clinicians 9:317-321, 2005.

Famciclovir (Famvir)

Drug Class: Antiviral
Usual Dose:
HSV ½: Herpes labialis: 500 mg (PO) q12h x 7 days. Genital herpes: *Initial therapy:* 500 mg (PO) q12h x 7-10 days. *Recurrent/intermittent therapy* (< 6 episodes/year): normal host: 125 mg (PO) q12h x 5 days; HIV-positive: 500 mg (PO) q12h x 7 days. *Chronic suppressive therapy* (> 6 episodes/year): 250 mg (PO) q12h x 1 year. Encephalitis: 500 mg (PO) q8h x 10 days
VZV: Chickenpox: 500 mg (PO) q8h x 5 days. Herpes zoster (shingles) (dermatomal/disseminated): 500 mg (PO) q8h x 7-10 days
Pharmacokinetic Parameters:
Peak serum level: 3.3 mcg/mL
Bioavailability: 77%
Excreted unchanged (urine): 60%
Serum half-life (normal/ESRD): 2.5/13 hrs
Plasma protein binding: 20%

Volume of distribution (V_d): 1.1 L/kg
Primary Mode of Elimination: Renal
Dosage Adjustments for HSV/VZV* (based on 250 mg [PO] q8h/500 mg [PO] q8h)

CrCl 40–60 mL/min	No change 500 mg (PO) q12h
CrCl 20-40 mL/min	125 mg (PO) q24h 500 mg (PO) q24h
CrCl < 20 mL/min	125 mg (PO) q24h 250 mg (PO) q24h
Post–HD dose	125 mg (PO) 250 mg (PO)
Post–PD dose	No information
CVVH dose	No information
Moderate hepatic insufficiency	No change
Severe hepatic insufficiency	No information

Drug Interactions: Digoxin (↑ digoxin levels)
Adverse Effects: Headache, seizures/tremors (dose related), nausea, diarrhea
Allergic Potential: Low
Safety in Pregnancy: B
Comments: 99% converted to penciclovir in liver/GI tract.
Meningeal dose = VZV dose
Cerebrospinal Fluid Penetration: 50%

REFERENCES:
Alrabiah FA, Sacks SL. New anti-herpesvirus agents. Their targets and therapeutic potential. Drugs 52:17-32, 1996.
Chakrabarty A, Tyring SK, Beutner K, et al. Recent clinical experience with famciclovir-a "third generation" nucleoside prodrug. Antivir Chem Chemother 15:251-3, 2004.
Luber AD, Flaherty JF Jr. Famciclovir for treatment of herpesvirus infections. Ann Pharmacother 30:978-85, 1996.
Website: www.famvir.com

Foscarnet (Foscavir)

Drug Class: Antiviral (HSV,CMV, VZV)
Usual Dose: <u>HSV</u>: 40 mg/kg (IV) q12h x 2-3 weeks; <u>CMV</u>: 90 mg/kg (IV) q12h x 2 weeks (induction dose), then 90-120 mg/kg (IV) q24h (maintenance dose) for life-long suppression. Relapse/reinduction dose: 120 mg/kg (IV) q24h x 2 weeks. <u>Acyclovir-resistant mucocutaneous HSV/VZV</u>: 60 mg/kg (IV) x 3 weeks
Pharmacokinetic Parameters:
Peak serum level: 150 mcg/ml
Bioavailability: Not applicable
Excreted unchanged (urine): 85%
Serum half-life (normal/ESRD): 2-4/25 hrs
Plasma protein binding: 17%
Volume of distribution (V_d): 0.5 L/kg
Primary Mode of Elimination: Renal /hepatic
Dosage Adjustments*

Induction	
CrCl 50-80 mL/min	40-50 mg/kg (IV) q8h
CrCl 20-50 mL/min	20-30 mg/kg (IV) q8h
CrCl < 20 mL/min	Avoid
Maintenance	
CrCl 50-80 mL/min	60-70 mg/kg (IV) q24h
CrCl 20-50 mL/min	65-80 mg/kg (IV) q48h
CrCl < 20 mL/min	Avoid
Post–HD dose	60 mg/kg (IV)
Post–PD dose	None
CVVH dose	Induction: 20-30 mg/kg (IV) q8h; maintenance: 65-80 mg/kg (IV) q48h
Moderate hepatic insufficiency	No change
Severe hepatic insufficiency	No change

Infusion pump must be used. Adequate hydration is recommended to prevent renal toxicity

Drug Interactions: Ciprofloxacin (↑ risk of seizures); amphotericin B, aminoglycosides, cis-platinum, cyclosporine, other nephrotoxic drugs (↑ nephrotoxicity); pentamidine IV (severe hypocalcemia reported; do not combine); zidovudine (↑ incidence/severity of anemia)
Adverse Effects: Major side effects include nephrotoxicity and tetany (from ↓ Ca⁺⁺). Others include anemia, nausea, vomiting, GI upset, headache, seizures, peripheral neuropathy, hallucinations, tremors, nephrogenic DI, ↓ Ca⁺⁺, ↓ Mg⁺⁺, ↓ PO₄⁼, oral/genital ulcers
Allergic Potential: Low
Safety in Pregnancy: C
Comments: Renal failure prevented/minimized by adequate hydration. Dilute with 150 cc normal saline per 1 gm foscarnet. Administer by IV slow infusion ≤ 1 mg/kg/min using an infusion pump. Meningeal dose = usual dose
Cerebrospinal Fluid Penetration:
Non-inflamed meninges = 90%
Inflamed meninges = 100%

REFERENCES:
Chrisp P, Clissold SP. Foscarnet: A review of its antiviral activity, pharmacokinetic properties, and therapeutic use in immunocompromised patients with cytomegalovirus retinitis. Drugs 41:104-29, 1991.
De Clercq E. Antiviral drugs in current clinical use. J Clin Virol 30:115-33, 2004.
Derary G, Martinez F, Katlama C, et al. Foscarnet nephrotoxicity: Mechanism, Incidence and prevention. Am J Nephrol 9:316-21, 1989.
Mattes FM, Hainsworth EG, Geretti AM, et al. A randomized, controlled trial comparing ganciclovir plus foscarnet (each at half dose) preemptive therapy of cytomegalovirus infection in transplant recipients. J Infect Dis 189:1355-61, 2004.
Whitley RJ, Jacobson MA, Friedberg DN, et al. Guidelines for the treatment of cytomegalovirus diseases in patients with AIDS in the era of potent antiretroviral therapy. Arch Intern Med 158:957-69, 1998.
Website: www.pdr.net

Ganciclovir (Cytovene)

Drug Class: Antiviral, nucleoside inhibitor/analogue
Usual Dose: 5 mg/kg (IV) q12h x 2 weeks (induction), then 5 mg/kg (IV) q24h or 1 gm

---

"Usual dose" assumes normal renal/hepatic function. * For renal insufficiency, give usual dose x 1 followed by maintenance dose per CrCl. For dialysis patients, dose the same as for CrCl < 10 mL/min and give supplemental (post-HD/PD dose) immediately after dialysis. CrCl = creatinine clearance; CVVH = continuous veno-venous hemo-filtration; HD/PD = hemodialysis/peritoneal dialysis. See pp. 275-278 for explanations, p. 1 for abbreviations

(PO) q8h (maintenance) for CMV retinitis (see comments)

Pharmacokinetic Parameters:
Peak serum level: 8.3 (IV)/1.2 (PO) mcg/ml
Bioavailability: 5%
Excreted unchanged (urine): 90%
Serum half-life (normal/ESRD): 3.6/28 hrs
Plasma protein binding: 1%
Volume of distribution (V_d): 0.74 L/kg
Primary Mode of Elimination: Renal
Dosage Adjustments*

CrCl 50–80 mL/min	2.5 mg/kg (IV) q12h (induction); 2.5 mg/kg (IV) q24h (maintenance); 500 mg (PO) q8h
CrCl 25–50 mL/min	2.5 mg/kg (IV) q24h (induction); 1.25 mg/kg (IV) q24h (maintenance); 500 mg (PO) q12h
CrCl 10-25 mL/min	1.25 mg/kg (IV) q24h (induction); 0.625 mg/kg (IV) q24h (maintenance); 500 mg (PO) q24h
CrCl < 10 mL/min	1.25 mg/kg (IV) 3x/week (induction); 0.625 mg/kg (IV) 3x/week (maintenance); 500 mg (PO) 3x/week
Post–HD dose	1.25 mg/kg (IV) (induction); 0.625 mg/kg (IV) (maintenance); 500 mg (PO)
Post–PD dose	None
CVVH dose	see CrCl 50–80 mL/min
Moderate hepatic insufficiency	No change
Severe hepatic insufficiency	No change

Drug Interactions: Cytotoxic drugs (may produce additive toxicity: stomatitis, bone marrow depression, alopecia); imipenem (↑ risk of seizures); probenecid (↑ ganciclovir levels); zidovudine (↓ ganciclovir levels, ↑ zidovudine levels, possible neutropenia)

Adverse Effects: Headaches, hallucinations, seizures/tremor (dose related), drug fever/rash, diarrhea, nausea/vomiting, GI upset, leukopenia, thrombocytopenia, anemia, retinal detachment
Allergic Potential: High
Safety in Pregnancy: C
Comments: Induction doses are always given IV. Maintenance doses may be given IV or PO. For CMV encephalitis, use same dosing regimen as for CMV retinitis (CNS penetration = 70%). For CMV pneumonitis, give 2.5 mg/kg (IV) q8h x 20 doses plus IVIG 500 mg/kg (IV) q48h x 10 doses; then follow with 5 mg/kg (IV) 3-5x/week x 20 doses plus IVIG 500 mg/kg (IV) 2x/week x 8 doses. For CMV colitis/esophagitis, use same dose for CMV retinitis induction x 3-6 weeks. Continue maintenance doses for CMV retinitis, encephalitis, and colitis/esophagitis until CD_4 cell count > 100–200. Reduce dose with neutropenia/thrombocytopenia. Bioavailability increased with food: 5% fasting; 6-9% with food; 28-31% with fatty food. Na^+ content = 4.0 mEq/g.
Meningeal dose = CMV retinitis dose
Cerebrospinal Fluid Penetration: 41%

REFERENCES:
Czock D, Scholle C, Rasche FM, et al. Pharmacokinetics of valganciclovir and ganciclovir in renal impairment. Clin Pharmacol Ther 72:142-50, 2002.
Matthews T, Boehme R. Antiviral activity and mechanism of action of ganciclovir. Rev Infect Dis 10:490-4, 1988.
Paya CV, Wilson JA, Espy MJ, et al. Preemptive use of oral ganciclovir to prevent cytomegalovirus infection in liver transplant patients: a randomized, placebo-controlled trial J Infect Dis 185:861-7, 2002.
Singh N. Preemptive therapy for cytomegalovirus with oral ganciclovir after liver transplantation. Transplantation 73:1977-78, 2002.
Tokimasa S, Hara J, Osugi Y, et al. Ganciclovir is effective for prophylaxis and treatment of human herpesvirus-6 in allogeneic stem cell transplantation. Bone Marrow Transplant 29:595-8, 2002.
Whitley RJ, Jacobson MA, Friedberg DN, et al. Guidelines for the treatment of cytomegalovirus diseases in patients with AIDS in the era of potent antiretroviral therapy. Arch Intern Med 158:957-69, 1998.

Website: www.rocheusa.com/products/

Gemifloxacin (Factive)

Drug Class: Fluoroquinolone
Usual Dose: 320 mg (PO) q24h
Pharmacokinetic Parameters:
Peak serum level: 1.6 mcg/ml
Bioavailability: 71%
Excreted unchanged (urine): 36%; 36%
excreted as active metabolites
Serum half-life (normal/ESRD): 7/10 hrs
Plasma protein binding: 55-73%
Volume of distribution (V_d): 4.2 L/kg
Primary Mode of Elimination: Renal
Dosage Adjustments*

CrCl > 40 mL/min	No change
CrCl < 40 mL/min	160 mg (PO) q24h
CrCl < 10 mL/min	160 mg (PO) q24h
Post–HD dose	160 mg (PO)
Post–PD dose	None
Post–CVVH dose	160 mg (PO) q24h
Moderate hepatic insufficiency	No change
Severe hepatic insufficiency	No change

Drug Interactions: Al^{++}, Fe^{++}, Mg^{++}, Zn^{++} antacids/multivitamins, didanosine, sucralfate (↓ gemifloxacin levels only if taken together); probenecid (↑ gemifloxacin levels); amiodarone, quinidine, procainamide, sotalol (may ↑ QTc interval, torsade de pointes; avoid)
Adverse Effects: Rash, ↑ LFTs (doses > 320 mg/d). Does not lower seizure threshold or cause seizures
Allergic Potential: Low
Safety in Pregnancy: C
Comments: Take at least 3 hours before or 2 hours after calcium/magnesium containing antacids. Take at least 2 hours before sucralfate. May ↑ QT_c interval > 3 msec.; avoid taking with other medications that prolong the QT_c interval,

and in patients with prolonged QT interval/heart block. Do not exceed usual dose
Cerebrospinal Fluid Penetration: < 10%

REFERENCES:
Chagan L. Gemifloxacin for the treatment of acute bacterial exacerbation of chronic bronchitis and community-acquired pneumonia. P&T 28:769-79, 2003.
File TM Jr, Tillotson GS. Gemifloxacin: a new, potent fluoroquinolone for the therapy of lower respiratory tract infections. Expert Rev Anti Infect Ther 2:831-43, 2004.
Gemifloxacin (factive). Med Lett Drugs Ther 46:78-9, 2004.
Goldstein EJ. Review of the in vitro activity of gemifloxacin against gram-positive and gram-negative anaerobic pathogens. J Antimicrob Chemother 45:55-65, 2000.
Hammerschlag MR. Activity of gemifloxacin and other new quinolones against Chlamydia pneumoniae: A review. J Antimicrob Chemother 45:35-9, 2000.
Islinger F, Bouw R, Stahl M, et al. Concentrations of gemifloxacin at the target site in healthy volunteers after a single oral dose. Antimicrob Agents Chemother 48:4246-9, 2004.
Santos J, Aguilar L, Garcia-Mendez E, et al. Clinical characteristics and response to newer quinolones in Legionella pneumonia: a report of 28 cases. J Chemother 15:461-5, 2003.
Saravolatz LD, Leggett J. Gatifloxacin, gemifloxacin, and moxifloxacin: the role of 3 newer fluoroquinolones. Clin Infect Dis 37:1210-5, 2003.
Waites KB, Crabb DM, Duffy LB. Inhibitory and bactericidal activities of gemifloxacin and other antimicrobials against Mycoplasma pneumoniae. Int J Antimicrob Agents 21:574-7, 2003.
Wilson R, Langan C, Ball P, et al. Oral gemifloxacin once daily for 5 days compared with sequential therapy with I.V. ceftriaxone/oral cefuroxime (maximum of 10 days) in the treatment of hospitalized patients with acute exacerbations of chronic bronchitis. Respir Med 97:242-9, 2003.
Wilson R, Schentag JJ, Ball P, et al. A comparison of gemifloxacin and clarithromycin in acute exacerbations of chronic bronchitis and long-term clinical outcomes. Clin Ther 24:639-52, 2002.
Website: www.factive.com

"Usual dose" assumes normal renal/hepatic function. * For renal insufficiency, give usual dose x 1 followed by maintenance dose per CrCl. For dialysis patients, dose the same as for CrCl < 10 mL/min and give supplemental (post-HD/PD dose) immediately after dialysis. CrCl = creatinine clearance; CVVH = continuous veno-venous hemo-filtration; HD/PD = hemodialysis/peritoneal dialysis. See pp. 275-278 for explanations, p. 1 for abbreviations

Gentamicin (Garamycin)

Drug Class: Aminoglycoside
Usual Dose: 5-7 mg/kg (IV) q24h or 240 mg (IV) q24h (preferred over q8h dosing) (see comments)
Pharmacokinetic Parameters:
Peak serum levels: 4-8 mcg/ml (q8h dosing); 16-24 mcg/ml (q24h dosing)
Bioavailability: Not applicable
Excreted unchanged (urine): 95%
Serum half-life (normal/ESRD): 2.5/48 hrs
Plasma protein binding: < 5%
Volume of distribution (V_d): 0.3 L/kg
Primary Mode of Elimination: Renal
Dosage Adjustments (based on 5 mg/kg)*

CrCl 50–80 mL/min	2.5 mg/kg (IV) q24h or 120 mg (IV) q24h
CrCl 10–50 mL/min	2.5 mg/kg (IV) q48h or 120 mg (IV) q48h
CrCl < 10 mL/min	1.25 mg/kg (IV) q48h or 80 mg (IV) q48h
Post–HD dose	1 mg/kg (IV) or 80 mg (IV)
Post–PD dose	0.5 mg/kg (IV) or 40 mg (IV)
CVVH dose	2.5 mg/kg (IV) or 120 mg (IV) q24h
Moderate hepatic insufficiency	No change
Severe hepatic insufficiency	No change

Drug Interactions: Amphotericin B, cephalothin, cyclosporine, enflurane, methoxyflurane, NSAIDs, polymyxin B, radiographic contrast, vancomycin (↑ nephrotoxicity); cis-platinum (↑ nephrotoxicity, ↑ ototoxicity); loop diuretics (↑ ototoxicity); neuromuscular blocking agents, magnesium sulfate (↑ apnea, prolonged paralysis); non-polarizing muscle relaxants (↑ apnea)

Adverse Effects: Neuromuscular blockade with rapid infusion/absorption. Nephrotoxicity only with prolonged/extremely high serum trough levels; may cause reversible non–oliguric renal failure (ATN). Ototoxicity associated with prolonged/extremely high peak serum levels (usually irreversible): Cochlear toxicity (1/3 of ototoxicity) manifests as decreased high frequency hearing, but deafness is unusual. Vestibular toxicity (2/3 of ototoxicity) develops before ototoxicity, and typically manifests as tinnitus
Allergic Potential: Low
Safety in Pregnancy: C
Comments: Dose for synergy = 2.5 mg/kg (IV) q24h or 120 mg (IV) q24h. Single daily dosing greatly reduces nephrotoxic/ototoxic potential. Incompatible with solutions containing β–lactams, erythromycin, chloramphenicol, furosemide, sodium bicarbonate. IV infusion should be given slowly over 1 hour. May be given IM. Avoid intraperitoneal infusion due to risk of neuromuscular blockade. Avoid intratracheal/aerosolized intrapulmonary instillation, which predisposes to antibiotic resistance. V_d increases with edema/ascites, trauma, burns, cystic fibrosis; may require ↑ dose. V_d decreases with dehydration, obesity; may require ↓ dose. Renal cast counts are the best indicator of aminoglycoside nephrotoxicity, not serum creatinine. Dialysis removes ~ 1/3 of gentamicin from serum. CAPD dose: 2-4 mg/L dialysate (IP) with each exchange
Therapeutic Serum Concentrations
(for therapeutic efficacy, not toxicity):
Peak (q24h/q8h dosing) = 16-24/8-10 mcg/ml
Trough (q24h/q8h dosing) = 0/1-2 mcg/ml
Intrathecal (IT) dose = 5 mg (IT) q24h
Cerebrospinal Fluid Penetration:
Non-inflamed meninges = 0%
Inflamed meninges = 20%
Bile Penetration: 30%

REFERENCES:
Cornely OA, Bethe U, Seifert H, et al. A randomized monocentric trial in febrile neutropenic patients: ceftriaxone and gentamicin vs cefepime and gentamicin. Ann Hematol 81:37-43, 2002.

"Usual dose" assumes normal renal/hepatic function. * For renal insufficiency, give usual dose x 1 followed by maintenance dose per CrCl. For dialysis patients, dose the same as for CrCl < 10 mL/min and give supplemental (post-HD/PD dose) immediately after dialysis. CrCl = creatinine clearance; CVVH = continuous veno-venous hemofiltration; HD/PD = hemodialysis/peritoneal dialysis. See pp. 275-278 for explanations, p. 1 for abbreviations

Cunha BA. Aminoglycosides: Current role in antimicrobial therapy. Pharmacotherapy 8:334-50, 1988.

Edson RS, Terrell CL. The aminoglycosides. Mayo Clin Proc 74:519-28, 1999.

Freeman CD, Nicolau DP, Belliveau PP, et al. Once-daily dosing of aminoglycosides: Review and recommendations for clinical practice. J Antimicrob Chemother 39:677-86, 1997.

Imipenem/Cilastatin (Primaxin)

Drug Class: Carbapenem
Usual Dose: 500 mg (IV) q6h (see comments)
Pharmacokinetic Parameters:
Peak serum level: 21-58 mcg/ml (500 mg dose)
Bioavailability: Not applicable
Excreted unchanged (urine): 70%
Serum half-life (normal/ESRD): 1/4 hrs
Plasma protein binding: 20% / 40% (cilastatin)
Volume of distribution (V_d): 0.2 L/kg
Primary Mode of Elimination: Renal
Dosage Adjustments* (based on 500 mg q6h and weight > 70 kg):

CrCl 50–80 mL/min	500 mg (IV) q6h
CrCl 10–50 mL/min	500 mg (IV) q8h
CrCl < 10 mL/min[†]	250 mg (IV) q12h
Post–HD dose	250 mg (IV)
Post–PD dose	250 mg (IV)
CVVH dose	500 mg (IV) q8h
Moderate hepatic insufficiency	No change
Severe hepatic insufficiency	No change

† *Avoid if CrCl ≤ 5 mL/min unless dialysis is instituted within 48 hours*

Drug Interactions: Cyclosporine (↑ cyclosporine levels); ganciclovir (↑ risk of seizures); probenecid (↑ imipenem levels)
Adverse Effects: Seizures, phlebitis
Allergic Potential: Low

Safety in Pregnancy: C
Comments: Imipenem:cilastatin (1:1). Infuse 500 mg (IV) over 20-30 minutes; 1 gm (IV) over 40-60 minutes. Imipenem is renally metabolized by dehydropeptidase I; cilastatin is an inhibitor of this enzyme, effectively preventing the metabolism of imipenem. Imipenem/cilastatin can be given IM (IM absorption: imipenem 75%; cilastatin 100%). For fully susceptible organisms, use 500 mg (IV) q6h; for moderately susceptible organisms (e.g., P. aeruginosa), use 1 gm (IV) q6-8h. Incompatible in solutions containing vancomycin or metronidazole. Seizures more likely in renal insufficiency/high doses (> 2 gm/d). Inhibits endotoxin release from gram-negative bacilli. May cross react with beta-lactams. Na^+ content = 3.2 mEq/gm
Cerebrospinal Fluid Penetration:
Non-inflamed meninges = 10%
Inflamed meninges = 15%
Bile Penetration: 1%

REFERENCES:
Balfour JA, Bryson HM, Brogden RN. Imipenem/cilastatin: An update of its antibacterial activity, pharmacokinetics, and therapeutic efficacy in the treatment of serious infections. Drugs 51:99-136, 1996.

Barza M. Imipenem: First of a new class of beta-lactam antibiotics. Ann Intern Med 103:552-60, 1985.

Bernabeu-Wittel M, Pichardo C, Garcia-Curial A, et al. Pharmacokinetic/pharmacodynamic assessment of the in-vivo efficacy of imipenem alone or in combination with amikacin for the treatment of experimental multiresistant Acinetobacter baumannii pneumonia. Clin Microbiol Infect 11:319-25, 2005.

Choi JY, Soo Park Y, Cho CH, et al. Synergic in-vitro activity of imipenem and sulbactam against Acinetobacter baumannii. Clin Microbiol Infect 10:1089-1104, 2004.

Fish DN, Teitelbaum, I, Abraham E. Pharmacokinetics and pharmacodynamics of imipenem during continuous renal replacement therapy in critically ill patients. Antimicrobial Agents and Chemotherapy 49:2421-2428, 2005.

Helinger WC, Brewer NS. Carbapenems and monobactams: Imipenem, meropenem, and aztreonam. Mayo Clin Proc 74:420-34, 1999.

Website: www.pdr.net

"Usual dose" assumes normal renal/hepatic function. * For renal insufficiency, give usual dose x 1 followed by maintenance dose per CrCl. For dialysis patients, dose the same as for CrCl < 10 mL/min and give supplemental (post-HD/PD dose) immediately after dialysis. CrCl = creatinine clearance; CVVH = continuous veno-venous hemo-filtration; HD/PD = hemodialysis/peritoneal dialysis. See pp. 275-278 for explanations, p. 1 for abbreviations

Isoniazid (INH)

Drug Class: Anti–TB drug
Usual Dose: 5 mg/kg or 300 mg (PO) q24h
(see comments)
Pharmacokinetic Parameters:
Peak serum level: 7 mcg/ml
Bioavailability: 90%
Excreted unchanged (urine): 50-70%
Serum half-life (normal/ESRD): 1/1 hr
Plasma protein binding: 15%
Volume of distribution (V_d): 0.75 L/kg
Primary Mode of Elimination: Hepatic
Dosage Adjustments*

CrCl 50–80 mL/min	No change
CrCl 10–50 mL/min	No change
CrCl < 10 mL/min	No change
Post–HD dose	300 mg
Post–PD dose	300 mg
CVVH dose	None
Moderate hepatic insufficiency	No change
Severe hepatic insufficiency	No change

Drug Interactions: Alcohol, rifampin (↑ risk of hepatic injury); alfentanil (↑ duration of alfentanil effect); aluminum salts (↓ isoniazid absorption); carbamazepine, phenytoin (↑ interacting drug levels); itraconazole (↓ itraconazole levels); warfarin (↑ INR)
Adverse Effects: ↑ SGOT/SGPT, drug fever/rash, age-dependent hepatotoxicity (after age 40), drug–induced ANA/SLE, hemolytic anemia, neuropsychiatric changes in the elderly. Transient/reversible ↑ SGOT/SGPT frequently occur early (< 3 weeks) after INH use. If ↑ SGOT/SGPT, monitor twice weekly until levels peak, then monitor weekly until levels return to within normal range. Stop INH only if ↑ SGOT/SGPT ≥ 10 x upper limit of normal
Allergic Potential: Low
Safety in Pregnancy: C

Comments: Administer with 50 mg of pyridoxine daily to prevent peripheral neuropathy. Increased blood pressure/rash with tyramine–containing products, e.g., cheese/wine. ↑ hepatotoxicity in slow acetylators. Slow acetylator dose: 150 mg (PO) q24h. TB D.O.T. dose: 15 mg/kg or 900 mg (PO) 3x/week. Meningeal dose = usual dose
Cerebrospinal Fluid Penetration:
Non-inflamed meninges = 90%
Inflamed meninges = 90%

REFERENCES:
Ahn C, Oh KH, Kim K, et al. Effect of peritoneal dialysis on plasma and peritoneal fluid concentrations of isoniazid, pyrazinamide, and rifampin. Perit Dial Int. 23:362-7, 2003.
Colebunders R, Apers L, Shamputa IC. Treatment of multidrug-resistant tuberculosis. Lancet 10:1240, 2004.
Ena J, Valls V. Short-course therapy with rifampin plus isoniazid, compared with standard therapy with isoniazid, for latent tuberculosis infection: A meta-analysis. Clinical Infectious Diseases 40:670-6, 2005.
Schaller A, Sun Z, Yang Y, et al. Salicylate reduces susceptibility of Mycobacterium tuberculosis to multiple antituberculosis drugs. Antimicrob Agents Chemother 46:2533-9, 2002.
Schlossberg D. Treatment of multi-drug resistant tuberculosis. Antibiotics for Clinicians 9:317-321, 2005
Van Scoy RE, Wilkowske CJ. Antituberculous agents. Mayo Clin Proc 67:179-87, 1992.

Itraconazole (Sporanox)

Drug Class: Antifungal
Usual Dose: 200 mg (PO, capsules or solution, solution produces better absorption) q12h or q24h depending on disease; due to enhanced drug delivery, IV therapy begins with 200 mg IV q12h x 2 days (4 doses) and then continues with only 200 mg (IV) q24h; PO follow-up to IV therapy for serious infection is at 200 mg PO q12h. Each IV dose should be infused over 1 hour (see comments)
Pharmacokinetic Parameters:
Peak serum level: 2.8 mcg/ml
Bioavailability: 55% (capsules)/90% (solution)
Excreted unchanged (urine): 1%
Serum half-life (normal/ESRD): 21-64/35 hrs
Plasma protein binding: 99.8%

"Usual dose" assumes normal renal/hepatic function. * For renal insufficiency, give usual dose x 1 followed by maintenance dose per CrCl. For dialysis patients, dose the same as for CrCl < 10 mL/min and give supplemental (post-HD/PD dose) immediately after dialysis. CrCl = creatinine clearance; CVVH = continuous veno-venous hemo-filtration; HD/PD = hemodialysis/peritoneal dialysis. See pp. 275-278 for explanations, p. 1 for abbreviations

Volume of distribution (V_d): 10 L/kg
Primary Mode of Elimination: Hepatic; metabolized predominantly by the cytochrome P450 3A4 isoenzyme system (CYP3A4)
Dosage Adjustments*

CrCl 10–80 mL/min	No change
CrCl < 10 mL/min	No change
Post–HD dose	100 mg (IV/PO)
Post–PD dose	None
Post–CVVH dose	None
Moderate or severe hepatic insufficiency	No change†

† ↑ $t_{1/2}$ of itraconazole in patients with hepatic insufficiency should be considered when given with medications metabolized by P450 isoenzymes. Also see Adverse Effects for information regarding patients who develop liver dysfunction.

Drug Interactions: *Itraconazole may ↑ plasma levels of:* alfentanil, buspirone, busulfan, carbamazepine, cisapride, cyclosporine, digoxin, dihydropyridines, docetaxel, dofetilide, methylprednisolone, oral hypoglycemics (↑ risk of hypoglycemia), pimozide, quinidine, rifabutin, saquinavir, sirolimus, tacrolimus, trimetrexate, verapamil, vinca alkaloids, warfarin; alprazolam, diazepam, midazolam, triazolam (↑ sedative/hypnotic effects); atorvastatin, lovastatin, simvastatin (↑ risk of rhabdomyolysis); indinavir, ritonavir, saquinavir; coadministration of oral midazolam, triazolam, lovastatin, or simvastatin with itraconazole is contraindicated; coadministration of cisapride, pimozide, quinidine, or dofetilide with itraconazole is contraindicated due to the risk of ↑ QTc/life-threatening ventricular arrhythmias. *Decreased itraconazole levels may occur with:* antacids, carbamazepine, H_2-receptor antagonists, isoniazid, nevirapine, phenobarbital, phenytoin, proton pump inhibitors, rifabutin, rifampin; coadministration of rifampin with itraconazole is not recommended. *Increased itraconazole levels*

may occur with: clarithromycin, erythromycin, indinavir, ritonavir
Adverse Effects: ≥ 2%: nausea, diarrhea, vomiting, headache, abdominal pain, bilirubinemia, rash, ↑ SGPT/SGOT, hypokalemia, ↑ serum creatinine. Rarely, itraconazole has been associated with serious hepatotoxicity (liver failure/death). If liver disease develops, discontinue treatment, perform liver function testing, and reevaluate risk/benefit of further treatment. Use itraconazole with caution in patients with ↑ liver enzymes, active liver disease, or previous drug-induced hepatotoxicity. Life-threatening ventricular arrhythmias/sudden death have occurred in patients using cisapride, pimozide, or quinidine concomitantly with itraconazole; coadministration of these drugs with itraconazole is contraindicated. Use itraconazole with caution in patients with ventricular dysfunction. IV itraconazole may cause transient, asymptomatic ↓ in ejection fraction for ≤ 12 hours. If CHF develops, consider discontinuation of itraconazole
Allergic Potential: Low
Safety in Pregnancy: C
Comments: *Oral itraconazole:* Requires gastric acidity for absorption. When antacids are required, administer ≥ 1 hour before or 2 hours after itraconazole capsules. Oral solution is better absorbed without food; capsules are better absorbed with food. Capsule bioavailability is food dependent: 40% fasting/90% post-prandial. For oral therapy, bioavailability of 10 ml of solution without food = 100 mg capsule with food. Administer with a cola beverage in patients with achlorhydria or taking H_2-receptor antagonists/other gastric acid suppressors. Oral solution produces more reliable blood levels and is preferred for oral/esophageal candidiasis where the local effect of the solution on the infection seem helpful. *IV itraconazole:* Hydroxypropyl-β-cyclodextrin stabilizer in IV formulation accumulates in renal failure. IV itraconazole should not be used in patients with CrCl < 30 mL/min; if possible, use the oral preparation. Infuse 60 ml of dilute solution (3.33 mg/ml = 200 mg itraconazole, pH ~ 4.8) IV over 60

"Usual dose" assumes normal renal/hepatic function. * For renal insufficiency, give usual dose x 1 followed by maintenance dose per CrCl. For dialysis patients, dose the same as for CrCl < 10 mL/min and give supplemental (post-HD/PD dose) immediately after dialysis. CrCl = creatinine clearance; CVVH = continuous veno-venous hemo-filtration; HD/PD = hemodialysis/peritoneal dialysis. See pp. 275-278 for explanations, p. 1 for abbreviations

minutes, using infusion set provided. After administration, flush the infusion set with 15-20 ml of normal saline injection. The compatibility of IV itraconazole with flush solutions other than normal saline is unknown.
Cerebrospinal Fluid Penetration: < 10%

REFERENCES:
Conte JE Jr, Golden JA, Kipps J, et al. Intrapulmonary pharmacokinetics and pharmacodynamics of itraconazole and 14-hydroxyitraconazol steady state. Antimicrob Agents Chemother 48:3823-7, 2004.
Go J, Cunha BA. Itraconazole. Antibiotics for Clinicians 3:61-70, 1999.
Lewis, RE, Wiederhold NP, Klepser ME. In vitro pharmacodynamics of amphotericin B, itraconazole, and voriconazole against candida, fusarium, and scedosporium spp. Antimicrobial Agents and Chemotherapy 49:945-951, 2005.
Mosquera J, Shartt A, Moore CB, et al. In vitro interaction of terbinafine with itraconazole, fluconazole, amphotericin B and 5-flucytosine against Aspergillus spp. J Antimicrob Chemother 50:189-94, 2002.
Rubin MA, Carroll KC, Cahill BC. Caspofungin in combination with itraconazole for the treatment of invasive aspergillosis in humans. Clin Infect Dis 34:1160-1, 2002.
Terrell CL. Antifungal agents Part II. The azoles. Mayo Clin Proc 74:78-100, 1999.
Winston DJ, Busuttil RW. Randomized controlled trial of oral itraconazole solution versus intravenous/oral fluconazole for prevention of fungal infections in liver transplant recipients. Transplantation 74:688-95, 2002.
Website: www.pdr.net

Ketoconazole (Nizoral)

Drug Class: Antifungal
Usual Dose: 200 mg (PO) q24h
Pharmacokinetic Parameters:
Peak serum level: 3.5 mcg/ml
Bioavailability: 82%
Excreted unchanged (urine): 70%
Serum half-life (normal/ESRD): 6/20 hrs
Plasma protein binding: 99%
Volume of distribution (V_d): 2 L/kg
Primary Mode of Elimination: Hepatic

Dosage Adjustments*

CrCl > 40 mL/min	No change
CrCl < 40 mL/min	No change
Post–HD/Post-PD dose	None
CVVH dose	No change
Moderate hepatic insufficiency	No information
Severe hepatic insufficiency	Avoid

Drug Interactions: Astemizole, cisapride, terfenadine (may ↑ QT interval, torsades de pointes); carbamazepine, INH (↓ ketoconazole levels); cimetidine, famotidine, nizatidine, ranitidine, omeprazole, INH (↓ ketoconazole absorption); cyclosporine, digoxin, loratadine, tacrolimus (↑ interacting drug levels with possible toxicity); didanosine (↓ ketoconazole levels); midazolam, triazolam (↑ interacting drug levels, ↑ sedative effects); oral hypoglycemics (severe hypoglycemia); phenytoin, rifabutin, rifampin (↓ ketoconazole levels, ↑ interacting drug); statins (↑ statin levels; rhabdomyolysis reported); warfarin (↑ INR)
Adverse Effects: Nausea, vomiting, abdominal pain, pruritus
Allergic Potential: Low
Safety in Pregnancy: C
Comments: Dose-dependent reduction in gonadal (androgenic) function. Decreased cortisol production with doses ≥ 800 mg/day, but does not result in adrenal insufficiency. Give oral doses with citric juices
Cerebrospinal Fluid Penetration: < 10%

REFERENCES:
Como JA, Dismukes WE. Oral azole drugs as systemic antifungal therapy. N Engl J Med 330:263-72, 1993.
Lyman CA, Walsh TJ. Systemically administered antifungal agents : A review of their clinical pharmacology and therapeutic applications. Drugs 44:9-35, 1992.
Terrell CL. Antifungal agents: Part II. The azoles. Mayo Clin Proc 74:78-100, 1999.
Website: www.pdr.net

"Usual dose" assumes normal renal/hepatic function. * For renal insufficiency, give usual dose x 1 followed by maintenance dose per CrCl. For dialysis patients, dose the same as for CrCl < 10 mL/min and give supplemental (post-HD/PD dose) immediately after dialysis. CrCl = creatinine clearance; CVVH = continuous veno-venous hemofiltration; HD/PD = hemodialysis/peritoneal dialysis. See pp. 275-278 for explanations, p. 1 for abbreviations

Levofloxacin (Levaquin)

Drug Class: Fluoroquinolone
Usual Dose: 500-750 mg (IV/PO) q24h (see comments)
Pharmacokinetic Parameters:
Peak serum level: 5-8 mcg/ml
Bioavailability: 99%
Excreted unchanged (urine): 87%
Serum half-life (normal/ESRD): 7 hrs/prolonged
Plasma protein binding: 30%
Volume of distribution (V_d): 1.3 L/kg
Primary Mode of Elimination: Renal
Dosage Adjustments* (based on 500 mg q24h)

CrCl 50–80 mL/min	No change
CrCl 10–50 mL/min	250 mg (IV/PO) q24h
CrCl < 10 mL/min	250 mg (IV/PO) q48h
HD/CAPD	250 mg (IV/PO) q48h
Post–HD dose	250 mg (IV/PO)
Post–PD dose	250 mg (IV/PO)
CVVH dose	250 mg (IV/PO) q24h
Moderate hepatic insufficiency	No change
Severe hepatic insufficiency	No change

Drug Interactions: Al^{++}, Fe^{++}, Mg^{++}, Zn^{++} antacids (↓ absorption of levofloxacin if taken together); NSAIDs (CNS stimulation); probenecid (↑ levofloxacin levels); warfarin (↑ INR)
Adverse Effects: Mild nausea, diarrhea, rash. Does not lower seizure threshold or cause seizures
Allergic Potential: Low
Safety in Pregnancy: C
Comments: Low incidence of GI side effects. Take 2 hours before or after aluminum/magnesium-containing antacids. Does not increase digoxin concentrations. May potentially lower seizure threshold or prolong the QTc interval, particularly in patients with predisposing conditions. Acute bacterial sinusitis dose: 750 mg (PO) q24h x 5 days. Community-acquired pneumonia dose: 750 mg (IV/PO) q24h x 5 days. Nosocomial pneumonia dose: 750 mg (IV/PO) q24h x 7-14 days.
Cerebrospinal Fluid Penetration: 16%

REFERENCES:
Alvarez-Lerma F, Palomar M, Olaechea P, et al. Levofloxacin in the treatment of pneumonia in intensive care unit patients. Journal of Chemotherapy 16:549-556, 2004.
Benko R, Matuz M, Doro P, et al. Pharmacokinetics and pharmacodynamics of levofloxacin in critically ill patients with ventilator-associated pneumonia. Int J Antimicrob Agents 30:162-168, 2007.
Burgess DS, Hall RG 2nd. Simulated comparison of the pharmacodynamics of ciprofloxacin and levofloxacin against Pseudomonas aeruginosa using pharmacokinetic data from healthy volunteers and 2002 minimum inhibitory concentration data. Clin Ther 29:1421-1427, 2007.
Croom KF, Goa KL. Levofloxacin: a review of its use in the treatment of bacterial infections in the United States. Drugs 63:2769-802, 2003.
Dunbar LM, Wunderink RG, Habib MP, et al. High-dose, short-course levofloxacin for community-acquired pneumonia: a new treatment paradigm. Clin Infect Dis 37:752-60, 2003.
File TM Jr, Milkovich G, Tennenberg AM, et al. Clinical implications of 750 mg, 5-day levofloxacin for the treatment of community-acquired pneumonia. Curr Med Res Opin 20:1473-81, 2004.
Fish DN. Levofloxacin: update and perspectives on one of the original 'respiratory quinolones'. Expert Rev Anti Infect Ther 1:371-87, 2004.
Furlanut M, Brollo L, Lugatti E, et al. Pharmacokinetic aspects of levofloxacin 500 mg once daily during sequential intravenous/oral therapy in patients with lower respiratory tract infections. J Antimicrob Chemother 51:101-6, 2003.
Garrison MW. Comparative antimicrobial activity of levofloxacin and ciprofloxacin against Streptococcus pneumoniae. J Antimicrob Chemother 52:503-6, 2003.
Golini G, Favari F, Marchetti F, Fontana R. Bacteriostatic and bactericidal activity of levofloxacin against clinical isolates from cystic fibrosis patients. Eur J Clin Microbiol Infect Dis 23:772-5, 2004.
Lee CK, Boyle MP, Diener-West M, et al. Levofloxacin pharmacokinetics in adult cystic fibrosis. Chest 131:796-802, 2007.
Marchetti F, Viale P. Current and future perspectives for levofloxacin in severe Pseudomonas aeruginosa infections. J Antimicrob Chemother 15:315-22, 2003.

"Usual dose" assumes normal renal/hepatic function. * For renal insufficiency, give usual dose x 1 followed by maintenance dose per CrCl. For dialysis patients, dose the same as for CrCl < 10 mL/min and give supplemental (post-HD/PD dose) immediately after dialysis. CrCl = creatinine clearance; CVVH = continuous veno-venous hemo-filtration; HD/PD = hemodialysis/peritoneal dialysis. See pp. 275-278 for explanations, p. 1 for abbreviations

Noreddin Am, Marras TK, Sanders K, et al. Pharmacodynamics target attainment analysis against Streptococcus pneumoniae using levofloxacin 500 mg, 750 mg and 1000 mg once daily in plasma (P) and epithelial lining fluid (ELF) of hospitalized patients with community acquired pneumonia (CAP). Int J Antimicrob Agents 24:479-84, 2004.

Pea F, Di Qual E, Cusenza A, et al. Pharmacokinetics and pharmacodynamics of intravenous levofloxacin in patients with early-onset ventilator-associated pneumonia. Clin Pharmacokinet 42:589-98, 2003.

Pea F, Marioni G, Pavan F, et al. Penetration of levofloxacin into paranasal sinuses mucosa of patients with chronic rhinosinusitis after a single 500 mg oral dose. Pharmacol Res 55:38-41, 2007.

Poole M, Anon J, Paglia M, et al. A trial of high dose, short-course levofloxacin for the treatment of acute bacterial sinusitis. Otolaryngol Head Neck Surg 134:10-17, 2006.

Schlossberg D. Treatment of multi-drug resistant tuberculosis. Antibiotics for Clinicians 9:317-321, 2005.

Website: www.levaquin.com

Linezolid (Zyvox)

Drug Class: Oxazolidinone
Usual Dose: 600 mg (IV/PO) q12h
Pharmacokinetic Parameters:
Peak serum level: 15-21 mcg/ml
Bioavailability: 100% (IV and PO)
Excreted unchanged (urine): 30%
Serum half-life (normal/ESRD): 6.4/7.1 hrs
Plasma protein binding: 31%
Volume of distribution (V_d): 0.64 L/kg
Primary Mode of Elimination:
Hepatic/metabolized
Dosage Adjustments*

CrCl 50–80 mL/min	No change
CrCl 10–50 mL/min	No change
CrCl < 10 mL/min	No change
Post–HD dose	600 mg (IV/PO)
Post–PD dose	None
CVVH dose	No change
Moderate hepatic insufficiency	No change

Severe hepatic insufficiency	No information

Drug Interactions: Pseudoephedrine, tyramine-containing foods (↑ risk of hypertensive crisis); serotonergic agents, e.g., SSRI's, tricyclic antidepressants (↑ risk of serotonin syndrome)
Adverse Effects: Mild, readily reversible thrombocytopenia, anemia, or leukopenia may occur after ≥ 2 weeks of therapy. Lactic acidosis (rare), optic/peripheral neuropathy (> 28 days of therapy, rare). Monitor visual function if symptomatic or therapy ≥ 2 weeks; monitor CBC weekly if therapy > 2 weeks
Allergic Potential: Low
Safety in Pregnancy: C
Comments: May be taken with or without food. Ideal for IV-to-PO switch programs. Unlike vancomycin, linezolid does not increase VRE prevalence and is available orally for MRSA, MRSE, and E. faecalis infections. Unlike quinupristin/dalfopristin, linezolid is active against E. faecalis and is available orally for MRSA, MRSE, and E. faecium (VRE) infections. Meningeal dose = usual dose
Cerebrospinal Fluid Penetration: 70%

REFERENCES:
Andes D, van Ogtrop ML, Peng J, et al. In vivo pharmacodynamics of a new oxazolidinone (linezolid). Antimicrob Agents Chemother 46:3484-3489, 2002.

Bolstrom A, Ballow CH, Qwarnstrom A, et al. Multicentre assessment of linezolid antimicrobial activity and spectrum in Europe: report from the Zyvox antimicrobial potency study (ZAPS-Europe). Clin Microbiol Infect 8:791-800, 2002.

Cercenado E, Garcia-Garrote F, Bouza E. In vitro activity of linezolid against multiple resistant gram-positive clinical isolates. J Antimicrob Chemother 47:77-81, 2001.

Conte JE Jr, Golden JA, Dipps J, et al. Intrapulmonary pharmacokinetics of linezolid. Antimicrob Agents Chemother 46:1475-80, 2000.

Go J, Cunha BA. Linezolid: A review. Antibiotics for Clinicians 4:82-88, 2000.

Hamel JC, Stapert D, Moerman JK, et al. Linezolid, critical characteristics. Infection 28:60-4, 2000.

Johnson JR. Linezolid versus vancomycin for methicillin-resistant Staphylococcus aureus infections. Clin Infect Dis. 36:236-7, 2003.

Li JZ, Willke RJ, Rittenhouse BE, et al. Approaches to analysis of length of hospital stay related to antibiotic

"Usual dose" assumes normal renal/hepatic function. * For renal insufficiency, give usual dose x 1 followed by maintenance dose per CrCl. For dialysis patients, dose the same as for CrCl < 10 mL/min and give supplemental (post-HD/PD dose) immediately after dialysis. CrCl = creatinine clearance; CVVH = continuous veno-venous hemofiltration; HD/PD = hemodialysis/peritoneal dialysis. See pp. 275-278 for explanations, p. 1 for abbreviations

therapy in a randomized clinical trial: linezolid versus vancomycin for treatment of known or suspected methicillin-resistant Staphylococcus species infections. Pharmacotherapy 22(2 Pt 2):45S-54S, 2002.

Moylett EH, Pacheco SE, Brown-Elliott BA, et al. Clinical experience with linezolid for the treatment of nocardia infection. Clin Infect Dis. 36:313-8, 2003.

Nasraway SA, Shorr AF, Kuter DJ, et al. Linezolid does not increase the risk of thrombocytopenia in patients with nosocomial pneumonia: comparative analysis of linezolid and vancomycin use. Clin Infect Dis 11:1609-16, 2003.

Paterson DL, Pasculle AW, McCurry K. Linezolid: the first oxazolidinone antimicrobial. Ann Intern Med. 139:863-4, 2003.

Plouffe JF. Emerging therapies for serious gram-positive bacterial infections: a focus on linezolid. Clin Infect Dis 4:144-9, 2000.

Saiman L, Goldfarb J, Kaplan SA, et al. Safety and tolerability of linezolid in children. Pediatr Infect Dis J. 22:S193-200, 2003.

San Pedro GS, Cammarata SK, Oliphant TH, Todisco T. Linezolid versus ceftriaxone/cefpodoxime in patients hospitalized for the treatment of Streptococcus pneumoniae pneumonia. Scand J Infect Dis 34:720-8, 2002.

Siegel RE. Linezolid to decrease length of stay in the hospital for patients with methicillin-resistant Staphylococcus aureus infection. Clin Infect Dis. 36:124-5, 2003.

Stalker DJ, Jungbluth GL. Clinical pharmacokinetics of linezolid, a novel oxazolidinone antibacterial. Clin Pharmacokinet. 42:1129-40, 2003.

Stevens DL, Dotter B, Madaras-Kelly K. A review of linezolid: the first oxazolidinone antibiotic. Expert Rev Anti Infect Ther 2:51-9, 2004.

Stevens DL, Herr D, Lampiris H, et al. Linezolid versus vancomycin for the treatment of methicillin-resistant Staphylococcus aureus infections. Clin Infect Dis 34:1481-90, 2002.

Wunderink RG, Rello J, Cammarata SK, et al. Linezolid vs vancomycin: analysis of two double-blind studies of patients with methicillin-resistant Staphylococcus aureus nosocomial pneumonia. Chest. 124:1789-97, 2003.

Website: www.zyvox.com

Loracarbef (Lorabid)

Drug Class: 2nd generation oral cephalosporin
Usual Dose: 400 mg (PO) q12h (see comments)
Pharmacokinetic Parameters:
Peak serum level: 14 mcg/mL
Bioavailability: 90%
Excreted unchanged (urine): 90%
Serum half-life (normal/ESRD): 1.2/32 hrs
Plasma protein binding: 25%
Volume of distribution (V_d): 0.35 L/kg
Primary Mode of Elimination: Renal
Dosage Adjustments*

CrCl 50–80 mL/min	No change
CrCl 10–50 mL/min	200 mg (PO) q24h
CrCl < 10 mL/min	200 mg (PO) q72h
Post–HD dose	400 mg (PO)
Post–PD dose	200 mg (PO)
CVVH dose	200 mg (PO) q12h
Moderate hepatic insufficiency	No change
Severe hepatic insufficiency	No change

Drug Interactions: None
Adverse Effects: Drug fever/rash, diarrhea
Allergic Potential: Low
Safety in Pregnancy: B
Comments: Take 1 hour before or 2 hours after meals. Community-acquired pneumonia dose: 400 mg (PO) q12h. Sinusitis/tonsillitis dose: 200 mg (po) q12h
Cerebrospinal Fluid Penetration: < 10%

REFERENCES:

Bandak SI, Turnak MR, Allen BS, et al. Assessment of the susceptibility of Streptococcus pneumoniae to cefaclor and loracarbef in 13 cases. J Chemother 12:299-305, 2000.

Gooch WM 3rd, Adelglass J, Kelsey DK, et al. Loracarbef versus clarithromycin in children with acute otitis media with effusion. Clin her 21:711-22, 1999.

Paster RZ, McAdoo MA, Keyserling CH. A comparison of a five-day regimen of cefdinir with a seven-day regimen of loracarbef for the treatment of acute exacerbations of chronic bronchitis. Int J Clin Pract 64:293-9, 2000.

Vogel F, Ochs HR, Wettich K, et al. Effect of step-down therapy of ceftriaxone plus loracarbef versus parenteral therapy of ceftriaxone on the intestinal

---

"Usual dose" assumes normal renal/hepatic function. * For renal insufficiency, give usual dose x 1 followed by maintenance dose per CrCl. For dialysis patients, dose the same as for CrCl < 10 mL/min and give supplemental (post-HD/PD dose) immediately after dialysis. CrCl = creatinine clearance; CVVH = continuous veno-venous hemo-filtration; HD/PD = hemodialysis/peritoneal dialysis. See pp. 275-278 for explanations, p. 1 for abbreviations

microflora in patients with community-acquired pneumonia. Clin Microbiol Infect 7:376-9, 2001. Website: www.pdr.net

Meropenem (Merrem)

Drug Class: Carbapenem
Usual Dose: 1 gm (IV) q8h (see comments)
Pharmacokinetic Parameters:
Peak serum level: 49 mcg/ml
Bioavailability: Not applicable
Excreted unchanged (urine): 70%
Serum half-life (normal/ESRD): 1/7 hrs
Plasma protein binding: 2%
Volume of distribution (V_d): 0.35 L/kg
Primary Mode of Elimination: Renal
Dosage Adjustments*

CrCl 25–50 mL/min	1 gm (IV) q12h
CrCl 10–25 mL/min	500 mg (IV) q12h
CrCl < 10 mL/min	500 mg (IV) q24h
Post–HD dose	500 mg (IV)
Post–PD dose	500 mg (IV)
CVVH dose	500 mg (IV) q12h
Moderate hepatic insufficiency	No change
Severe hepatic insufficiency	No change

Drug Interactions: Probenecid (↑ meropenem half-life by 40%)
Adverse Effects: Rarely, mild infusion site inflammation
Allergic Potential: Low
Safety in Pregnancy: B
Comments: No adverse effects with 2 gm (IV) q8h regimen used for cystic fibrosis/meningitis. No cross allergenicity with penicillins/β–lactams; safe to use in penicillin allergic patients. Meropenem (1 gm) may be given by rapid IV infusion over 15-30 minutes (C_{max} = 49 mcg/ml) or as a bolus IV injection over 3-5 minutes (C_{max} = 112 mcg/ml). Inhibits endotoxin release from gram-negative bacilli. Na^+ content = 3.92 mEq/g. Meningeal dose = 2 gm (IV) q8h
Cerebrospinal Fluid Penetration:
Non-inflamed meninges = 10%
Inflamed meninges = 15%

REFERENCES:
Berman SJ, Fogarty CM, Fabian T, et al. Meropenem monotherapy for the treatment of hospital-acquired pneumonia: results of a multicenter trial. J Chemother 16:362-71, 2004.
Cunha BA: The safety of meropenem in elderly and renally impaired patients. Intern J Antimicrob Ther 10:109-117, 1998.
Cunha BA. Cross allergenicity of penicillin with carbapenems and monobactams. J Crit Illness 13:344,1998.
Cunha BA. Pseudomonas aeruginosa: Resistance and therapy. Semin Respir Infect 17:231-9, 2002
Cunha BA. The use of meropenem in critical care. Antibiotics for Clinicians 4:59-66, 2000.
Erdem I, Kucukercan M, Ceran N. In vitro activity of combination therapy with cefepime, piperacillin-tazobactam, or meropenem with ciprofloxacin against multidrug-resistant Pseudomonas aeruginosa strains. Chemotherapy 49:294-7, 2003.
Fish DN, Singletary TJ. Meropenem: A new carba-penem antibiotic. Pharmacotherapy 17:644-69, 1997.
Garcia-Rodriguez JA, Jones RN. Antimicrobial resistance in gram-negative isolates from European intensive care units: data from the Meropenem Yearly Susceptibility Test Information Collection (MYSTIC) programme. J Chemother 14:25-32, 2002.
Hellinger WC, Brewer NS. Carbapenems and monobactams: Imipenem, meropenem, and aztreonam. Mayo Clin Proc 74:420-34, 1999.
Jaruratanasirikul S, Sriwiriyajan, Punyo J. Comparison of the pharmacodynamics of meropenem in patients with ventilator-associated pneumonia following administration by 3-hour infusion or bolus injection. Antimicrobial Agents and Chemotherapy 49:1337-39, 2005.
Kitzes-Cohen R, Farin D, Piva G, et al. Pharmacokinetics and pharmacodynamics of meropenem in critically ill patients. Int J Antimicrob Agents 19:105-10, 2002.
Lomaestro BM, Drusano GL. Pharmacodynamic evaluation of extending the administration time of meropenem using a Monte Carlo simulation. Antimicrobial Agents and Chemotherapy 49:461-463, 2005.
Mattoes HM, Kuti JL, Drusano GL, et al. Optimizing antimicrobial pharmacodynamics: dosage strategies for meropenem. Clin Ther 26:1187-98, 2004.
Rhomberg PR, Jones RN, Sades HS, et al. Antimicrobial resistance rates and clonality results from the

---

"Usual dose" assumes normal renal/hepatic function. * For renal insufficiency, give usual dose x 1 followed by maintenance dose per CrCl. For dialysis patients, dose the same as for CrCl < 10 mL/min and give supplemental (post-HD/PD dose) immediately after dialysis. CrCl = creatinine clearance; CVVH = continuous veno-venous hemo-filtration; HD/PD = hemodialysis/peritoneal dialysis. See pp. 275-278 for explanations, p. 1 for abbreviations

meropenem yearly susceptibility test information collection (MYSTIC) programed: report of year five (2003). Diagn Microbiol Infect Dis 49:273-81, 2004.

Sodhi M, Axtell SS, Callahan J, et al. Is it safe to use carbapenems in patients with a history of allergy to penicillin? J Antimicrob Chemother 54:1155-7, 2004.

Website: www.MerremIV.com

Minocycline (Minocin)

Drug Class: 2nd generation tetracycline
Usual Dose: 100 mg (IV/PO) q12h or 200 mg (IV/PO) q24h (see comments)
Pharmacokinetic Parameters:
Peak serum level: 4 mcg/mL
Bioavailability: 95%
Excreted unchanged (urine): 10%
Serum half-life (normal/ESRD): 15/18-69 hrs
Plasma protein binding: 75%
Volume of distribution (V_d): 1.5 L/kg
Primary Mode of Elimination: Hepatic
Dosage Adjustments*

CrCl > 50 mL/min	No change
CrCl 10–50 mL/min	No change
CrCl < 10 mL/min	No change
Post–HD/PD dose	None
CVVH dose	No change
Moderate hepatic insufficiency	No change
Severe hepatic insufficiency	100 mg (IV/PO) q24h

Drug Interactions: Antacids, Al^{++}, Ca^{++}, Fe^{++}, Mg^{++}, Zn^{++}, multivitamins, sucralfate (↓ minocycline absorption); isotretinoin (pseudotumor cerebri); warfarin (↑ INR)
Adverse Effects: Nausea, GI upset if not taken with food, hyperpigmentation of skin with prolonged use, vestibular toxicity (dizziness), photosensitivity rare
Allergic Potential: Low
Safety in Pregnancy: X
Comments: Infuse slowly over 1 hour. Dizziness due to high inner ear levels. Also effective

against Nocardia. Neuroborreliosis dose: 100 mg (PO) q12h (may be preferable to doxycycline). Meningeal dose = usual dose
Cerebrospinal Fluid Penetration:
Non-inflamed meninges = 50%
Inflamed meninges = 50%
Bile Penetration: 1000%

REFERENCES:
Klein NC, Cunha BA. New uses for older antibiotics. Med Clin North Am 85:125-32, 2001.
Lewis KE, Ebden P, Wooster SL, et al. Multi-system Infection with Nocardia farcinica-therapy with linezolid and minocycline. J Infect. 46:199-202, 2003.
Website: www.pdr.net

Moxifloxacin (Avelox)

Drug Class: Fluoroquinolone
Usual Dose: 400 mg (IV/PO) q24h (see comments)
Pharmacokinetic Parameters:
Peak serum level: 4.4 (IV)/4.5 (PO) mcg/mL
Bioavailability: 90%
Excreted unchanged (urine): 20%
Serum half-life (normal/ESRD): 12/12 hrs
Plasma protein binding: 50%
Volume of distribution (V_d): 2.2 L/kg
Primary Mode of Elimination: Hepatic
Dosage Adjustments*

CrCl 50–80 mL/min	No change
CrCl 10–50 mL/min	No change
CrCl < 10 mL/min	No change
Post–HD dose	None
Post–PD dose	None
CVVH dose	No change
Moderate hepatic insufficiency	No change
Severe hepatic insufficiency	No information

Drug Interactions: Al^{++}, Fe^{++}, Mg^{++}, Zn^{++} antacids, citrate/citric acid, dairy products (↓ absorption of fluoroquinolones only if taken

---

"Usual dose" assumes normal renal/hepatic function. * For renal insufficiency, give usual dose x 1 followed by maintenance dose per CrCl. For dialysis patients, dose the same as for CrCl < 10 mL/min and give supplemental (post-HD/PD dose) immediately after dialysis. CrCl = creatinine clearance; CVVH = continuous veno-venous hemo-filtration; HD/PD = hemodialysis/peritoneal dialysis. See pp. 275-278 for explanations, p. 1 for abbreviations

together); amiodarone, procainamide, sotalol (may ↑ QTc interval, torsade de pointes)

Adverse Effects: May ↑ QT_c interval > 3 msec. (as with other quinolones); avoid taking with medications that prolong the QT_c interval, and in patients with cardiac arrhythmias/heart block. Does not lower seizure threshold or cause seizures

Allergic Potential: Low

Safety in Pregnancy: C

Comments: Only quinolone with anti–B. fragilis activity. Metabolized to microbiologically-inactive glucuronide (M1)/sulfate (M2) conjugates. Take 4 hours before or 8 hours after calcium or magnesium containing antacids or didanosine. No interactions with oral hypoglycemics. C8-methoxy group increases activity and decreases resistance potential. TB dose (alternate drug in multidrug-resistant TB drug regimen): 400 mg (PO) q24h

Cerebrospinal Fluid Penetration: < 10%

REFERENCES:

Anzueto A, Niederman MS, Pearle J, et al. Community-Acquired Pneumonia Recovery in the Elderly Study Group. Community-Acquired Pneumonia Recovery in the Elderly (CAPRIE): efficacy and safety of moxifloxacin therapy versus that of levofloxacin therapy. Clin Infect Dis. 42:73-81, 2006.

Behra-Miellet J, Dubreuil L, Jumas-Bilak E. Antianaerobic activity of moxifloxacin compared with that of ofloxacin, ciprofloxacin, clindamycin, metronidazole and beta-lactams. Int J Antimicrob Agents 20:366-74, 2002.

Balfour JA, Wiseman LR. Moxifloxacin. Drugs 57:363-73, 1999.

Caeiro JP, Iannini PB. Moxifloxacin (Avelox): a novel fluoroquinolone with a broad spectrum of activity. Expert Rev Anti Infect Ther 1:363-70, 2004.

Drummond MF, Becker DL, Hux M, et al. An economic evaluation of sequential I.V./PO moxifloxacin therapy compared to I.V./PO co-amoxiclav with or without clarithromycin in the treatment of community-acquired pneumonia. Chest. 124:526-35, 2003.

Hoeffken G, Talan D, Larsen LS, et al. Efficacy and safety of sequential moxifloxacin for treatment of community-acquired pneumonia associated with atypical pathogens. Eur J Clin Microbiol Infect Dis 23:772-5, 2004.

Katz E, Larsen LS, Fogarty CM, et al. Safety and efficacy of sequential I.V. to P.O. moxifloxacin versus conventional combination therapies the treatment of community-acquired pneumonia in patients requiring initial I.V. therapy. J Emerg Med 27:554-9, 2004.

Klutman NE, Culley CM, Lacy ME, et al. Moxifloxacin. Antibiotics for Clinicians. 5:17-27, 2001.

Lode H, Grossman C, Choudhri S, et al. Sequential IV/PO moxifloxacin treatment of patients with severe community-acquired pneumonia. Respir Med. 97:1134-42, 2003.

Rijnders BJ. Moxifloxacin for community-acquired pneumonia. Antimicrob Agents Chemother 47:444-445, 2003.

Saravolatz LD, Leggett J. Gatifloxacin, gemifloxacin, and moxifloxacin: the role of 3 newer fluoroquinolones. Clin Infect Dis 37:1210-5, 2003.

Schentag JJ. Pharmacokinetic and pharmacodynamic predictors of antimicrobial efficacy: moxifloxacin and Streptococcus pneumoniae. J Chemother 14(Suppl 2):13-21, 2002.

Schlossberg D. Treatment of multi-drug resistant tuberculosis. Antibiotics for Clinicians 9:317-321, 2005

Speciale A, Musumeci R, Blandino G, et al. Minimal inhibitory concentrations and time-kill determination of moxifloxacin against aerobic and anaerobic isolates. Int J Antimicrob Agents 19:111-8, 2002.

Torres A, Muir JF, Corris P, et al. Effectiveness of oral moxifloxacin in standard first-line therapy in community-acquired pneumonia. Eur Respir J. 21:135-43, 2003.

Website: www.avelox.com

Nafcillin (Unipen)

Drug Class: Antistaphylococcal penicillin

Usual Dose: 2 gm (IV) q4h

Pharmacokinetic Parameters:

Peak serum level: 80 mcg/ml

Bioavailability: Not applicable

Excreted unchanged (urine): 10-30%

Serum half-life (normal/ESRD): 0.5/4 hrs

Plasma protein binding: 90%

Volume of distribution (V_d): 0.24 L/kg

Primary Mode of Elimination: Hepatic

Dosage Adjustments*

CrCl 10–80 mL/min	No change
CrCl < 10 mL/min	No change
Post–HD/PD dose	None
CVVH dose	No change

"Usual dose" assumes normal renal/hepatic function. * For renal insufficiency, give usual dose x 1 followed by maintenance dose per CrCl. For dialysis patients, dose the same as for CrCl < 10 mL/min and give supplemental (post-HD/PD dose) immediately after dialysis. CrCl = creatinine clearance; CVVH = continuous veno-venous hemo-filtration; HD/PD = hemodialysis/peritoneal dialysis. See pp. 275-278 for explanations, p. 1 for abbreviations

Moderate or severe hepatic insufficiency	No change

Drug Interactions: Cyclosporine (↓ cyclosporine levels); nifedipine, warfarin (↓ interacting drug effect)
Adverse Effects: Drug fever/rash, leukopenia
Allergic Potential: High
Safety in Pregnancy: B
Comments: Avoid oral formulation (not well absorbed/erratic serum levels). Na^+ content = 3.1 mEq/g. Meningeal dose = usual dose
Cerebrospinal Fluid Penetration:
Non-inflamed meninges = 1%
Inflamed meninges = 20%
Bile Penetration: 100%

REFERENCES:
Donowitz GR, Mandell GL. Beta-lactam antibiotics. N Engl J Med 318:419-26 and 318:490-500, 1993.
Wright AJ. The penicillins. Mayo Clin Proc 74:290-307, 1999.
Website: www.pdr.net

Oxacillin (Prostaphlin)

Drug Class: Antistaphylococcal penicillin
Usual Dose: 1-2 gm (IV) q4h
Pharmacokinetic Parameters:
Peak serum level: 43 mcg/ml
Bioavailability: Not applicable
Excreted unchanged (urine): 39-66%
Serum half-life (normal/ESRD): 0.5/1 hrs
Plasma protein binding: 94%
Volume of distribution (V_d): 0.2 L/kg
Primary Mode of Elimination: Renal
Dosage Adjustments* (based on 2 gm q4h):

CrCl 10–80 mL/min	No change
CrCl < 10 mL/min	No change
Post–HD dose	None
Post–PD dose	None
CVVH dose	No change
Moderate hepatic insufficiency	No change

Severe hepatic insufficiency	No change

Drug Interactions: Cyclosporine (↓ cyclosporine levels); nifedipine, warfarin (↓ interacting drug effect)
Adverse Effects: Drug fever/rash, leukopenia, ↑ SGOT/SGPT, interstitial nephritis
Allergic Potential: High
Safety in Pregnancy: B
Comments: Avoid oral formulation (not well absorbed/erratic serum levels). Na^+ content = 3.1 mEq/g. Meningeal dose = usual dose
Cerebrospinal Fluid Penetration:
Non-inflamed meninges = 1%
Inflamed meninges = 10%
Bile Penetration: 25%

REFERENCES:
Al-Homaidhi H, Abdel-Haq NM, El-Baba M, et al. Severe hepatitis associated with oxacillin therapy. South Med J 95:650-2, 2002.
Donowitz GR, Mandell GL. Beta-lactam antibiotics. N Engl J Med 318:419-26 and 318:490-500, 1993.
Jensen AG, Wachmann CH, Espersen F, et al. Treatment and outcome of Staphylococcus aureus bacteremia: a prospective study of 278 cases. Arch Intern Med 162:25-32, 2002.
Jones ME, Mayfield DC, Thronsberry C, et al. Prevalence of oxacillin resistance in Staphylococcus aureus among inpatients and outpatients in the United States during 2000. Antimicrob Agents Chemother 46:3104-5, 2002.
Wright AJ. The penicillins. Mayo Clin Proc 74:290-307, 1999.
Website: www.pdr.net

Penicillin G (various)

Drug Class: Natural penicillin
Usual Dose: 2-4 mu (IV) q4h (see comments)
Pharmacokinetic Parameters:
Peak serum level: 20-40 mcg/ml
Bioavailability: Not applicable
Excreted unchanged (urine): 80%
Serum half-life (normal/ESRD): 0.5/5.1 hrs
Plasma protein binding: 60%
Volume of distribution (V_d): 0.3 L/kg
Primary Mode of Elimination: Renal

"Usual dose" assumes normal renal/hepatic function. * For renal insufficiency, give usual dose x 1 followed by maintenance dose per CrCl. For dialysis patients, dose the same as for CrCl < 10 mL/min and give supplemental (post-HD/PD dose) immediately after dialysis. CrCl = creatinine clearance; CVVH = continuous veno-venous hemofiltration; HD/PD = hemodialysis/peritoneal dialysis. See pp. 275-278 for explanations, p. 1 for abbreviations

Dosage Adjustments*

CrCl 50–80 mL/min	2–4 mu (IV) q4h
CrCl 10–50 mL/min	1–2 mu (IV) q4h
CrCl < 10 mL/min	1 mu (IV) q6h
Post–HD dose	2 mu (IV)
Post–PD dose	0.5 mu (IV)
CVVH dose	2 mu (IV) q6h
Moderate hepatic insufficiency	No change
Severe hepatic insufficiency	No change

Drug Interactions: Probenecid (↑ penicillin G levels)
Adverse Effects: Drug fever/rash, E. multiforme/Stevens–Johnson syndrome; anaphylactic reactions (hypotension, laryngospasm, bronchospasm), hives, serum sickness
Allergic Potential: High
Safety in Pregnancy: B
Comments: Incompatible in solutions containing erythromycin, aminoglycosides, calcium bicarbonate, or heparin. Jarisch–Herxheimer reactions when treating spirochetal infections, e.g., Lyme disease, syphilis, yaws. Penicillin G (potassium): K^+ content = 1.7 mEq/g; Na^+ content = 0.3 mEq/g. Penicillin G (sodium): Na^+ content = 2 mEq/g. Syphilis doses: 1°, 2°, early latent syphilis: PCN benzathine 2.4 mu (IM) x 1 dose. Late latent syphilis: PCN benzathine 2.4 mu (IM) q8h once weekly x 3. Neurosyphilis PCN G 4 mu (IV) q4h x 2 weeks. Meningeal dose = 4 mu (IV) q4h
Cerebrospinal Fluid Penetration:
Non-inflamed meninges ≤ 1%
Inflamed meninges = 5%
Bile Penetration: 500%

REFERENCES:
Falco V, Almirante B, Jordano Q, et al. Influence of penicillin resistance of outcome in adult patients with invasive pneumococcal pneumonia. Is penicillin useful against intermediately resistant strains? J Antimicrob Chemother 54:481-8, 2004.
Giachetto G, Pirez MC, Nanni L, et al. Ampicillin and penicillin concentration in serum and pleural fluid of hospitalized children with community-acquired pneumonia. Pediatr Infect Dis J 7:625-9, 2004.
Steininger C, Allerberger F, Gnaiger E. Clinical significance of inhibition kinetics for Streptococcus pyogenes in response to penicillin. J Antimicrob Chemother 50:517-23, 2002.
Wright AJ. The penicillins. Mayo Clin Proc 74:290-307, 1999.

Pentamidine (Pentam 300, NebuPent)

Drug Class: Antiparasitic
Usual Dose: 4 mg/kg (IV) q24h (see comments)
Pharmacokinetic Parameters:
Peak serum level: 0.6-1.5 mcg/ml
Bioavailability: Not applicable
Excreted unchanged (urine): 50%
Serum half-life (normal/ESRD): 6.4/90 hrs
Plasma protein binding: 69%
Volume of distribution (V_d): 5 L/kg
Primary Mode of Elimination: Metabolized
Dosage Adjustments*

CrCl 50–80 mL/min	No change
CrCl 10–50 mL/min	No change
CrCl < 10 mL/min	No change
Post–HD dose	None
Post–PD dose	None
CVVH dose	No change
Moderate or severe hepatic insufficiency	No change

Drug Interactions: Alcohol, valproic acid, didanosine, (↑ risk of pancreatitis); foscarnet (severe hypocalcemia reported; do not combine); amphotericin B, aminoglycosides, capreomycin, cis-platinum, colistin, methoxyflurane, polymyxin B, vancomycin, other nephrotoxic drugs (↑ nephrotoxicity)

Adverse Effects: Rash, hypotension, hypocalcemia, hypoglycemia, ↑ creatinine, pancreatitis, local injection site reactions, severe leukopenia, anemia, thrombocytopenia, may ↑ QT_c interval with IV administration
Allergic Potential: High
Safety in Pregnancy: C
Comments: Well absorbed IM, but painful. Administer IV slowly in D_5W over 1 hour, not saline. Adverse effects with aerosolized pentamidine include chest pain, arrhythmias, dizziness, wheezing, coughing, dyspnea, headache, anorexia, nausea, diarrhea, rash, pharyngitis. If PCP patient also has pulmonary TB, aerosolized pentamidine treatments may expose medical personnel to TB via droplet inhalation. Nebulizer dose: Inhaled pentamidine isethionate (NebuPent) 300 mg monthly via Respirgard II nebulizer can be used for PCP prophylaxis, but is less effective than IV/IM pentamidine and is not effective against extrapulmonary P. carinii.
Cerebrospinal Fluid Penetration: < 10%

REFERENCES:
Chan C, Montaner J, LeFebvre BA, et al. Atovaquone suspension compared with aerosolized pentamidine for prevention of Pneumocystis carinii pneumonia in human immunodeficiency virus infected subsets intolerant of trimethoprim or sulfamethoxazole. J Infect Dis 180:369-376, 1999.
Goa KL, Campoli-Richards DM. Pentamidine isethionate: A review of its antiprotozoal activity, pharmacokinetic properties and therapeutic use in Pneumocystis carinii pneumonia. Drugs 33:242-58, 1987.
Guerin PJ, Alar P, Sundar S, et al. Visceral leishmaniasis: current status of control, diagnosis, and treatment, and a proposed research and development agenda. Lancet Infect Dis. 2:494-501, 2002.
Lionakis MS, Lewis RE, Samonis G, et al. Pentamidine is active in vitro against Fusarium species. Antimicrob Agents Chemother. 47:3252-9, 2003.
Monk JP, Benfield P. Inhaled pentamidine: An overview of its pharmacological properties and a review of its therapeutic use in Pneumocystis carinii pneumonia. Drugs 39:741-56, 1990.
Rodriquez M, Fishman JA. Prevention of infection due to Pneumocystis spp. in human immunodeficiency virus-negative immunocompromised patients. Clin Microbiol Rev 17:770-82, 2004.
Sattler FR, Cowam R. Nielsen DM, et al. Trimethoprim-sulfamethoxazole compared with pentamidine for treatment of Pneumocystis carinii pneumonia in the acquired immunodeficiency syndrome. Ann Intern Med 109:280-7, 1988.
Website: www.pdr.net

Piperacillin (Pipracil)

Drug Class: Antipseudomonal penicillin
Usual Dose: 3 gm (IV) q4-6h (see comments)
Pharmacokinetic Parameters:
Peak serum level: 412 mcg/ml
Bioavailability: Not applicable
Excreted unchanged (urine): 50-70%
Serum half-life (normal/ESRD): 1/3 hrs
Plasma protein binding: 16%
Volume of distribution (V_d): 0.24 L/kg
Primary Mode of Elimination: Renal
Dosage Adjustments* (based on 4 gm q8h):

CrCl 50–80 mL/min	No change
CrCl 10–50 mL/min	3 gm (IV) q8h
CrCl < 10 mL/min	3 gm (IV) q12h
Post–HD dose	1 gm (IV)
Post–PD dose	2 gm (IV)
CVVH dose	3 gm (IV) q8h
Moderate or severe hepatic insufficiency	No change

Drug Interactions: Aminoglycosides (inactivation of piperacillin in renal failure); warfarin (↑ INR); oral contraceptives (↓ oral contraceptive effect); cefoxitin (↓ piperacillin effect)
Adverse Effects: Drug fever/rash, anaphylactic reactions (hypotension, laryngospasm, broncho-spasm), hives, serum sickness, leukopenia
Allergic Potential: High
Safety in Pregnancy: B
Comments: 75% absorbed when given IM. Do not mix/administer with aminoglycosides. Most active antipseudomonal penicillin against P. aeruginosa. Na^+ content = 1.8 mEq/g. Nosocomial pneumonia/P. aeruginosa dose: 3 gm (IV) q4h. Meningeal dose = usual dose
Cerebrospinal Fluid Penetration:

"Usual dose" assumes normal renal/hepatic function. * For renal insufficiency, give usual dose x 1 followed by maintenance dose per CrCl. For dialysis patients, dose the same as for CrCl < 10 mL/min and give supplemental (post-HD/PD dose) immediately after dialysis. CrCl = creatinine clearance; CVVH = continuous veno-venous hemo-filtration; HD/PD = hemodialysis/peritoneal dialysis. See pp. 275-278 for explanations, p. 1 for abbreviations

Non-inflamed meninges = 1%
Inflamed meninges = 30%
Bile Penetration: 1000%

REFERENCES:
Donowitz GR, Mandell GL. Beta-lactam antibiotics. N Engl J Med 318:419-26 and 318:490-500, 1993.
Kim MK, Capitano B, Mattoes HM, et al. Pharmacokinetic and pharmacodynamic evaluation of two dosing regimens for piperacillin-susceptible organisms. Pharmacotherapy 22:569-77, 2002.
Tan JS, File TM, Jr. Antipseudomonal penicillins. Med Clin North Am 79:679-93, 1995.
Website: www.pdr.net

Piperacillin/tazobactam (Zosyn, Tazocin)

Drug Class: Antipseudomonal penicillin
Usual Dose: 3.375 gm (IV) q6h (see comments)
Pharmacokinetic Parameters:
Peak serum level: 298/34 mcg/ml
Bioavailability: Not applicable
Excreted unchanged (urine): 60/80%
Serum half-life (normal/ESRD): [1.5/8] / [1/7] hrs
Plasma protein binding: 30/30%
Volume of distribution (V_d): 0.3/0.21 kg
Primary Mode of Elimination: Renal
Dosage Adjustments (see comments):

CrCl > 40 mL/min	No change
CrCl 20–40 mL/min	2.25 gm (IV) q6h
CrCl < 20 mL/min	2.25 gm (IV) q8h
Hemodialysis	2.25 gm (IV) q8h
Post–HD dose	0.75 gm (IV)
Post–PD dose	None
CVVH dose	2.25 gm (IV) q6h
Moderate or severe hepatic insufficiency	No change

Drug Interactions: Aminoglycosides (↓ aminoglycoside levels); vecuronium (↑ vecuronium effect); probenecid (↑ piperacillin/tazobactam levels); methotrexate (↑ methotrexate levels)

Adverse Effects: Drug fever/rash, eosinophilia, ↓/↑ platelets, leukopenia (with prolonged use > 21 days), ↑ PT/PTT, mild transient ↑ SGOT/SGPT, insomnia, headache, constipation, nausea, hypertension
Allergic Potential: High
Safety in Pregnancy: B
Comments: Dosage adjustments for P. aeruginosa/nosocomial pneumonia: For CrCl > 40 mL/min use 4.5 gm (IV) q6h. For CrCl 20-40 mL/min use 3.375 gm (IV) q6h. For CrCl < 20 mL/min use 2.25 gm (IV) q6h. For hemodialysis (HD) use 2.25 gm (IV) q8h; give 0.75 gm (IV) post-HD on HD days. Do not mix with Ringers lactate. Minimizes emergence of multi-drug resistant gram-negative rods and VRE. Na⁺ content = 2.4 mEq (54 mg)/g
Cerebrospinal Fluid Penetration:
Non-inflamed meninges = 1%
Inflamed meninges = 30%
Bile Penetration: 6000%

REFERENCES:
Buck C, Bertram N, Ackermann T, et al. Pharmacokinetics of piperacillin/tazobactam: intermittent dosing vs. continuous infusion. Int J Antimicrob Agents 25:62-7, 2005.
Florea NR, Kotapati S, Kuti JL, et al. Cost analysis of continuous versus intermittent infusion of piperacillin-tazobactam: a time-motion study. Am J Health Syst Pharm. 60:2321-7, 2003.
Fonseca AP, Extremina C, Fonseca AF, et al. Effect of subinhibitory concentration of piperacillin/tazobactam on Pseudomonas aeruginosa. J Med Microbiol 53(Pt 9):903-10, 2004.
Mattoes HM, Capitano B, Kim MK, et al. Comparative pharmacokinetic and pharmacodynamic profile of piperacillin/tazobactam 3.375 G Q4H and 4.5 G Q6H. Chemotherapy 458:59-63, 2002.
Minnaganti VR, Cunha BA. Piperacillin/tazobactam. Antibiotics for Clinicians 3:101-8, 1999.
Sanders WE Jr, Sanders CC. Piperacillin/tazobactam: A critical review of the evolving clinical literature. Clin Infect Dis 22:107-23, 1996.
Schoonover LL, Occhipinti DJ, Rodvold KA, et al. Piperacillin/tazobactam: A new beta-lactam/beta-lactamase inhibitor combination. Ann Pharmacother 29:501-14, 1995.
Winston LG, Charlebois ED, Pang S, et al. Impact of a formulary switch from ticarcillin-clavulanate to piperacillin-tazobactam on colonization with

---

"Usual dose" assumes normal renal/hepatic function. * For renal insufficiency, give usual dose x 1 followed by maintenance dose per CrCl. For dialysis patients, dose the same as for CrCl < 10 mL/min and give supplemental (post-HD/PD dose) immediately after dialysis. CrCl = creatinine clearance; CVVH = continuous veno-venous hemofiltration; HD/PD = hemodialysis/peritoneal dialysis. See pp. 275-278 for explanations, p. 1 for abbreviations

vancomycin-resistant enterococci. Am J Infect Control 32:462-9, 2004.
Website: www.zosyn.com

Polymyxin B

Drug Class: Cell membrane-altering antibiotic
Usual Dose: 1-1.25 mg/kg (IV) q12h (1 mg = 10,000 units) (see comments)
Pharmacokinetic Parameters:
Peak serum level: 8 mcg/ml
Bioavailability: Not applicable
Excreted unchanged (urine): 60%
Serum half-life (normal/ESRD): 6/48 hrs
Plasma protein binding: < 10%
Volume of distribution (V_d): No data
Primary Mode of Elimination: Renal
Dosage Adjustments*

CrCl 50–80 mL/min	0.5-1 mg/kg (IV) q12h
CrCl 10–50 mL/min	0.5 mg/kg (IV) q12h
CrCl < 10 mL/min	0.2 mg/kg (IV) q12h
Post–HD/PD dose	No information
CVVH dose	0.5 mg/kg (IV) q12h
Moderate or severe hepatic insufficiency	No change

Drug Interactions: Amphotericin B, amikacin, gentamicin, tobramycin, vancomycin (↑ nephrotoxicity)
Adverse Effects: Renal failure. Neurotoxicity associated with very prolonged/high serum levels; neuromuscular blockade potential with renal failure/neuromuscular disorders
Allergic Potential: Low
Safety in Pregnancy: B
Comments: Inhibits endotoxin release from gram-negative bacilli. Avoid intraperitoneal infusion due to risk of neuromuscular blockade. Increased risk of reversible non–oliguric renal failure (ATN) when used with other nephrotoxic drugs. No ototoxic potential. May be given IM with procaine, but painful. Nebulizer dose for multidrug resistant P. aeruginosa in cystic fibrosis/bronchiectasis: 80 mg in saline via aerosol/nebulizer q8h (for recurrent infection use 160 mg). Intrathecal (IT) polymyxin B dose = 5 mg (50,000 u) q24h x 3 days, then q48h x 2 weeks. Dissolve 50 mg (500,000 u) into 10 ml for IT administration
Cerebrospinal Fluid Penetration: < 10%

REFERENCES:
Bratu S, Quale J, Cebular S, et al. Multidrug-resistant Pseudomonas aeruginosa in Brooklyn, New York: molecular epidemiology and in vitro activity of polymyxin B. Eur J Clin Microbiol Infect Dis 24:196-201, 2005.
Evans ME, Feola DJ, Rapp RP. Polymyxin B sulfate and colistin: Old antibiotics for emerging multiresistant gram-negative bacteria. Ann Pharmacother 33:960-7, 1999.
Falagas ME, Kasiakou SK. Colistin: the revival of polymyxins for the management of multidrug-resistant gram-negative bacterial infections. Clin Infect Dis 40:1333-41, 2005.
Menzies D, Minnaganti VR, Cunha BA. Polymyxin B. Antibiotics for Clinicians 4:33-40, 2000.
Parchuri S, Mohan S, Young S, Cunha BA. Chronic ambulatory peritoneal dialysis associated peritonitis ESBL producing Klebsiella pneumoniae successfully treated with polymyxin B. Heart & Lung 34:360-363, 2005.
Segal-Maurer S, Mariano N, Qavi A, et al. Successful treatment of ceftazidime-resistant Klebsiella pneumoniae ventriculitis with intravenous meropenem and intraventricular polymyxin B: Case report and review. Clin Infect Dis 28:1134-8, 1999.

Posaconazole (Noxafil)

Drug Class: Antifungal (triazole)
Usual Dose: Available only as a 40 mg/mL oral solution. Daily dosage is 800 mg given in divided doses to optimize absorption. Usual regimen is 400 mg (PO) q12h with a meal or with 240 mL of a nutritional supplement. In patients who cannot tolerate oral feeding, dosing with 200 mg (PO) q6h produces adequate absorption. Concomitant antacid therapy should be avoided. Blood levels are not increased with higher dosages
Pharmacokinetic Parameters:
Peak serum level: steady state ~ 3 mcg/mL
Bioavailability: Unknown due to lack of IV formulation. Absorption is dramatically affected by food and dosing schedule. Administration

---

"Usual dose" assumes normal renal/hepatic function. * For renal insufficiency, give usual dose x 1 followed by maintenance dose per CrCl. For dialysis patients, dose the same as for CrCl < 10 mL/min and give supplemental (post-HD/PD dose) immediately after dialysis. CrCl = creatinine clearance; CVVH = continuous veno-venous hemo-filtration; HD/PD = hemodialysis/peritoneal dialysis. See pp. 275-278 for explanations, p. 1 for abbreviations

with food and in divided doses produces best systemic exposure
Excreted unchanged (feces): 66%
Serum half-life (normal/ESRD): 35 hrs (range 20–66 hrs)
Plasma protein binding: 98.2%
Volume of distribution (V_d): 1774 L
Primary Mode of Elimination: Principally excreted unchanged in feces. The major metabolite is a monoglucuronide of posaconazole. Posaconazole is not removed by dialysis

Dosage Adjustments*

CrCl 50–80 mL/min	No change
CrCl 10–50 mL/min	No change
CrCl < 10 mL/min	No change
Post–HD dose	None
Post–PD dose	None
CVVH dose	No information
Moderate or severe hepatic insufficiency	No guidance; exposure/half-life ↑ with hepatic impairment

Drug Interactions: Posaconazole is metabolized by hepatic glucuronidation. Inducers (e.g., rifampin, phenytoin) and inhibitors (e.g., cyclosporin, erythromycin) may alter disposition. Posaconazole also inhibits hepatic CYP3A4 and thus can increase exposure of drugs metabolized by that enzyme. Rifabutin, phenytoin (↓ posaconazole exposure 50%); H2 receptor antagonists (↓ posaconazole exposure); terfenadine, astemizole, cisapride, pimozide, halofantrine, quinidine (CYP3A4 substrates, ↑ interacting drug levels, ↑ risk of cardiac arrhythmias); ergot (↑ ergot levels and risk of ergotism); statins (↑ statin levels and risk of rhabdomyolysis); vinca alkaloids (↑ vinca alkaloid levels and risk of neurotoxicity); rifabutin (↑ rifabutin levels and risk of uveitis); cyclosporine, tacrolimus, sirolimus, midazolam and other benzodiazepines metabolized by CYP3A4, calcium channel blockers metabolized by CYP3A4 (diltiazem, verapamil, nifedipine, nisoldipine), digoxin, sulfonylureas (↑ interacting drug levels), HIV protease inhibitors (likely ↑ PI levels, not yet documented)
Adverse Effects: ↑ SGOT/SGPT; QTc/QT prolongation
Allergic Potential: Low
Safety in Pregnancy: C (likely to be D)
Comments: Clinical efficacy data based principally on open-label studies, although a recent study (Trends in Medical Mycology, 25 Oct 2005, Berlin) showed that posaconazole (200 mg 3x/d) significantly reduced the incidence of aspergillosis relative to fluconazole (400 mg daily) in hematopoietic stem cell transplant recipients with severe graft vs. host disease (and thus a high risk of invasive fungal infection). Registration is currently limited to the EU (marketing authorization granted Oct, 2005). Registration is pending with US FDA.
Cerebrospinal Fluid Penetration: Unknown

REFERENCES:
Chen A, Sobel JD. Emerging azole antifungals. Expert Opin Emerg Drugs 10:21-33, 2005.
Courtney R, Pai S, Laughlin M, et al. Pharmacokinetics, safety, and tolerability of oral posaconazole administered in single and multiple doses in healthy adults. Antimicrob Agents Chemother 47:2788-2795, 2003.
Courtney R, Radwanski E, Lim J, et al. Pharmacokinetics of posaconazole coadministered with antacid in fasting or nonfasting healthy men. Antimicrob Agents Chemother 48:804-808, 2004.
Courtney R, Sansone A, Smith W, et al. Posaconazole pharmacokinetics, safety, and tolerability in subjects with varying degrees of chronic renal disease. J Clin Pharmacol 45:185-192, 2005.
Courtney R, Wexler D, Radwanski E, et al. Effect of food on the relative bioavailability of two oral formulations of posaconazole in healthy adults. Brit J Clin Pharmacol 57:218-222, 2004.
Dodds Ashley ES, Alexander BD. Posaconazole. Drugs Today 41:393-400, 2005.
European Medicines Agency. Posaconazole SP European Public Assessment Report (EPAR). Accessed online at www.emae.eu.int on November 16, 2005.
Ezzet F, Wexler D, Courtney R, et al. Oral bioavailability of posaconazole in fasted healthy subjects - comparison between three regimens and basis for clinical dosage recommendations. Clin Pharmacokinet 44:211-220, 2005.

Golan Y. Overview of transplant mycology. Am J Health Syst Pharm 62:S17-21, 2005.

Herbrecht R, Nivoix Y, Fohrer C, et al. Management of systemic fungal infections: alternatives to itraconazole. J Antimicrob Chemother 56:139-148, 2005.

Keating GM. Posaconazole. Drugs 65:1553-69, 2005.

Krieter P, Flannery B, Musick T, et al. Disposition of posaconazole following single-dose oral administration in healthy subjects. Antimicrob Agents Chemother 48:3543-51, 2004.

Nagappan V, Deresinski S. Posaconazole: A broad-spectrum triazole antifungal agent. Clin Infect Dis 45:1610-1617, 2007.

Torres HA, Hachem RY, Chemaly RF, et al. Posaconazole: a broad-spectrum triazole antifungal. Lancet Infect Dis. 5:775-85, 2005.

van Burik JA. Role of new antifungal agents in prophylaxis of mycoses in high risk patients. Curr Opin Infect Dis 18:479-83, 2005.

Wexler D, Courtney R, Richards W, et al. Effect of posaconazole on cytochrome P450 enzymes: a randomized, open-label, two-way crossover study. Eur J Pharm Sci 21:645-653, 2004.

Pyrazinamide (PZA)

Drug Class: Anti-TB drug
Usual Dose: 25 mg/kg (PO) q24h (max. 2 gm) (see comments)
Pharmacokinetic Parameters:
Peak serum level: 30-50 mcg/ml
Bioavailability: 90%
Excreted unchanged (urine): 10%
Serum half-life (normal/ESRD): 9/26 hrs
Plasma protein binding: 10%
Volume of distribution (V_d): 0.9 L/kg
Primary Mode of Elimination: Hepatic
Dosage Adjustments*

CrCl < 80 mL/min	No change
Post–HD dose	25 mg/kg (PO) or 1 gm (PO)
Post–PD dose	No change
CVVH dose	No information
Moderate hepatic insufficiency	No information

Severe hepatic insufficiency	Avoid

Drug Interactions: INH, rifabutin, rifampin (may ↑ risk of hepatotoxicity)
Adverse Effects: Drug fever/rash, malaise, nausea, vomiting, anorexia, ↑ SGOT/SGPT, ↑ uric acid, sideroblastic anemia
Allergic Potential: Low
Safety in Pregnancy: C
Comments: Avoid in patients with gout (may precipitate acute attacks). TB D.O.T. dose: 4 gm (PO) 2x/week or 3 gm (PO) 3x/week. Meningeal dose = usual dose
Cerebrospinal Fluid Penetration: 100%

REFERENCES:
Ahn C, Oh KH, Kim K, et al. Effect of peritoneal dialysis on plasma and peritoneal fluid concentrations of isoniazid, pyrazinamide, and rifampin. Perit Dial Int. 23:362-7, 2003.

Davidson PT, Le HQ. Drug treatment of tuberculosis 1992. Drugs 43:651-73, 1992.

Drugs for tuberculosis. Med Lett Drugs Ther 35:99-101,1993.

Havlir DV, Barnes PF. Tuberculosis in patients with human immunodeficiency virus infection. N Engl J Med 340:367-73, 1999.

Iseman MD. Treatment of multidrug-resistant tuberculosis. N Engl J Med 329:784-91, 1993.

Ijaz K, McElroy PD, Navin TR. Short course rifampin and pyrazinamide compared with isoniazid for latent tuberculosis infection: a cost-effectiveness analysis based on a multicenter clinical trial. Clin Infect Dis 39:289, 2004.

Van Scoy RE, Wilkowske CJ. Antituberculous agents. Mayo Clin Proc 67:179-87, 1992.

Quinupristin/dalfopristin (Synercid)

Drug Class: Streptogramin
Usual Dose: 7.5 mg/kg (IV) q8h
Pharmacokinetic Parameters:
Peak serum level: 3.2/8 mcg/ml
Bioavailability: Not applicable
Excreted unchanged: 20% (urine); 80% (feces)
Serum half-life (normal/ESRD): [3.1/1]/[3.1/1] hrs
Plasma protein binding: 55/15%

Volume of distribution (V_d): 0.45/0.24 L/kg
Primary Mode of Elimination: Hepatic
Dosage Adjustments*

CrCl 50–80 mL/min	No change
CrCl 10–50 mL/min	No change
CrCl < 10 mL/min	No change
Post–HD dose	None
Post–PD dose	None
CVVH dose	No change
Moderate hepatic insufficiency	No change
Severe hepatic insufficiency	No information

Drug Interactions: Amlodipine (↑ amlodipine toxicity); astemizole, cisapride (may ↑ QT interval, torsades de pointes); carbamazepine (↑ carbamazepine toxicity: ataxia, nystagmus, diplopia, headache, seizures); cyclosporine, delavirdine, indinavir, nevirapine (↑ interacting drug levels); diazepam, midazolam (↑ interacting drug effect); diltiazem, felodipine, isradipine (↑ interacting drug toxicity: dizziness, hypotension, headache, flushing); disopyramide (↑ disopyramide toxicity: arrhythmias, hypotension, syncope); docetaxel (↑ interacting drug toxicity: neutropenia, anemia, neuropathy); lidocaine (↑ lidocaine toxicity: neurotoxicity, arrhythmias, seizures); methylprednisolone (↑ methylprednisolone toxicity: myopathy, diabetes mellitus, cushing's syndrome); nicardipine, nifedipine, nimodipine (↑ interacting drug toxicity: dizziness, hypotension, flushing, headache); statins (↑ risk of rhabdomyolysis)
Adverse Effects: Pain, inflammation, and swelling at infusion site (dose related), severe/prolonged myalgias, hyperbilirubinemia. Hepatic insufficiency increases concentration (AUC) of metabolites by 180%/50%
Allergic Potential: Low
Safety in Pregnancy: B

Comments: Administer in D_5W or sterile water, not in saline. Requires central IV line for administration. Does not cover E. faecalis
Cerebrospinal Fluid Penetration: < 10%

REFERENCES:
Abb J. Comparative activity of linezolid, quinupristin-dalfopristin and newer quinolones against Streptococcus pneumoniae. Int J Antimicrob Agents. 21:289-91, 2003.
Blondeau JM, Sanche Se. Quinupristin/dalfopristin. Expert Opin Pharmacother 3:1341-64, 2002.
Bryson HM, Spencer CM. Quinupristin/dalfopristin. Drugs 52:406-15, 1996.
Chant C, Ryback MH. Quinupristin/dalfopristin (RP 59500): A new streptogramin antibiotic. Ann Pharmacother 29:1022-7, 1995.
Goff DA, Sierawski SJ. Clinical experience of quinupristin-dalfopristin for the treatment of antimicrobial-resistant gram-positive infections. Pharmacotherapy 22:748-58, 2002.
Griswold MW, Lomaestro BM, Briceland LL. Quinupristin-dalfopristin (RP 59500): An injectable streptogramin combination. Am J Health Syst Pharm. 53:2045-53, 1996.
Nadler H, Dowzicky MJ, Feger C, et al. Quinupristin/dalfopristin: A novel selective-spectrum antibiotic for the treatment of multi-resistant and other gram-positive pathogens. Clin Microbiol Newslett 21:103-12, 1999.
Scotton PG, Rigoli R, Vaglia A. Combination of quinupristin/dalfopristin and glycopeptide in severe methicillin-resistant staphylococcal infections failing previous glycopeptide regimen. Infection 30:161-3, 2002.
Website: www.synercid.com

Rifampin (Rifadin, Rimactane)

Drug Class: Antibiotic/anti-TB drug
Usual Dose: 600 mg (PO) q24h (see comments)
Pharmacokinetic Parameters:
Peak serum level: 7 mcg/ml
Bioavailability: 95%
Excreted unchanged (urine): 15%
Serum half-life (normal/ESRD): 3.5/11 hrs
Plasma protein binding: 80%
Volume of distribution (V_d): 0.93 L/kg
Primary Mode of Elimination: Hepatic

"Usual dose" assumes normal renal/hepatic function. * For renal insufficiency, give usual dose x 1 followed by maintenance dose per CrCl. For dialysis patients, dose the same as for CrCl < 10 mL/min and give supplemental (post-HD/PD dose) immediately after dialysis. CrCl = creatinine clearance; CVVH = continuous veno-venous hemo-filtration; HD/PD = hemodialysis/peritoneal dialysis. See pp. 275-278 for explanations, p. 1 for abbreviations

Dosage Adjustments*

CrCl 50–80 mL/min	No change
CrCl 10–50 mL/min	No change
CrCl < 10 mL/min	No change
Post–HD dose	None
Post–PD dose	None
CVVH dose	No change
Moderate hepatic insufficiency	No change; use caution
Severe hepatic insufficiency	Avoid

Drug Interactions: Amprenavir, indinavir, nelfinavir (↑ rifampin levels); beta-blockers, clofibrate, cyclosporine, oral contraceptives, quinidine, sulfonylureas, tocainamide, warfarin (↓ interacting drug effect); caspofungin (↓ caspofungin levels, may ↓ caspofungin effect); clarithromycin, ketoconazole (↑ rifampin levels, ↓ interacting drug levels); corticosteroids (↑ corticosteroid requirement); delavirdine (↑ rifampin levels, ↓ delavirdine levels; avoid); disopyramide, itraconazole, phenytoin, propafenone, theophylline, methadone, nelfinavir, ritonavir, tacrolimus, drugs whose metabolism is induced by rifampin, e.g., ACE inhibitors, dapsone, diazepam, digoxin, diltiazem, doxycycline, fluconazole, fluvastatin, haloperidol, nifedipine, progestins, triazolam, tricyclics, zidovudine (↓ interacting drug levels); fluconazole, TMP-SMX (↑ rifampin levels); INH (INH converted into toxic hydrazine); mexiletine (↑ mexiletine clearance); nevirapine (↓ nevirapine levels; avoid)
Adverse Effects: Red/orange discoloration of body secretions, flu–like symptoms, ↑ SGOT/SGPT, drug fever, rash, thrombocytopenia
Allergic Potential: Moderate
Safety in Pregnancy: Probably safe
Comments: Potent CYP 3A4 inducer. Contraindicated in HIV. For anti–TB therapy, monitor potential hepatotoxicity with serial SGOT/SGPTs weekly x 3, then monthly x 3. Take 1 hour before or 2 hours after meals. TB D.O.T. dose: 10 mg/kg or 600 mg (PO) 2-3x/week. As an anti-staphylococcal drug (with another anti-staph antibiotic); give as 300 mg (PO) q12h. MSSA nasal carriage dose: 600 mg (PO) q12h x 72 hours. Meningeal dose = usual dose
Cerebrospinal Fluid Penetration:
Non-inflamed meninges = 50%
Inflamed meninges = 50%
Bile Penetration: 7000%

REFERENCES:
Castahneira D. Rifampin. Antibiotics for Clinicians 6:89-100, 2001.
Centers for Disease Control and Prevention. Notice to readers: Updated guidelines for the use of rifabutin or rifampin for the treatment and prevention of tuberculosis among HIV-infected patients taking protease inhibitors or nonnucleoside reverse transcriptase inhibitors. MMWR 49:183-189, 2000.
Davidson PT, Le HQ. Drug treatment of tuberculosis 1992. Drugs 43:651-73, 1992.
Ena J, Valls V. Short-course therapy with rifampin plus isoniazid compared with standard therapy with isoniazid, for latent tuberculosis infection: a meta-analysis. Clin Infect Dis 40:670-6, 2005.
Giamarellos-Bourboulis EJ, Sambatakou H, Galani I, et al. In vitro interaction of colistin and rifampin on multidrug-resistant Pseudomonas aeruginosa. J Chemother. 15:235-8, 2003.
Havlir DV, Barnes PF. Tuberculosis in patients with human immunodeficiency virus infection. N Engl J Med 340:367-73, 1999.
Ijaz K, McElroy PD, Navin TR. Short course rifampin and pyrazinamide compared with isoniazid for latent tuberculosis infection: a cost-effectiveness analysis based on a multicenter clinical trial. Clin Infect Dis 39:289, 2004.
Lundstrom TS, Sobel JD. Vancomycin, trimethoprim - sulfamethoxazole, and rifampin. Infect Dis Clin North Am 9:747-67, 1995.
Panel on Clinical Practices for Treatment of HIV Infection. Guidelines for the use of antiretroviral agents in HIV-infected adults and adolescents. Department of Health and Human Services. www.aidsinfo.nih.gov/guidelines/. October 6, 2005.
Perlman DC, Segal Yoniah, Rosenkranz S, et al. The clinical pharmacokinetics of rifampin and ethambutol in HIV-infected persons with tuberculosis. Clin Infect Dis 41:1638-47, 2005.
Schlossberg D. Treatment of multi-drug resistant tuberculosis. Antibiotics for Clinicians 9:317-321, 2005.

"Usual dose" assumes normal renal/hepatic function. * For renal insufficiency, give usual dose x 1 followed by maintenance dose per CrCl. For dialysis patients, dose the same as for CrCl < 10 mL/min and give supplemental (post-HD/PD dose) immediately after dialysis. CrCl = creatinine clearance; CVVH = continuous veno-venous hemo-filtration; HD/PD = hemodialysis/peritoneal dialysis. See pp. 275-278 for explanations, p. 1 for abbreviations

Van Scoy RE, Wilkowske CJ. Antituberculous agents. Mayo Clin Proc 67:179-87, 1992.

Vesely JJ, Pien FD, Pien BC. Rifampin, a useful drug for nonmyocobacterial infections. Pharmacotherapy 18:345-57, 1998.

Website: www.pdr.net

Rimantadine (Flumadine)

Drug Class: Antiviral
Usual Dose: 100 mg (PO) q12h (see comments)
Pharmacokinetic Parameters:
Peak serum level: 0.7 mcg/ml
Bioavailability: 90%
Excreted unchanged (urine): 25%
Serum half-life (normal/ESRD): 25/38 hrs
Plasma protein binding: 40%
Volume of distribution (V_d): 4.5 L/kg
Primary Mode of Elimination: Hepatic
Dosage Adjustments*

CrCl 50–80 mL/min	No change
CrCl 10–50 mL/min	No change
CrCl < 10 mL/min	100 mg (PO) q24h
Post–HD dose	None
Post–PD dose	None
CVVH dose	None
Moderate hepatic insufficiency	No change
Severe hepatic insufficiency	100 mg (PO) q24h

Drug Interactions: Alcohol (↑ CNS effects); benztropine, trihexyphenidyl, scopolamine (↑ interacting drug effect: dry mouth, ataxia, blurred vision, slurred speech, toxic psychosis); cimetidine (↓ rimantadine clearance); CNS stimulants (additive stimulation); digoxin (↑ digoxin levels); trimethoprim (↑ rimantadine and trimethoprim levels)
Adverse Effects: Dizziness, headache, insomnia, anticholinergic effects (blurry vision, dry mouth, orthostatic hypotension, urinary retention, constipation)
Allergic Potential: Low
Safety in Pregnancy: C
Comments: Less anticholinergic side effects than amantadine. Patients ≥ 60 years old or with a history of seizures should receive 100 mg (PO) q24h. Influenza dose (prophylaxis): 100 mg (PO) q12h for duration of exposure/outbreak. Influenza dose (therapy): 100 mg (PO) q12h x 7 days. May improve peripheral airway function/oxygenation in influenza A
Cerebrospinal Fluid Penetration: No data

REFERENCES:
Antiviral drugs for prophylaxis and treatment of influenza. Med Lett Drugs Ther 46:85-7, 2004.

Dolin R, Reichman RC, Madore HP, et al. A controlled trial of amantadine and rimantadine in the prophylaxis of Influenza A infection. N Engl J Med 307:580-4, 1982.

Gravenstein S, Davidson HE. Current strategies for management of influenza in the elderly population. Clin Infect Dis 35:729-37, 2002.

Jefferson T, Deeks JJ, Demicheli V, et al. Amantadine and rimantadine for preventing and treating influenza A in adults. Cochrane Database Syst Rev 3:CD001169, 2004.

Keating MR. Antiviral agents. Mayo Clin Proc 67:160-78, 1992.

Schmidt AC. Antiviral therapy for influenza : a clinical and economic comparative review. Drugs 64:2031-46, 2004.

Wintermeyer SM, Nahata MC. Rimantadine: A clinical perspective. Ann Pharmacotherapy 29:299-310, 1995.

Website: www.pdr.net

Streptomycin

Drug Class: Anti-TB aminoglycoside
Usual Dose: 15 mg/kg (IM) q24h or 1 gm (IM) q24h (see comments)
Pharmacokinetic Parameters:
Peak serum level: 25-50 mcg/ml
Bioavailability: Not applicable
Excreted unchanged (urine): 90%
Serum half-life (normal/ESRD): 2.5/100 hrs
Plasma protein binding: 35%
Volume of distribution (V_d): 0.26 L/kg
Primary Mode of Elimination: Renal
Dosage Adjustments*

CrCl 50–80 mL/min	No change

"Usual dose" assumes normal renal/hepatic function. * For renal insufficiency, give usual dose x 1 followed by maintenance dose per CrCl. For dialysis patients, dose the same as for CrCl < 10 mL/min and give supplemental (post-HD/PD dose) immediately after dialysis. CrCl = creatinine clearance; CVVH = continuous veno-venous hemo-filtration; HD/PD = hemodialysis/peritoneal dialysis. See pp. 275-278 for explanations, p. 1 for abbreviations

CrCl 10–50 mL/min	15 mg/kg (IM) q72h or 1 gm (IM) q72h
CrCl < 10 mL/min	15 mg/kg (IM) q72h or 1 gm (IM) q72h
Post–HD dose	7.5 mg/kg (IM) or 500 mg (IM) 2-3 x/week
Post–PD dose	7.5 mg/kg (IM) or 500 mg (IM) or 20-40 mg/ml in dialysate q24h
CVVH dose	15 mg/kg (IM) or 1 gm (IM) q72h
Moderate hepatic insufficiency	No change
Severe hepatic insufficiency	No change

Drug Interactions: Amphotericin B, cephalothin, cyclosporine, enflurane, methoxyflurane, NSAIDs, polymyxin B, radiographic contrast, vancomycin (↑ nephrotoxicity); cis-platinum (↑ nephrotoxicity, ↑ ototoxicity); loop diuretics (↑ ototoxicity); neuromuscular blocking agents (↑ apnea, prolonged paralysis); non-polarizing muscle relaxants (↑ apnea)
Adverse Effects: Most ototoxic aminoglycoside (usually vestibular ototoxicity); least nephrotoxic aminoglycoside
Allergic Potential: Low
Safety in Pregnancy: D
Comments: May be given IV slowly over 1 hour. TB D.O.T. dose: 20-30 mg/kg (IM) 2-3x/week. Dose for tularemia: 1 gm (IV/IM) q12h. Dose for plague: 2 gm (IV/IM) q12h.
Cerebrospinal Fluid Penetration: 20%

REFERENCES:
Akaho E, Maekawa T, Uchinashi M. A study of streptomycin blood level information of patients undergoing hemodialysis. Biopharm Drug Dispos 23:47-52, 2002.
Davidson PT, Le HQ. Drug treatment of tuberculosis 1992. Drugs 43:651-73, 1992.
Morris JT, Cooper RH. Intravenous streptomycin: A useful route of administration. Clin Infect Dis 19:1150-1, 1994.
Van Scoy RE, Wilkowske CJ. Antituberculous agents. Mayo Clin Proc 67:179-87, 1992.
Ormerod P. The clinical management of the drug-resistant patient. Ann NY Acad Sci 953:185-91, 2001.

Telithromycin (Ketek)

Drug Class: Ketolide
Usual Dose: <u>Acute sinusitis/AECB</u>: 800 mg (PO) q24h x 5 days. <u>Community-acquired pneumonia</u>: 800 mg (PO) q24h x 7-10 days. 800 mg (PO) dose taken as two 400-mg tablets (PO) at once

Pharmacokinetic Parameters:
Peak serum level: 2.27 mcg/ml
Bioavailability: 57%
Excreted unchanged (urine): 13%
Serum half-life (normal/ESRD): 9.8/11 hrs
Plasma protein binding: 65%
Volume of distribution (V_d): 2.9 L/kg
Primary Mode of Elimination: Hepatic
Dosage Adjustments*

CrCl 30–80 mL/min	No change
CrCl 10–30 mL/min	600 mg (PO) q24h
CrCl < 10 mL/min	600 mg (PO) q24h
CrCl < 30 mL/min + hepatic impairment	400 mg (PO) q24h
Post–HD dose	No information
Post–PD dose	No information
CVVH dose	No information
Moderate hepatic insufficiency	No change
Severe hepatic insufficiency	No change

Drug Interactions: Digoxin (↑ interacting drug levels); ergot derivatives (acute ergot toxicity); itraconazole, ketoconazole (↑ telithromycin level); midazolam, triazolam (↑ interacting drug levels, sedation); oral anticoagulants (may ↑

"Usual dose" assumes normal renal/hepatic function. * For renal insufficiency, give usual dose x 1 followed by maintenance dose per CrCl. For dialysis patients, dose the same as for CrCl < 10 mL/min and give supplemental (post-HD/PD dose) immediately after dialysis. CrCl = creatinine clearance; CVVH = continuous veno-venous hemo-filtration; HD/PD = hemodialysis/peritoneal dialysis. See pp. 275-278 for explanations, p. 1 for abbreviations

anticoagulant effects; monitor PT/INR); simvastatin (↑ risk of rhabdomyolysis; giving simvastatin 12h after telithromycin decreases the ↑ in simvastatin levels ~ 50%); theophylline (additive nausea). CYP 3A4 inhibitor/substate. Telithromycin is contraindicated with cisapride and pimozide

Adverse Effects: Nausea, diarrhea, dizziness, syncope. Contraindicated in patients with history of hepatitis/jaundice (rarely fatal acute/fulminant hepatitis or acute liver failure). Avoid with myasthenia gravis (↑ risk of respiratory failure)

Resistance Potential: Low
Allergic Potential: Low
Safety in Pregnancy: C
Comments: May take with or without food. New smaller tablets minimize potential GI upset

REFERENCES:
Aubier M, Aldons PM, Leak A, et al. Telithromycin is as effective as amoxicillin/clavulanate in acute exacerbations of chronic bronchitis. Respir Med 96:862-71, 2002.
Brown SD, Farrell DJ. Antibacterial susceptibility among streptococcus pneumoniae isolated from paediatric and adult patients as part of the PROTECT US study in 2001-2002. Journal of Antimicrobial Chemotherapy 54 (Suppl. S1):23-29, 2004.
Brown SD, Rybak MJ. Antimicrobial susceptibility of streptococcus pneumoniae, streptococcus pyogenes and haemophilus influenzae collected from patients across the USA, in 2001-2002, as part of the PROTECT US study. Journal of Antimicrobial Chemotherapy 54 (Suppl. S1):7-15, 2004.
Carbon C, Moola S, Velancsics I, et al. Telithromycin 800 mg once daily for seven to ten days is an effective and well-tolerated treatment for community-acquired pneumonia. Clin Microbiol Infect 9:691-703, 2003.
Doern GV, Brown SD. Antimicrobial susceptibility among community acquired respiratory pathogens in the USA: data from PROTEKT US 2000-01. J Inf 48:56-65, 2004.
Dunbar LM, Carbon C, van Rensburg D, et al. Efficacy of telithromycin in community-acquired pneumonia caused by atypical and intracellular pathogens. Infect Dis Clin Pract 13:10-16, 2005 .
Ferguson BJ, Guzzetta RV, Spector SL, et al. Efficacy and safety of oral telithromycin once daily for 5 days versus moxifloxacin one daily for 10 days in the treatment of acute bacterial rhinosinusitis. Otolaryngol Head Neck Surg 131:207-14, 2004.
Hagberg L, Torres A, van Rensburg D, et al. Efficacy and tolerability of once-daily telithromycin compared with high-dose amoxicillin for treatment of community-acquired pneumonia. Infection 30:378-386, 2002.
Jacobs MR. In vivo veritas: in vitro macrolide resistance in systemic S. pneumoniae infections does result in clinical failure. Clin Infect Dis 35;565-9, 2002.
Klugman KP, Lonks JR. Hidden epidemic of macrolide-resistant pneumococci. Emerg Infect Dis 11:802-807, 2005.
Low DE, Brown S, Felmingham D. Clinical and bacteriology efficacy of the ketolide telithromycin against isolates of key respiratory pathogens: a pooled analysis of phase III studies. Clin Microbiol Infect 10:27-36, 2004.
Ortega M, Marco F, Almela M, et al. Activity of telithromycin against erythromycin-susceptible and -resistant Streptococcus pneumoniae is from adults with invasive infections. Int J Antimicrob Agents 24:616-8, 2004.
Roos K, Tellier G, Baz M, et al. Clinical and bacteriological efficacy of 5-day telithromycin in acute maxillary sinusitis: a pooled analysis. www.elsevierhealth.com/journals/jinf.
Tellier G, Niederman MS, Nusrat R, et al. Clinical and bacteriological efficacy and safety of 5 and 7 day regimens of telithromycin once daily compared with a 10 day regimen of clarithromycin twice daily in patients with mild to moderate community-acquired pneumonia. Journal of Antimicrobial Chemotherapy 54:515-523, 2004.
van Rensburg D, Fogarty C, De Salvo MC, et al. Efficacy of oral telithromycin in community-acquired pneumonia caused by resistant Streptococcus pneumoniae. Journal of Infection 51:201-5, 2005.
Zervos MJ, Heyder AM, Leroy B. Oral telithromycin 800 mg once daily for 5 days versus cefuroxime axetil 500 mg twice daily for 10 days in adults with acute exacerbations of chronic bronchitis. J Int Med Res 31:157-69, 2003.
Website: www.ketek.com

Ticarcillin (Ticar)

Drug Class: Antipseudomonal penicillin
Usual Dose: 3 gm (IV) q6h
Pharmacokinetic Parameters:
Peak serum level: 118-300 mcg/ml
Bioavailability: Not applicable
Excreted unchanged (urine): 95%
Serum half-life (normal/ESRD): 1/5 hrs
Plasma protein binding: 45%
Volume of distribution (V_d): 0.2 L/kg

"Usual dose" assumes normal renal/hepatic function. * For renal insufficiency, give usual dose x 1 followed by maintenance dose per CrCl. For dialysis patients, dose the same as for CrCl < 10 mL/min and give supplemental (post-HD/PD dose) immediately after dialysis. CrCl = creatinine clearance; CVVH = continuous veno-venous hemo-filtration; HD/PD = hemodialysis/peritoneal dialysis. See pp. 275-278 for explanations, p. 1 for abbreviations

Primary Mode of Elimination: Renal
Dosage Adjustments*

CrCl 50–80 mL/min	No change
CrCl 10–50 mL/min	2 gm (IV) q8h
CrCl < 10 mL/min	2 gm (IV) q12h
Post–HD dose	2 gm (IV)
Post–PD dose	3 gm (IV)
CVVH dose	2 gm (IV) q8h
Moderate hepatic insufficiency	No change
Severe hepatic insufficiency	No change

Drug Interactions: Aminoglycosides (inactivation of ticarcillin in renal failure); warfarin (↑ INR); oral contraceptives (↓ oral contraceptive effect); cefoxitin (↓ ticarcillin effect)
Adverse Effects: Drug fever/rash; E. multiforme/Stevens–Johnson syndrome, anaphylactic reactions (hypotension, laryngospasm, bronchospasm), hives, serum sickness. Dose-dependent inhibition of platelet aggregation is minimal/absent (usual dose is less than carbenicillin)
Allergic Potential: High
Safety in Pregnancy: B
Comments: Administer 1 hour before or after aminoglycoside. Na^+ content = 5.2 mEq/g. Meningeal dose = usual dose
Cerebrospinal Fluid Penetration:
Non-inflamed meninges = 1%
Inflamed meninges = 30%

REFERENCES:
Donowitz GR, Mandell GL. Beta-lactam antibiotics. N Engl J Med 318:419-26 and 318:490-500, 1993.
Tan JS, File TM, Jr. Antipseudomonal penicillins. Med Clin North Am 79:679-93, 1995.
Wright AJ. The penicillins. Mayo Clin Proc 74:290-307, 1999.

Ticarcillin/clavulanate (Timentin)

Drug Class: Antipseudomonal penicillin
Usual Dose: 3.1 gm (IV) q6h
Pharmacokinetic Parameters:
Peak serum level: 330 mcg/ml
Bioavailability: Not applicable
Excreted unchanged (urine): 95/45%
Serum half-life (normal/ESRD): [1/13]/[½] hrs
Plasma protein binding: 45/25%
Volume of distribution (V_d): 0.2/0.3 L/kg
Primary Mode of Elimination: Renal
Dosage Adjustments*

CrCl 50–80 mL/min	2 gm (IV) q4h
CrCl 10–50 mL/min	2 gm (IV) q8h
CrCl < 10 mL/min	2 gm (IV) q12h
Post–HD dose	2 gm (IV)
Post–PD dose	3.1 gm (IV)
CVVH dose	3.1 gm (IV) q8h
Moderate hepatic insufficiency	If CrCl < 10 mL/min: 2 gm (IV) q24h
Severe hepatic insufficiency	If CrCl < 10 mL/min: 2 gm (IV) q24h

Drug Interactions: Aminoglycosides (↓ aminoglycoside levels); methotrexate (↑ methotrexate levels); vecuronium (↑ vecuronium effect)
Adverse Effects: Drug fever/rash, E. multiforme/Stevens–Johnson syndrome, anaphylactic reactions (hypotension, laryngospasm, bronchospasm), hives, serum sickness
Allergic Potential: High
Safety in Pregnancy: B
Comments: 20% of clavulanate removed by dialysis. Na^+ content = 4.75 mEq/g. K^+ content = 0.15 mEq/g
Cerebrospinal Fluid Penetration: < 10%

REFERENCES:
Donowitz GR, Mandell GL. Beta-lactam antibiotics. N Engl J Med 318:419-26 and 318:490-500, 1993.
Itokazu GS, Danziger LH. Ampicillin-sulbactam and ticarcillin-clavulanic acid: A comparison of their in vitro activity and review of their clinical efficacy. Pharmacotherapy 11:382-414, 1991.
Wright AJ. The penicillins. Mayo Clin Proc 74:290-307, 1999.
Website: www.timentin.com

Tigecycline (Tygacil)

Drug Class: Glycylcycline
Usual Dose: 100 mg (IV) x 1 dose, then 50 mg q12h (IV)
Pharmacokinetic Parameters:
Peak serum level: 1.45 mcg/ml (100 mg dose); 0.87 mcg/ml (50 mg dose)
Bioavailability: Not applicable
Excreted unchanged (urine): 22%
Serum half-life (normal/ESRD): 42/42 hrs
Plasma protein binding: 89%
Volume of distribution (V_d): 8 L/kg
Primary Mode of Elimination: Biliary
Dosage Adjustments:

CrCl 50–80 mL/min	No change
CrCl 10–50 mL/min	No change
CrCl < 10 mL/min	No change
Post–HD dose	None
Post–PD dose	None
CVVH dose	No change
Moderate hepatic insufficiency	No change
Severe hepatic insufficiency (Child Pugh C)	100 mg (IV) x 1 dose, then 25 mg (IV) q12h

Drug Interactions: Warfarin (↑ INR). Does not inhibit and is not metabolized by CYP450
Adverse Effects: N/V, dyspepsia, diarrhea, dizziness, asthenia, ↑ SGOT, ↑ alkaline phosphatase, ↑ amylase, ↑ LDH, ↑ BUN, ↓ total protein

Allergic Potential: Low
Safety in Pregnancy: D
Comments: Use for complicated skin/skin structure infections and for complicated intraabdominal infections. Avoid use in patients < 18 years of age. Infuse over 30-60 minutes; mix with D5W or 0.9% NaCl. Safe to use in penicillin/sulfa-allergic patients
Cerebrospinal Fluid Penetration: No data
Bile Penetration: 3800%

REFERENCES:
Bendu C, Culebras E, Gomez M, et al. In vitro activity of tigecycline against Bacteroides species. J Antimicrob Chemother 56:349-52, 2005.
Biedenbach DJ, Beach ML, Jones RN. In vitro antimicrobial activity of GAR-936 tested against antibiotic-resistant gram-positive blood stream infection isolates and strains producing extended-spectrum beta-lactamases. Diagn Microbiol Infect Dis 40:173-7, 2001.
Bouchillon SK, Hoban DJ, Johnson BM, et al. In vitro evaluation of tigecycline and comparative agents in 3049 clinical isolates: 2001 to 2002. Diagn Microbiol Infect Dis 51:291-5, 2005.
Bradford PA. Tigecycline: A first in class glycylcycline. Clinical Microbiology Newsletter 26:163-168, 2004.
Bratu S, Tolaney P, Karumudi U, et al. Carbapenemase-producing Klebsiella pneumoniae in Brooklyn, NY: molecular epidemiology and in vitro activity of polymyxin B and other agents. J Antimicrob Chemother 56:128-32, 2005.
Cercenado E, Cercenado S, Gomez JA, et al. In vitro activity of tigecycline (GAR-936), a novel glycylcycline, against vancomycin-resistant enterococci and staphylococci with diminished susceptibility to glycopeptides. J Antimicrob Chemother 52:138-9, 2003.
Fritache TR, Kirby JT, Jones RN. In vitro activity of tigecycline (GAR-936) tested against 11,859 recent clinical isolates associated with community-acquired respiratory tract and gram-positive cutaneous infections. Diagn Microbiol Infect Dis. 49:201-9, 2004
Garrison MW, Neumiller JJ, Setter SM. Tigecycline: an investigational glycylcycline antimicrobial with activity against resistant gram-positive organisms. Clin Ther 27:12-22, 2005.
Kitzis MD, Ly A, Goldstein FW. In vitro activities of tigecycline (GAR-936) against multidrug-resistant Staphylococcus aureus and Streptococcus pneumoniae. Antimicrob Agents Chemother 48:366-7, 2004.

Meagher AK, Ambrose PG, Grasela TH, et al. The pharmacokinetic and pharmacodynamic profile of tigecycline. Clin Infect Dis 41(Suppl 5):S333-40, 2005.

Milarovic D, Schmitz FJ, Verhoef, et al. Activities of the glycylcycline tigecycline (GAR-936) against 1,924 recent European clinical bacterial isolates. Antimicrob Agents Chemother 47:400-4, 2003.

Muralidharan G, Fruncillo RJ, Micalizzi M, et al. Effects of age and sex on single-dose pharmacokinetics of tigecycline in healthy subjects. Antimicrob Agents Chemother 49:1656-1659, 2005.

Muralidharan G, Micalizzi M, Speth J, et al. Pharmacokinetics of tigecycline after single and multiple doses in healthy subjects. Antimicrob Agents Chemother 49:220-9, 2005.

Noskin GA. Tigecycline: a new glycylcycline for treatment of serious infections. Clin Infect Dis 41(Suppl 5):S303-14, 2005.

Pachon-Ibanez ME, Jimenez-Melias MF, Pichardo C, et al. Activity of tigecycline (GAR-936) against Acinetobacter baumanni strains, including those resistant to imipenem. Antimicrob Agents Chemother 48:4479-81, 2004.

Pankey GA. Tigecycline. J Antimicrob Chemother 53:470-80, 2005

Rubinstein E, Vaughan D. Tigecycline: a novel glycylcycline. Drugs 65:1317-36, 2005.

Zinner SH. Overview of antibiotic use and resistance: setting the stage for tigecycline. Clin Infect Dis 41(Suppl 5):S289-92, 2005.

Website: www.tygacil.com

TMP–SMX (Bactrim, Septra)

Drug Class: Folate antagonist/sulfonamide
Usual Dose: 2.5-5 mg/kg (IV/PO) q6h
Pharmacokinetic Parameters:
Peak serum level: 2-8/40-80 mcg/ml
Bioavailability: 98%
Excreted unchanged (urine): 67/85%
Serum half-life (normal/ESRD): (10/8)/40-80 hrs
Plasma protein binding: 44-70%
Volume of distribution (V$_d$): 1.8/0.3 L/kg
Primary Mode of Elimination: Renal
Dosage Adjustments*

CrCl 50–80 mL/min	No change
CrCl 10–50 mL/min	1.25-2.5 mg/kg (IV/PO) q6h
CrCl < 10 mL/min	Avoid (except for PCP use 1.25-2.5 mg/kg [IV/PO] q8h)
Post–HD dose	5 mg/kg (IV/PO)
Post–PD dose	0.16 mg/kg (IV/PO)
CVVH dose	2.5 mg/kg (IV/PO) q6h
Moderate hepatic insufficiency	No change
Severe hepatic insufficiency	No change

Drug Interactions: *TMP component:* Azathioprine (leukopenia); amantadine, dapsone, digoxin, methotrexate, phenytoin, rifampin, zidovudine (↑ interacting drug levels, nystagmus with phenytoin); diuretics (↑ serum K$^+$ with K$^+$-sparing diuretics, ↓ serum Na$^+$ with thiazide diuretics); warfarin (↑ INR, bleeding). *SMX component:* Cyclosporine (↓ cyclosporine levels); phenytoin (↑ phenytoin levels, nystagmus, ataxia); methotrexate (↑ antifolate activity); sulfonylureas, thiopental (↑ interacting drug effect); warfarin (↑ INR, bleeding)
Adverse Effects:
TMP: Folate deficiency, hyperkalemia
SMX: Leukopenia, thrombocytopenia, hemolytic anemia ± G6PD deficiency, aplastic anemia, ↑ SGOT/SGPT, severe hypersensitivity reactions (E. multiforme/Stevens–Johnson syndrome), ↑ risk of hypoglycemia in chronic renal failure
Allergic Potential: Very high (SMX); none (TMP)
Safety in Pregnancy: C
Comments: Drug fever/rash increased in HIV/AIDS. Excellent bioavailability (IV = PO).
1 SS tablet = 80 mg TMP + 400 mg SMX.
1 DS tablet = 160 mg TMP + 800 mg SMX.
1 SS tablet (PO) q6h = 10 mg/kg (IV) q24h.
1 DS tablet (PO) q6h = 20 mg/kg (IV) q24h.
Meningeal dose = 5 mg/kg (IV/PO) q6h
Cerebrospinal Fluid Penetration:
Non-inflamed meninges = 40%
Inflamed meninges = 40%
Bile Penetration: 100%

"Usual dose" assumes normal renal/hepatic function. * For renal insufficiency, give usual dose x 1 followed by maintenance dose per CrCl. For dialysis patients, dose the same as for CrCl < 10 mL/min and give supplemental (post-HD/PD dose) immediately after dialysis. CrCl = creatinine clearance; CVVH = continuous veno-venous hemo-filtration; HD/PD = hemodialysis/peritoneal dialysis. See pp. 262-265 for explanations, p. 1 for abbreviations

REFERENCES:

Cockerill FR, Edson RS. Trimethoprim-sulfamethoxazole. Mayo Clin Proc 66:1260-9, 1991.

El-Sadr W, Luskin-Hawk R, Yurik TM, et al. A randomized trial of daily and thrice weekly trimethoprim-sulfamethoxazole for the prevention of Pneumocystis carinii pneumonia in HIV infected individuals. Clin Infect Dis 29:775-83, 1999.

Francis P, Patel VB, Bill PL, et al. Oral trimethoprim-sulfamethoxazole in the treatment of cerebral toxoplasmosis in AIDS patients-a prospective study. S Afr Med J 94:51-3, 2004.

Giannakopoulos G, Johnson ES. TMP-SMX. Antibiotics for Clinicians 1:63-9, 1997.

Lundstrom TS, Sobel JD. Vancomycin, trimethoprim-sulfamethoxazole, and rifampin. Infect Dis Clin North Am 9:747-67, 1995.

Masters PA, O'Bryan TA, Zurlo JM, et al. Trimethoprim-sulfamethoxazole revisited. Arch Intern Med 163:402-10, 2003.

Nicolle LE. Urinary tract infection: traditional pharmacologic therapies. Am J Med 113(Suppl 1A):35S-44S, 2002.

Para MF, Dohn M, Frame P, et al, for the ACTG 268 dapsone study Team. Reduced toxicity with gradual initiation of trimethoprim-sulfamethoxazole as primary prophylaxis for Pneumocystis carinii pneumonia: AIDS Clinical Trials Group 268. J Acquire Immune Defic Syndr 24:337-43, 2000.

Smith LG, Sensakovic J. Trimethoprim-sulfamethoxazole. Med Clin North Am 66:143-56, 1982.

Thomas CF Jr, Limper AH. Pneumocystis pneumonia. N Engl J Med 350:2487-98, 2004.

Website: www.pdr.net

Tobramycin (Nebcin)

Drug Class: Aminoglycoside
Usual Dose: 5 mg/kg (IV) q24h or 240 mg (IV) q24h (preferred over q8h dosing) (see comments)
Pharmacokinetic Parameters:
Peak serum levels: 4-8 mcg/ml (q8h dosing); 16-24 mcg/ml (q24h dosing)
Bioavailability: Not applicable
Excreted unchanged (urine): 95%
Serum half-life (normal/ESRD): 2.5/56 hrs
Plasma protein binding: 10%
Volume of distribution (V_d): 0.24 L/kg
Primary Mode of Elimination: Renal

Dosage Adjustments*

CrCl 50–80 mL/min	2.5 mg/kg (IV) q24h or 120 mg (IV) q24h
CrCl 10–50 mL/min	2.5 mg/kg (IV) q48h or 120 mg (IV) q48h
CrCl < 10 mL/min	1.25 mg/kg (IV) q48h or 60 mg (IV) q48h
Post–HD dose	1 mg/kg (IV) or 80 mg (IV)
Post–PD dose	0.5 mg/kg (IV) or 40 mg (IV) or 2-4 mg/L in dialysate q24h
CVVH dose	2.5 mg/kg (IV) or 120 mg (IV) q48h
Moderate hepatic insufficiency	No change
Severe hepatic insufficiency	No change

Drug Interactions: Amphotericin B, cyclosporine, enflurane, methoxyflurane, NSAIDs, polymyxin B, radiographic contrast, vancomycin (↑ nephrotoxicity); cis-platinum (↑ nephrotoxicity, ↑ ototoxicity); loop diuretics (↑ ototoxicity); neuromuscular blocking agents (↑ apnea, prolonged paralysis); non-polarizing muscle relaxants (↑ apnea)
Adverse Effects: Neuromuscular blockade with rapid infusion/absorption. Nephrotoxicity only with prolonged/extremely high serum trough levels; may cause reversible non–oliguric renal failure (ATN). Ototoxicity associated with prolonged/extremely high peak serum levels (usually irreversible): Cochlear toxicity (1/3 of ototoxicity) manifests as decreased high frequency hearing, but deafness is unusual. Vestibular toxicity (2/3 of ototoxicity) develops before ototoxicity, and typically manifests as tinnitus
Allergic Potential: Low
Safety in Pregnancy: C

"Usual dose" assumes normal renal/hepatic function. * For renal insufficiency, give usual dose x 1 followed by maintenance dose per CrCl. For dialysis patients, dose the same as for CrCl < 10 mL/min and give supplemental (post-HD/PD dose) immediately after dialysis. CrCl = creatinine clearance; CVVH = continuous veno-venous hemofiltration; HD/PD = hemodialysis/peritoneal dialysis. See pp. 262-265 for explanations, p. 1 for abbreviations

Comments: Single daily dosing greatly reduces nephrotoxic/ototoxic potential. Incompatible with solutions containing β–lactams, erythromycin, chloramphenicol, furosemide, sodium bicarbonate. IV infusion should be given slowly over 1 hour. May be given IM. Avoid intraperitoneal infusion due to risk of neuromuscular blockade. Avoid intratracheal/aerosolized intrapulmonary instillation, which predisposes to antibiotic resistance. V_d increases with edema/ascites, trauma, burns, cystic fibrosis; may require ↑ dose. V_d decreases with dehydration, obesity; may require ↓ dose. Renal cast counts are the best indicator of aminoglycoside nephrotoxicity, not serum creatinine. Dialysis removes ~ 1/3 of tobramycin from serum. Tobramycin nebulizer dose: 300 mg via nebulizer q12h (not recommended due to ↑ risk of resistance). CAPD dose: 2-4 mg/L in dialysate (I.P.) with each exchange

Therapeutic Serum Concentrations (for therapeutic efficacy, not toxicity):
Peak (q24h/q8h dosing) = 16-24/8-10 mcg/ml
Trough (q24h/q8h dosing) = 0/1-2 mcg/ml
Dose for synergy = 2.5 mg/kg (IV) q24h or 120 mg (IV) q24h
Intrathecal (IT) dose = 5 mg (IT) q24h
Cerebrospinal Fluid Penetration:
Non-inflamed meninges = 0%
Inflamed meninges = 20%
Bile Penetration: 30%

REFERENCES:
Begg EJ, Barclay ML. Aminoglycosides - 50 years on. Br J Clin Pharmacol 39:597-603, 1995.
Buijk SE, Mouton JW, Gyssens IC, et al. Experience with a once-daily dosing program of aminoglycosides in critically ill patients. Intensive Care Med 28:936-42, 2002.
Cheer SM, Waugh J, Noble S. Inhaled tobramycin (TOBI): a review of its use in the management of Pseudomonas aeruginosa infections in patients with cystic fibrosis. Drugs. 63:2501-20, 2003.
Cunha BA. Aminoglycosides: Current role in antimicrobial therapy. Pharmacotherapy 8: 334-50, 1988.
Edson RS, Terrel CL. The aminoglycosides. Mayo Clin Proc 74:519-28, 1999.
Geller DE, Pistlick WH, Nardella PA, et al. Pharmacokinetics and bioavailability of aerosolized tobramycin in cystic fibrosis. Chest 122:219-26, 2002.
Gilbert DN. Once-daily aminoglycoside therapy. Antimicrob Agents Chemother 35:399-405, 1991.
Hustinx WN, Hoepelman IM. Aminoglycoside dosage regimens: Is once a day enough? Clin Pharmacokinet 25:427-32, 1993.
Kahler DA, Schowengerdt KO, Fricker FJ, et al. Toxic serum trough concentrations after administration of nebulized tobramycin. Pharmacotherapy. 23:543-5, 2003.
Lortholary O, Tod M, Cohen Y, et al. Aminoglycosides. Med Clin North Am 79:761-87, 1995.
McCormack JP, Jewesson PJ. A critical reevaluation of the "therapeutic range" of aminoglycosides. Clin Infect Dis 14:320-39, 1992.
Moss RB. Long-term benefits of inhaled tobramycin in adolescent patients with cystic fibrosis. Chest 121:55-63, 2002.
Whitehead A, Conway SP, Etherington C, et al. Once-daily tobramycin in the treatment of adult patients with cystic fibrosis. Eur Respir J 19:303-9, 2002.
Website: www.pdr.net

Trimethoprim-Sulfamethoxazole, see TMP–SMX (Bactrim, Septra)

Valacyclovir (Valtrex)

Drug Class: Antiviral (HSV, VZV)
Usual Dose:
HSV ½: Herpes labialis: 2 gm (PO) q12h x 1 day.
Genital herpes: Initial therapy: 1 gm (PO) q12h x 7-10 days. Recurrent/intermittent therapy (< 9 episodes/year): normal host: 500 mg (PO) q24h x 5 days; HIV-positive: 1 gm (PO) q12h x 5-10 days. Chronic suppressive therapy (> 9 episodes/year): normal host: 1 gm (PO) q24h x 1 year; HIV-positive: 500 mg (PO) q12h x 1 year.
Encephalitis: 1 gm (PO) q8h x 10 days
VZV: Chickenpox: 1 gm (PO) q8h x 5 days.
Herpes zoster (shingles) (dermatomal/disseminated): 1 gm (PO) q8h x 7-10 days
Pharmacokinetic Parameters:
Peak serum level: 3.7-.5 mcg/ml
Bioavailability: 55%
Excreted unchanged (urine): 1%

Serum half-life (normal/ESRD): 3/14 hrs
Plasma protein binding: 15%
Volume of distribution (V$_d$): 0.7 L/kg
Primary Mode of Elimination: Renal
Dosage Adjustments* (based on 1 gm q8h):

CrCl 10–50 mL/min	1 gm (PO) q12h
CrCl < 10 mL/min	500 mg (PO) q24h
Post–HD dose	1 gm (PO)
Post–PD dose	500 mg
CVVH dose	500 mg (PO) q24h
Moderate hepatic insufficiency	No change
Severe hepatic insufficiency	No change

Drug Interactions: Cimetidine, probenecid (↑ acyclovir levels)
Adverse Effects: Headache, nausea, diarrhea, abdominal pain, weakness
Allergic Potential: Low
Safety in Pregnancy: B
Comments: Converted to acyclovir in liver. Meningeal dose = HSV dose
Cerebrospinal Fluid Penetration: 50%

REFERENCES:
Acost EP, Fletcher CV. Valacyclovir. Ann Pharmacotherapy 31:185-91, 1997.
Alrabiah FA, Sacks SL. New antiherpesvirus agents: Their targets and therapeutic potential. Drugs 52:17-32, 1996.
Fiddian P, Sabin CA, Griffiths PD. Valacyclovir provides optimum acyclovir exposure for prevention of cytomegalovirus and related outcomes after argan transplantation. J Infect Dis 186(Suppl 1):S110-5, 2002.
Ljungman P, de La Camara R, Milpied N, et al. Randomized study of valacyclovir as prophylaxis against cytomegalovirus reactivation in recipients of allogeneic bone marrow transplants. Blood 99:3050-6, 2002.
MacDougall C, Guglielmo BJ. Pharmacokinetics of valacilovir. J Antimicrob Chemother 53:899-901, 2004.
Perry CM, Faulds D. Valacyclovir: A review of its antiviral activity, pharmacokinetic properties, and therapeutic efficacy in herpesvirus infections. Drugs 52:754-72, 1996.
Tyring SK, Baker D, Snowden W. Valacyclovir for herpes simplex virus infection: long-term safety and sustained efficacy after 20 years' experience with acyclovir. J Infect Dis 186(Suppl 1):S40-6, 2002.
Website: www.valtrex.com

Valganciclovir (Valcyte)

Drug Class: Antiviral, Nucleoside inhibitor/analogue
Usual Dose: 900 mg (PO) q12h x 21 days (induction), then 900 mg (PO) q24h for life (maintenance). 900 mg dose taken as two 450-mg tablets once daily with food
Pharmacokinetic Parameters:
Peak serum level: 5.6 mcg/ml
Bioavailability: 59.4%
Excreted unchanged (urine): 90%
Serum half-life (normal/ESRD): 4.1/67.5 hrs
Plasma protein binding: 1%
Volume of distribution (V$_d$): 15.3 L/kg
Primary Mode of Elimination: Renal
Dosage Adjustments*

CrCl 40–60 mL/min	450 mg (PO) q12h (induction), then 450 mg (PO) q24h (maintenance)
CrCl 25–40 mL/min	450 mg (PO) q24h (induction), then 450 mg (PO) q48h (maintenance)
CrCl 10–25 mL/min	450 mg (PO) q48h (induction), then 450 mg (PO) 2x/week (maintenance)
CrCl < 10 mL/min	Avoid
Post–HD dose	Avoid
Post–PD dose	Use CrCl 25–40 mL/min dose
CVVH dose	No information

"Usual dose" assumes normal renal/hepatic function. * For renal insufficiency, give usual dose x 1 followed by maintenance dose per CrCl. For dialysis patients, dose the same as for CrCl < 10 mL/min and give supplemental (post-HD/PD dose) immediately after dialysis. CrCl = creatinine clearance; CVVH = continuous veno-venous hemo-filtration; HD/PD = hemodialysis/peritoneal dialysis. See pp. 262-265 for explanations, p. 1 for abbreviations

Moderate hepatic insufficiency	No change
Severe hepatic insufficiency	No change

Drug Interactions: Cytotoxic drugs (may produce additive toxicity: stomatitis, bone marrow depression, alopecia); imipenem (↑ risk of seizures); probenecid (↑ valganciclovir levels); zidovudine (↓ valganciclovir levels, ↑ zidovudine levels, possible neutropenia)
Adverse Effects: Drug fever/rash, diarrhea, nausea, vomiting, GI upset, leukopenia, anemia, thrombocytopenia, paresthesias/peripheral neuropathy, retinal detachment, aplastic anemia
Allergic Potential: Low
Safety in Pregnancy: C
Comments: Valganciclovir exposures (AUC) larger than for IV ganciclovir. Tablets should be taken with food. Valganciclovir is rapidly hydrolyzed to ganciclovir. Not interchangeable on a tablet-to-tablet basis with oral ganciclovir. Much higher bioavailability than ganciclovir capsules; serum concentration equivalent to IV ganciclovir. Indicated for induction/maintenance therapy of CMV retinitis/infection. Preferred to ganciclovir for all indications except for CMV prophylaxis in liver transplants.
Meningeal dose = usual dose
Cerebrospinal Fluid Penetration: 70%

REFERENCES:
Cocohoba JM, McNicholl IR. Valganciclovir: an advance in cytomegalovirus therapeutics. Ann Pharmacother 36:1075-9, 2002.
Czock D, Scholle C, Rasche FM, et al. Pharmacokinetics of valganciclovir and ganciclovir in renal impairment. Clin Pharmacol Ther 72:142-50, 2002.
Jung D, Dorr A. Single-dose pharmacokinetics of valganciclovir in HIV and CMV seropositive subjects. J Clin Pharmacol 39:800-804, 1999.
Razonable RR, Paya CV. Valganciclovir for the prevention and treatment of cytomegalovirus disease in immunocompromised hosts. Expert Rev Anti Infect Ther 2:27-41, 2004.
Rubin RH. Cytomegalovirus infection in the liver transplant recipient. Epidemiology, pathogenesis, and clinical management. Clin Liver Dis 1:439-52, 2004.
Segarra-Newnham M, Salazar MI. Valganciclovir: A new oral alternative for cytomegalovirus retinitis in human immunodeficiency virus-seropositive individuals. Pharmacotherapy 22:1124-8, 2002.
Slifkin M, Doron S, Snydman DR. Viral prophylaxis in organ transplant patients. Drugs 64:2763-92, 2004.
Taber DJ, Ashcraft E, Baillie GM, et al. Valganciclovir prophylaxes in patients at high risk for the development of cytomegalovirus disease. Transpl Infect Dis 6:101-9, 2004.
Zamora MR, Nicolls MR, Hodges TN, et al. Following universal prophylaxis with intravenous ganciclovir and cytomegalovirus immune globulin, valganciclovir is safe and effective for prevention of CMV infection following lung transplantation. Am J Transplant 4:1635-42, 2004.
Website: www.rocheusa.com/products/

Vancomycin (Vancocin)

Drug Class: Glycopeptide
Usual Dose: 1 gm (IV) q12h (see comments)
Pharmacokinetic Parameters:
Peak serum level: 63 mcg/ml
Bioavailability: IV (not applicable)/PO (0%)
Excreted unchanged (urine): 90%
Serum half-life (normal/ESRD): 6/180 hrs
Plasma protein binding: 55%
Volume of distribution (V_d): 0.7 L/kg
Primary Mode of Elimination: Renal
Dosage Adjustments*

CrCl 50–80 mL/min	500 mg (IV) q12h
CrCl 10–50 mL/min	500 mg (IV) q24h
CrCl < 10 mL/min	1 gm (IV) qweek
Post–HD dose	None
Post–PD dose	None
CVVH dose	1 gm (IV) q24h
Moderate hepatic insufficiency	No change
Severe hepatic insufficiency	No change

Drug Interactions: Aminoglycosides, amphotericin B, polymyxin B (↑ nephrotoxicity)
Adverse Effects: "Red man/neck syndrome" with rapid IV infusion (histamine mediated), leukopenia, cardiac arrest, hypotension

---

"Usual dose" assumes normal renal/hepatic function. * For renal insufficiency, give usual dose x 1 followed by maintenance dose per CrCl. For dialysis patients, dose the same as for CrCl < 10 mL/min and give supplemental (post-HD/PD dose) immediately after dialysis. CrCl = creatinine clearance; CVVH = continuous veno-venous hemo-filtration; HD/PD = hemodialysis/peritoneal dialysis. See pp. 262-265 for explanations, p. 1 for abbreviations

Allergic Potential: Low
Safety in Pregnancy: C
Comments: Not nephrotoxic. "Red man/neck syndrome" can be prevented/minimized by infusing IV vancomycin slowly over 1–2 hours. Intraperitoneal absorption = 40%. IV vancomycin use increases prevalence of VRE. For C. difficile diarrhea, use oral vancomycin 250 mg (PO) q6h. Vancomycin (IV/PO) ineffective for C. difficile colitis. Intrathecal (IT) dose = 20 mg (IT) in preservative free NaCl
Therapeutic Serum Concentrations (for therapeutic efficacy, not toxicity):
Peak = 25-40 mcg/ml
Trough = 5-12 mcg/ml
There is no convincing data that vancomycin is ototoxic or nephrotoxic; therefore CrCl, not serum levels, should be used to adjust vancomycin dosing. Prolonged/high dose vancomycin (60 mg/kg/day or 2 gm [IV] q12h) has been useful in treating S. aureus osteomyelitis, S. aureus infections with high MICs (VISA), and infections in difficult-to-penetrate tissues without toxicity. In bone or CSF, vancomycin tissue concentrations are ~ 15% of serum levels
Cerebrospinal Fluid Penetration:
Non-inflamed meninges = 0%
Inflamed meninges = 15%
Bile Penetration: 50%

REFERENCES:
Cantu TG, Yamanaka-Yuen NA, Lietman PS. Serum vancomycin concentrations: Reappraisal of their clinical value. Clin Infect Dis 18:533-43, 1994.
Cosgrove SE, Carroll KC, Perl TM. Staphylococcus aureus with reduced susceptibility to vancomycin. Clin Infect Dis 39:539-45, 2004.
Cunha BA. Vancomycin serum levels: unnecessary, unhelpful, and costly. Antibiotics for Clinicians 8:273-77, 2004.
Cunha BA, Deglin J, Chow M, et al. Pharmacokinetics of vancomycin in patients undergoing chronic hemodialysis. Rev Infect Dis 3:269-72, 1981.
Cunha BA. Vancomycin. Med Clin North Am 79:817-31, 1995.
DelDot ME, Lipman J, Tett SE. Vancomycin pharmacokinetics in critically ill patients receiving continuous venovenous haemodiafiltration. Br J Clin Pharmacol 58:259-68, 2004.

Menzies D. Goel K, Cunha BA. Vancomycin. Antibiotics for Clinicians 2:97-9, 1998.
Moellering RC Jr. Monitoring serum vancomycin levels: climbing the mountain because it is there? Clin Infect Dis 18;544-6, 1994.
Rybak MJ. The pharmacokinetic and pharmacodynamic properties of vancomycin. Clin Infect Dis 42:S35-9, 2006.
Stevens DL. The role of vancomycin in the treatment paradigm. Clin Infect Dis 42:S51-7, 2006.
Website: www.pdr.net

Voriconazole (Vfend)

Drug Class: Triazole antifungal
Usual Dose: <u>IV dosing</u>: Loading dose of 6 mg/kg (IV) q12h x 1 day, then maintenance dose of 4 mg/kg (IV) q12h. Can switch to weight-based PO maintenance dosing anytime while on maintenance IV dose (see comments)
<u>PO dosing</u>: *Weight ≥ 40 kg*: Loading dose of 400 mg (PO) q12h x 1 day, then maintenance dose of 200 mg (PO) q12h. If response is inadequate, the dose may be increased to 300 mg (PO) q12h. *Weight < 40 kg*: Loading dose of 200 mg (PO) x 1 day, then maintenance dose of 100 mg (PO) q12h. If response is inadequate, the dose may be increased to 150 mg (PO) q12h. For chronic/non-life-threatening infections, loading dose may be given PO (see comments)
Pharmacokinetic Parameters:
Peak serum level: 2.3-4.7 mcg/ml
Bioavailability: 96%
Excreted unchanged (urine): 2%
Serum half-life (normal/ESRD): 6/6 hrs
Plasma protein binding: 58%
Volume of distribution (V_d): 4.6 L/kg
Primary Mode of Elimination: Hepatic
Dosage Adjustments*

CrCl 50–80 mL/min	No change
CrCl 10–50 mL/min	No change PO; do not use IV
CrCl < 10 mL/min	No change PO; do not use IV
Post–HD dose	Usual dose (IV/PO)

"Usual dose" assumes normal renal/hepatic function. * For renal insufficiency, give usual dose x 1 followed by maintenance dose per CrCl. For dialysis patients, dose the same as for CrCl < 10 mL/min and give supplemental (post-HD/PD dose) immediately after dialysis. CrCl = creatinine clearance; CVVH = continuous veno-venous hemofiltration; HD/PD = hemodialysis/peritoneal dialysis. See pp. 262-265 for explanations, p. 1 for abbreviations

Post–PD dose	No information
CVVH dose	Use 10–50 mL/min dosing
Moderate hepatic insufficiency	6 mg/kg (IV) q12h x 1 day or 200 mg (PO) q12h x 1 day, then 2 mg/kg (IV) q12h or 100 mg (PO) q12h (> 40 kg)
Severe hepatic insufficiency	No information

Drug Interactions: Benzodiazepines, vinca alkaloids (↑ interacting drug levels); carbamazepine, ergot alkaloids, rifampin, rifabutin, sirolimus, long-acting barbiturates (contraindicated with voriconazole); cyclosporine, omeprazole (↑ interacting drug levels, ↓ interacting drug dose by 50%); tacrolimus (↑ tacrolimus levels, ↓ tacrolimus dose by 66%); phenytoin (↓ voriconazole levels); ↑ voriconazole dose from 4 mg/kg [IV] to 5 mg/kg [IV] and from 200 mg [PO] to 400 mg [PO]; warfarin (↑ INR); statins (↑ risk of rhabdomyolysis); dihydropyridine calcium channel blockers (hypotension); sulfonylureas (hypoglycemia). Voriconazole has not been studied with protease inhibitors or NNRTIs, but ↑ voriconazole levels are predicted (↑ hepatotoxicity/adverse effects)
Adverse Effects: ↑ SGOT/SGPT; dose-dependent arrhythmias, hepatotoxicity, visual events (blurring vision, ↑ brightness, pain; effect on vision is not know > 28 days of therapy), hallucinations, hypoglycemia, ↑ QT_c interval; 20% incidence of rash noted in trials, including severe Stevens-Johnson Syndrome; photosensitivity reactions (avoid direct sunlight)
Allergic Potential: High
Safety in Pregnancy: D
Comments: If intolerance to therapy develops, the IV maintenance dose may be reduced to 3 mg/kg and the PO maintenance dose may be reduced in steps of 50 mg/d to a minimum of 200 mg/d q12h (weight ≥ 40 kg) or 100 mg q12h (weight < 40 kg). Non-linear kinetics

(doubling of oral dose = 2.8-fold increase in serum levels).
10-15% of patients have serum levels > 6 mcg/ml. Food decreases bioavailability; take 1 hour before or after meals. Do not use IV voriconazole if CrCl < 50 mL/min to prevent accumulation of voriconazole IV vehicle, sulphobutyl ether cyclodextrin (SBECD); instead use oral formulation, which has no SBECD. Loading dose may be given PO for chronic/non-life-threatening infections. Because of visual effects, do not drive or operate machinery. Monitor LFTs before and during therapy. May also be used following 7 days IV antifungal therapy with amphotericin formulations or echinocandins to complete oral antifungal therapy. Meningeal dose = usual dose
Cerebrospinal Fluid Penetration: 90%

REFERENCES:
Boucher HW, Groll AH, Chiou CC, et al. Newer systemic antifungal agents: pharmacokinetics, safety and efficacy. Drugs 64:1997-2020, 2004.
Castiglioni B, Sutton DA, Rinaldi MG, et al. Pseudallescheria boydii (Anamorph Scedosporium apiospermum). Infection in solid organ transplant recipients in a tertiary medical center and review of the literature. Medicine (Baltimore) 81:333-48, 2002.
Chandrasekar PH, Manavathu E. Voriconazole: A second-generation triazole. Drugs for Today 37:135-48, 2001.
Denning DW, Ribaud P, Milpied N, et al. Efficacy and safety of voriconazole in the treatment of acute invasive aspergillosis. Clin Infect Dis 34:563-71, 2002.
Espinel-Ingroff A, Boyle K, Sheehan DJ. In vitro antifungal activities of voriconazole and reference agents as determined by NCCLS methods: Review of the literature. Mycopathologia 150:101-115, 2001.
Gallagher JC, MacDougall C, Ashley ES, et al. Recent advances in antifungal pharmacotherapy for invasive fungal infections. Expert Rev Anti Infect Ther 2:253-68, 2004.
Ghannoum MA, Kuhn DM. Voriconazole – better chances for patients with invasive mycoses. Eur J Med Res 7:242-256, 2002.
Herbrecht R, Denning DW, Patterson TF, et al. Voriconazole versus amphotericin B for primary therapy of invasive aspergillosis. N Engl J Med 347:408-15, 2002.
Hoffman HL, Rathbun RC. Review of the safety and efficacy of voriconazole. Expert Opin Investig Drugs 11:409-29, 2002.

"Usual dose" assumes normal renal/hepatic function. * For renal insufficiency, give usual dose x 1 followed by maintenance dose per CrCl. For dialysis patients, dose the same as for CrCl < 10 mL/min and give supplemental (post-HD/PD dose) immediately after dialysis. CrCl = creatinine clearance; CVVH = continuous veno-venous hemo-filtration; HD/PD = hemodialysis/peritoneal dialysis. See pp. 262-265 for explanations, p. 1 for abbreviations

Lazaurs HM, Blumer JL, Yanovich, et al. Safety and pharmacokinetics of oral voriconazole in patients at risk of fungal infection: a dose escalation study. J Clin Pharmacol 42:395-402, 2002.

Poza G, Montoya J, Redondo C, et al. Meningitis caused by Pseudallescheria boydii treated with voriconazole. Clin Infect Dis 30:981-2, 2000.

Purkins L, Wood N, Ghahramani P, et al.

Pharmacokinetics and safety of voriconazole following intravenous- to oral-dose escalation regimens. Antimicrob Agents Chemother 46:2546-53, 2002.

Sabo JA, Abdel-Rahman SM. Voriconazole: A new antifungal. Ann Pharmacotherapy 34:1032-43, 2000.

Website: www.vfend.com

REFERENCES AND SUGGESTED READINGS

AAD-Sinusitis, Sinus and Allergy Health Partnership. Antimicrobial treatment guidelines for acute bacterial rhinosinusitis. Otolaryngol Head Neck Surg 130:1-45. 2004.

Acharya PS. Telithromycin: the first ketolide for the treatment of respiratory infections. Am J Health Syst Pharm 1;62:905-16:2005.

Cuenca-Estrella M. Combinations of antifungal agents in therapy - what value are they? J Antimicrob Chemother 54:854-69, 2004.

Cunha BA. Antimicrobial therapy. Medical Clinics of North America, 2006.

De Clercq E. Antiviral drugs in current clinical use. J Clin Virol 30:115-33, 2004.

Garau J. Role of beta-lactam agents in the treatment of community-acquired pneumonia. Eur J Clin Microbiol Infect Dis 24:83-99, 2005.

Grossman RF, Rotschafer JC, Tan JS. Antimicrobial treatment of lower respiratory tract infections in the hospital setting. Am J Med 118(Suppl 7A):29S-38S, 2005.

Jain R, Danziger LH. Multidrug-resistant Acinetobacter infections: an emerging challenge to clinicians. Ann Pharmacother 38:1449-59, 2004.

Klugman KP, Lonks JR. Hidden epidemic of macrolide-resistant pneumococci. Emerg Infect Dis 11:802-7, 2005.

Kunimoto D, Long R. Tuberculosis: still overlooked as a cause of community-acquired pneumonia–how not to miss it. Respir Care Clin N Am 11:25-34, 2005.

Marrie TJ. Therapeutic implications of macrolide resistance in pneumococcal community-acquired lower respiratory tract infections. Int J Clin Pract 58:769-76, 2004.

Marrie TJ. Nonresponses and treatment failures with conventional empiric regiment in patients with community-acquired pneumonia. Infect Dis Clin North Am 18:829-41, 2004.

Obach RS, Walsky RL, Venkatakrishnan K, Houston JB, Tremaine LM. In vitro cytochrome P450 inhibition data and the prediction of drug-drug interactions: Qualitative relationships, quantitative predictions, and the rank-order approach. Clin Pharmacol Ther 78:582-592, 2005.

Parnham MJ. Immunomodulatory effects of antimicrobials in the therapy of respiratory tract infections. Curr Opin Infect Dis 18:125-31, 2005.

Piscitelli SC, Gallicano KD. Interactions among drugs for HIV and opportunistic infections. N Engl J Med 344:984-996, 2001.

Poole M, Anon J, Paglia M, et al. A trial of high-dose, short-course levofloxacin for the treatment of acute bacterial sinusitis. Otolaryngol Head Neck Surg, 134:10-17, 2006.

Segreti J, House HR, Siegel RE. Principles of antibiotic treatment of community-acquired pneumonia in the outpatient setting. Am J Med 118(Suppl 7A):21S-28S, 2005.

TEXTBOOKS

Ambrose P, Nightingale AT (eds). Principles of Pharmacodynamics. Marcel Dekker, Inc., New York, 2001.

Anderson RJ, Schrier RW (eds). Clinical Use of Drugs in Patients with Kidney and Liver Disease. W. B. Saunders Company, Philadelphia, 1981.

Baddour L, Gorbach SL (eds). Therapy of Infectious Diseases. Saunders, Philadelphia, 2003.

Bartlett JG, Auwaerter PG, Pam PA (eds). The ABX Guide, 1st edition, Thomson PDR, Montvale, NJ, 2005.

Bartlett JG (ed). The Johns Hopkins Hospital Guide to Medical Care of Patients with HIV Infection, Lippincott Williams & Wilkins, Philadelphia, 2005.

Bennet WM, Aronoff GR, Golper TA, Morrison G, Brater DC, Singer I (eds). Drug Prescribing in Renal Failure, 2nd Edition. American College of Physicians, Philadelphia, 2000.

Bryskier A (ed). Antimicrobial Agents. ASM Press, Washington, D.C., 2005.

Cunha BA (ed). Antibiotic Essentials, 7th edition, Physicians' Press, Royal Oak, MI, 2008.

Dolin R, Masur H, Saag MS (eds). AIDS Therapy, 2nd edition. Churchill Livingstone, New York, 2003.

Finch RG, Greenwood D, Norrby SR, Whitley RJ (eds). Antibiotic and Chemotherapy. Churchill Livingstone, United Kingdom, 2003.

Gorbach SL, Bartlett JG, Blacklow NR (eds). Infectious Diseases, ed 3. Philadelphia, Lippincott, Williams & Wilkins, 2004.

Ieada CM, Keaten, Jr, BL, Goldman MP, Gray LD, Aberg JA (eds). Infectious Diseases Handbook, 4th Edition. Lexi-Comp, Inc., Hudson, 2001.

Kucers A, Crowe S, Grayson ML, Hoy J (eds). The Use of Antibiotics: A Clinical Review of Antibacterial, Antifungal, and Antiviral Drugs, 5th Edition. Butterworth-Heinemann, Oxford, 1997.

Mandell GL, Bennett JE, Dolin R (eds). Mandell, Douglas and Bennett's Principles and Practice of Infectious Disease, 6th Edition. Elsevier, Philadelphia, 2005.

O'Grady F, Lambert HP, Finch RG, Greenwood D (eds). Antibiotic and Chemotherapy, 2nd Edition. Churchill Livingstone, New York, 1997.

Physicians' Desk Reference, 60th Edition. Thompson PDR, Montvale, NJ, 2006.

Piscitelli SC, Rodvold KE (eds). Drug Interactions in Infectious Diseases. Humana Press, Totowa, 2001.

Pratt WB, Fekety R (eds). The Antimicrobial Drugs, Oxford University Press, New York, 1986.

Ristuccia AM, Cunha BA (eds). Antimicrobial Therapy. Raven Press, New York, 1984.

Root RK (ed). Clinical Infectious Diseases: A Practical Approach. Oxford University Press, New York, 1999.

Schlossberg D (eds). Current Therapy of Infectious Disease, 3rd Edition. Mosby-Yearbook, St. Louis, 2007.

Schlossberg D (ed). Tuberculosis and Non-Tuberculous Mycobacterial Infection, 6th Edition. McGraw-Hill, New York, 2006.

Scholar EM, Pratt WB (eds). The Antimicrobial Drugs, 2nd Edition. Oxford University Press, New York, 2000.

Wormser GP (ed). AIDS, 4th Edition. Elsevier, Philadelphia, 2004.

Yoshikawa TT, Norman DC (eds). Antimicrobial Therapy in the Elderly. Marcel Dekker, New York, 1994.

Yoshikawa TT, Rajagopalan S (eds). Antibiotic Therapy for Geriatric Patients. Taylor & Francis, New York, 2006.

Yu VL, Merigan, Jr. TC, Barrier SL (eds). Antimicrobial Therapy and Vaccines, 2nd edition. Williams & Wilkins, Baltimore, 2005.

Zinner SH, Young LS, Acar JF, Ortiz-Neu C (eds). New Considerations for Macrolides, Azalides, Streptogramins, and Ketolides. Marcel Dekker, Inc., New York, 2000.

INDEX